THE RANCHO LOS AMIGOS LEVELS OF COGNITIVE FUNCTIONING

Level I	No response	Appears to be in deep sleep, unresponsive to any stimuli
Level II	Generalized response	Responses are inconsistent and not specific to stimuli; often same response regardless of stimulus; response may be physiologic, gross body movement, or vocalization; response may be delayed; earliest response is to deep pain
Level III	Localized response	Responses remain inconsistent, but are specific to stimuli; may follow simple commands, but is still inconsistent and delayed; may pull at tubes or restraints; may respond more for family/close friends
Level IV	Confused Agitated	Heightened state of activity; agitation; wanders; poor attention span; poor short-term memory; may cry or scream to stimulus; may be aggressive/hostile; speech incoherent and inappropriate; confabulation; self-care requires maximum assistance
Level V	Confused Inappropriate	Responds to simple commands fairly consistently; responses random and nonpurposeful with complex commands or lack of structure; may be agitated with complex stimuli; wanders; easily distracted; memory severely impaired; unable to learn; inappropriate verbalizations; self-care requires moderate assistance or supervision
Level VI	Confused Appropriate	Goal-directed behavior depends on external input; tolerates unpleasant stimuli; follows simple directions consistently; carry-over for tasks relearned; responses may be incorrect due to memory but are appropriate to situation; oriented inconsistently; beginning awareness of situation; no anticipation; no longer wanders; self-care requires minimal assistance or supervision
Level VII	Automatic Appropriate	Responds appropriately and is oriented; adheres to daily routine automatically; minimal confusion; shallow recall; lacks insight; poor judgment and problem-solving; carry-over for new learning slow; minimal supervision for learning and safety; self-care independent; interest in social/recreational activities
Level VIII	Purposeful Appropriate	Alert and oriented; able to recall and integrate past and recent events; carry-over for new learning if meaningful; no supervision once activities learned; independent at home/community within physical capabilities; may still function below premorbid abilities; decreased tolerance for stress

(Adapted from Hagen.[63])

NEUROLOGIC DISORDERS

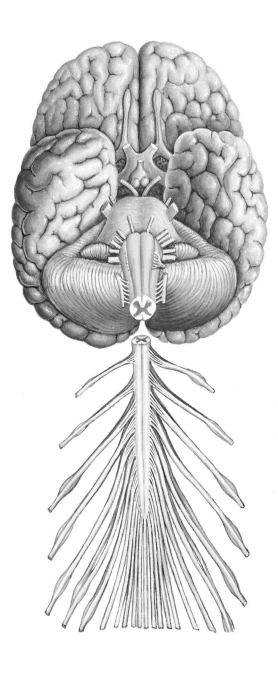

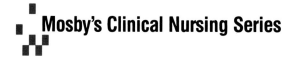

Mosby's Clinical Nursing Series

Mosby's Clinical Nursing Series

Cardiovascular Disorders

by Mary Canobbio

Respiratory Disorders

by Susan Wilson and June Thompson

Infectious Diseases

by Deanna Grimes

Orthopedic Disorders

by Leona Mourad

Renal Disorders

by Dorothy Brundage

Neurologic Disorders

by Esther Chipps, Norma Clanin, and Victor Campbell

Cancer Nursing

by Anne Belcher

Genitourinary Disorders

by Mikel Gray

Immunologic Disorders

by Christine Mudge-Grout

Gastrointestinal Disorders

by Dorothy Doughty and Debra Broadwell

NEUROLOGIC DISORDERS

ESTHER M. CHIPPS, RN, MS
Clinical Associate
The Ohio State University
College of Nursing, Columbus, Ohio

NORMA J. CLANIN, RN, MS, CRRN
Clinical Associate
The Ohio State University
College of Nursing, Columbus, Ohio

VICTOR G. CAMPBELL, RN, PHD
Assistant Professor
The Ohio State University
College of Nursing, Columbus, Ohio

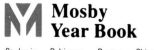 **Mosby Year Book**

St. Louis   Baltimore   Boston   Chicago   London   Philadelphia   Sydney   Toronto

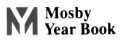
**Mosby
Year Book**

Dedicated to Publishing Excellence

Executive Editor: Don Ladig
Managing Editor: Sally Adkisson
Project Manager: Mark Spann
Senior Production Editor: Stephen Hetager
Designer: Liz Fett
Layout: Doris Hallas

The authors wish to acknowledge the contributions of The Ohio State
University Hospitals and Doctors Hospital, Columbus, Ohio.

Mosby–Year Book, Inc.
11830 Westline Industrial Drive
St. Louis, Missouri 63146

The authors and publisher have made a conscientious effort to ensure
that the drug information and recommended dosages in this book are
accurate and in accord with accepted standards at the time of
publication. However, pharmacology is a rapidly changing science, so
readers are advised to check the package insert provided by the
manufacturer before administering any drug.

ISBN 0-8016-1372-8

92 93 94 95 96 CL/VH 9 8 7 6 5 4 3 2

Contributors

Chapter 9, "Drug Therapy for Neurologic Disorders," contributed by

EVELYN SALERNO, Pharm.D., R.Ph.
Adjunct Professor, University of Miami School of Nursing, Miami, Florida;
Director of Pharmacy Services, Hospice, Inc., Miami, Florida

Original illustrations prepared by

GEORGE J. WASSILCHENKO
Tulsa, Oklahoma

and

DONALD P. O'CONNOR
St. Peters, Missouri

Photography by

PATRICK WATSON
Poughkeepsie, New York

Preface

Neurologic Disorders is the sixth volume in Mosby's Clinical Nursing Series, a new kind of resource for practicing nurses.

The Series is the result of the most elaborate market research ever undertaken by Mosby–Year Book. We first surveyed hundreds of working nurses to determine what kind of resources practicing nurses want in order to meet their advanced information needs. We then approached clinical specialists—proven authors and experts in 10 practice areas, from cardiovascular to orthopedics—and asked them to develop a common format that would meet the needs of nurses in practice, as specified by the survey respondents. This plan was then presented to 9 focus groups composed of working nurses over a period of 18 months. The plan was refined between each group, and in the later stages we published a 32-page full-color sample so that detailed changes could be made to improve the physical layout and appearance of the book, section by section and page by page. The result is a new genre of professional books for nursing professionals.

Neurologic Disorders begins with an innovative Color Atlas of Neurologic Structure and Function. This review of the anatomy and physiology contains a collection of detailed full-color drawings to depict normal structure and function.

Chapter 2 is a comprehensive guide to neurologic assessment. Clear, full-color photographs have been included to show proper patient positioning and assessment techniques in sharp detail. All photos are accompanied by concise instructions in the text. Special assessment tools for determining neurologic status and cognitive functioning are included inside the front cover.

Chapter 3 presents detailed information and full-color photographs of diagnostic tests and equipment. A consistent format for each diagnostic procedure gives nurses information about the purpose of the test; indications and contraindications; and nursing care associated with each test, including necessary patient teaching.

Chapters 4 and 5 present neurologic disorders of the central nervous system and the peripheral nervous system. Many detailed charts and illustrations accompany the text. The pathophysiology is comprehensive to aid in understanding the nature of the condition or disease. Potential complications of each disorder are highlighted in a box for quick and easy reference. Commonly prescribed diagnostic tests and medical management techniques are briefly reviewed for the nurse's

reference. The nursing process format provides detailed assessments and findings, nursing diagnoses, patient goals, nursing interventions with rationales, and expected outcomes. While concepts of acute care and rehabilitation have been integrated throughout the nursing process presentations, there is a special emphasis on their integration in the discussions of craniocerebral trauma, cerebrovascular accidents, and spinal cord trauma. An up-to-date and comprehensive discussion of the central nervous system complications of AIDS is also included. Patient teaching concerns are identified at the end of each disorder, thus enabling the nurse to anticipate questions often asked by the patient and family, and to maximize teaching efforts and time.

Chapter 6 focuses on frequently performed surgical procedures and therapeutic interventions for neurologic conditions. A discussion of cranial and spinal surgery, emphasizing the most common complications and nursing care is included. Plasmapheresis, a relatively new therapeutic procedure used in the treatment of neuromuscular diseases of immunologic origin, is included.

Chapter 7 provides further in-depth discussion of rehabilitation philosophy and goals, followed by special sections on adjustment, adaptation, and coping; sexuality; and stabilization and mobility. Other major concerns of rehabilitation are identified, and the reader is referred to the integrated content elsewhere in the text.

Chapter 8 presents numerous patient teaching guides. These are designed so that they can be copied, distributed to patients and their families, and used for a reference after discharge.

Chapter 9 reviews many of the pharmaceutical agents used to treat patients with neurologic disorders. Drugs are listed by trade and generic names and common dosages are identified.

This book is intended for use by nurses practicing in acute care as well as rehabilitation settings, including general medical-surgical practitioners as well as those nurses practicing in the neuroscience area. We also hope that this book will be a valuable adjunct to medical-surgical nursing texts for nursing students. It is our hope that this book will contribute to the overall advancement of neuroscience nursing. The nursing care of the patient with a neurologic condition requires an in-depth knowledge base, refined problem-solving skills, clinical technical skills, and a dedication to assisting patients and their families to adapt to challenging and complex changes in function and lifestyle.

Contents

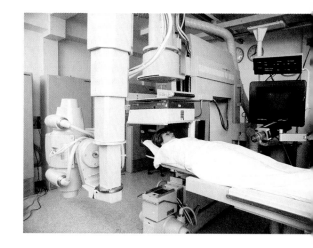

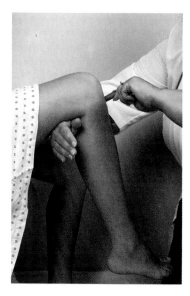

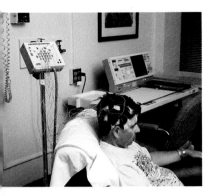

4 CENTRAL NERVOUS SYSTEM DISORDERS, 47

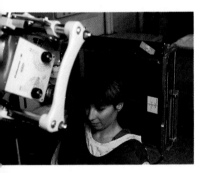

5 PERIPHERAL NERVOUS SYSTEM DISORDERS, 211

6 SURGICAL AND THERAPEUTIC INTERVENTIONS, 236

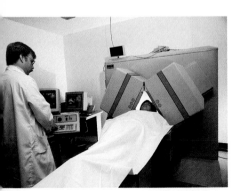

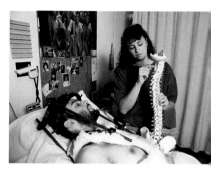
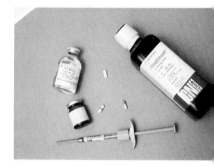

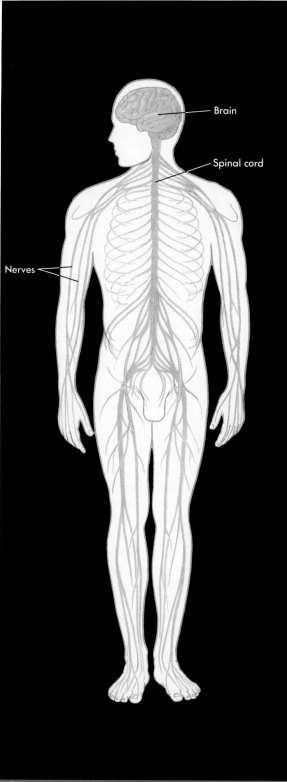

CHAPTER 1

Color Atlas of Neurologic Structure and Function

The human nervous system consists of complex structures and processes similar to an intricate circuit board, through which the various functions of the body are integrated. Because these functions are integrative, the physiologic and psychologic ramifications of a neurologic dysfunction can be devastating for both patients and their families.

The nervous system is divided into two fairly distinct structural categories: the central nervous system (CNS), which consists of the brain and the spinal cord, and the peripheral nervous system (PNS), which comprises 12 pairs of cranial nerves, 31 pairs of spinal nerves, and the sympathetic and parasympathetic subdivisions of the autonomic nervous system. Functionally, the central and peripheral nervous systems are interdependent in that each is made up of millions of shared neurons and neuroglial cells. The neuron is the basic unit of the nervous system; the neuroglial cells support the neuron.

Cerebrum

Corpus callosum

Thalamus

Hypo-thalamus

Cerebellum

Pituitary gland

Cervical enlargement

Spinal cord

Dural sheath

Lumbar enlargement

Conus medullaris

Filum terminale

MICROSTRUCTURE OF THE NERVOUS SYSTEM

NEUROGLIAL CELLS

About 40% of the structures of the brain and spinal cord are made up of **neuroglial cells.** These cells protect, support, and nourish the cell bodies and processes of the neurons. There are four distinct types of neuroglial cells: **astroglia (astrocyte), ependyma, microglia,** and **oligodendroglia** (Figure 1-1 and Table 1-1). Unlike neurons, neuroglial cells can divide and multiply by mitosis, and they are a main source of nervous system tumors.

NEURONS

Neurons come in many sizes and shapes, and each transmits specific nervous stimuli (Figure 1-2). Neurons have properties of excitation and electrical-chemical conductivity. In the central nervous system, groups of neurons are called **nuclei;** in the peripheral nervous system, they are called **ganglia.**

NERVES

In the peripheral nervous system, the neuron carries impulses to and from the central nervous system via the chainlike grouping of neuron cell fibers called nerves. The term **nerve** applies only to cell fibers in the peripheral nervous system; in the central nervous system, these groups of cell fibers are called **fiber tracts.**

The axon is the part of the nerve that conducts impulses. The myelin sheath around the axon insulates, protects, and nourishes the axon. Periodic interruptions of the myelin sheath are called **nodes of Ranvier.**

Fibrous astrocyte

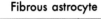

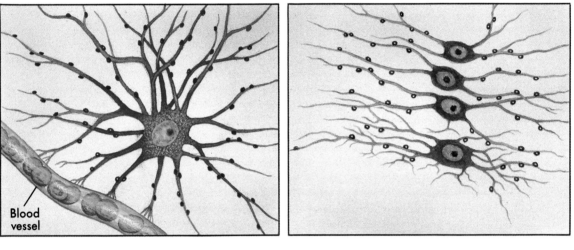

Oligodendrocytes

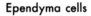

Microglia cells

Ependyma cells

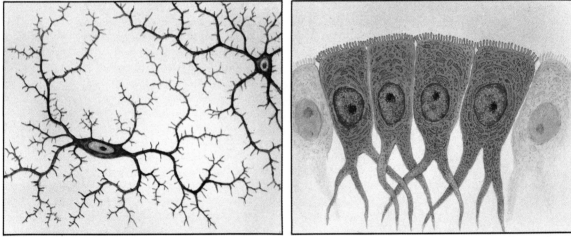

FIGURE 1-1
Types of neuroglial cells.

Table 1-1

TYPES OF NEUROGLIAL CELLS

Astroglia (astrocyte)

Supplies nutrients to neuron structure and supports framework for neurons and capillaries; forms part of the blood-brain barrier

Oligodendroglia

Forms the myelin sheath in the CNS

Ependyma

Lines the ventricular system; forms the choroid plexus, which produces CSF

Microglia

Occurs mainly in the white matter; phagocytizes waste products from injured neurons

From Thelan.[138]

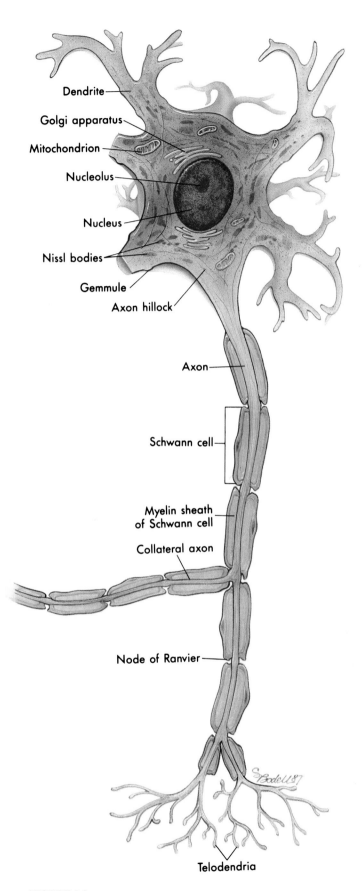

FIGURE 1-2
Structural features of neurons: dendrites, cell body, and axons. (From Seeley.[130])

PHYSIOLOGY OF NERVE TISSUE

NERVE IMPULSE

Nerve fibers are charged (**polarized**) in their resting state. In this state the cells have a resting membrane potential of −70 mV, meaning that the inside of the cell membrane has a negative charge in relation to the outside. There is a high concentration of sodium (Na^+) outside the cell and a high concentration of potassium (K^+) in the cell, resulting in unequal electrical charges across the cell membrane. This difference stems from the cell's relative impermeability to sodium and the sodium-potassium pump mechanism, whereby sodium is pumped continuously out of the cell and potassium is pumped in.

With an adequate stimulus (called the **threshold intensity**), the permeability of the cell membrane changes markedly and rapidly; this change results in a gain of sodium and a loss of potassium in the cell. With the gain of sodium, the cell becomes positively charged in relation to the interstitial space, and an action potential, or **depolarization**, results. The depolarization stimulus excites one area, which then excites adjacent parts of the cell membrane (**conduction**), until the entire membrane is stimulated at the same intensity. Thus the wave of depolarization moves cyclically along the entire length of the nerve. After depolariza-

tion, the ionic flow reverses: sodium is pumped out as potassium is pumped back into the cell. This is the **repolarization** process, whereby the membrane is returned to its resting potential. During depolarization and one third of the repolarization process, the neuron cell cannot be restimulated with another action potential. This interval, or **absolute refractory period,** prevents repeated excitation of the neuron (Figure 1-3).

SYNAPSE

Because neurons are arranged in chainlike pathways, impulses must travel from one cell to another via functional junctions called synapses (Figure 1-4). Actual synaptic transmission is a chemical process that occurs because of the release of neurotransmitters (see box). In addition, synapses are polarized so that the impulse flows in one direction only (e.g., from the axon of one neuron to the axon, dendrites, or cell body of another neuron in a pathway).

The anatomic structures of the synapse consist of **presynaptic terminals,** the **synaptic cleft,** and the **postsynaptic membrane.** The presynaptic terminals (also called **presynaptic knobs**) contain hundreds of very small circular vesicles that store excitatory or inhibitory neurotransmitters.

NEUROTRANSMITTER SUBSTANCES AND SUSPECTED NEUROTRANSMITTER SUBSTANCES

Neurotransmitters

Acetylcholine
Norepinephrine
Epinephrine
Glycine
Gamma-aminobutyric acid (GABA)
Glutamic acid
Substance P
Serotonin
Dopamine
Aspartic acid

Modified from Seeley.[130]

Neuromodulators

Enkephalins
Endorphins
Substance P

Other compounds (either neurotransmitters or neuromodulators)

Prostaglandins
Cyclic AMP
Histamine
Cholic acid

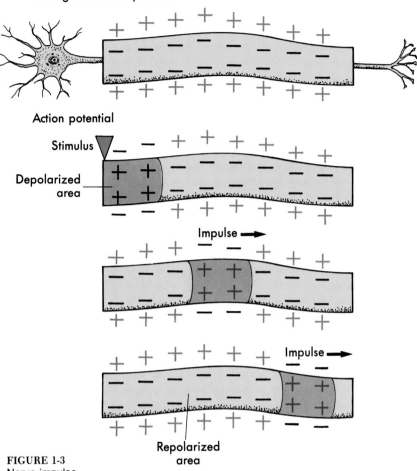

Resting membrane potential

Action potential

Stimulus

Depolarized area

Impulse →

Impulse →

Repolarized area

FIGURE 1-3
Nerve impulse.

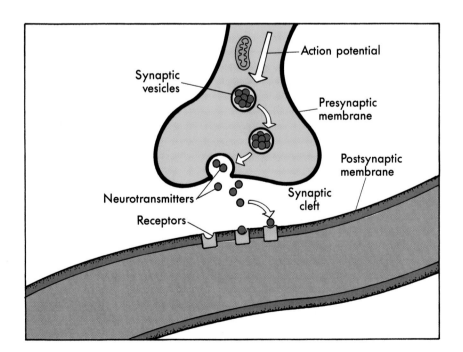

Action potential

Synaptic vesicles

Presynaptic membrane

Postsynaptic membrane

Neurotransmitters

Synaptic cleft

Receptors

FIGURE 1-4
Synaptic transmission.

CENTRAL NERVOUS SYSTEM

PROTECTIVE STRUCTURES OF THE CENTRAL NERVOUS SYSTEM

Skull

The brain is protected by the bony structure of the skull, which is divided into two primary sections, the cranium and the skeleton of the face (Figure 1-5). The cranial portion of the skull is made up of eight relatively flat, irregular bones joined by a series of fixed joints, called **sutures.**

At the base of the skull in the inferior-anterior portion of the occipital bone is a large, oval opening called the **foramen magnum.** It is here that the brain and spinal cord become continuous. Also at the base of the skull is a series of openings (called **foramina**) for the entrance and exit of paired cranial nerves and cerebral blood vessels.

Cranial Meninges

Between the skull and the brain lie three connective tissue layers called the **meninges** (Figure 1-6). Each meningeal layer is a continuous separate sheet that, like the skull, protects the soft brain tissue.

The outermost meninx is the fibrous, double-layered **dura mater.** The dura mater envelops the brain and separates the brain into compartments by its various folds. The **falx cerebri** is a vertical fold of the dura mater at the midsagittal line that separates the two cerebral hemispheres. The **tentorium cerebelli** is a horizontal double fold of dura that supports the temporal and occipital lobes and separates the cerebral hemispheres from the brainstem and the cerebellum. (The tentorium provides an important line of division.) Structures above the tentorium are called supratentorial, and those below it are called infratentorial. The **falx cerebelli** separates the two hemispheres of the cerebellum.

Between the dura mater and the middle meningeal layer is a narrow serous cavity called the **subdural space.** Vessels within the subdural space have few support structures and therefore are easily injured.

The middle layer of the meninges is called the **arachnoid.** It is composed of a two-layered, fibrous, elastic membrane that crosses over the folds and fissures of the brain. Between the arachnoid and the inner meningeal layer is the **subarachnoid space.** Within the subarachnoid space are cerebral arteries and veins of different sizes. At the base of the brain, dilations in the subarachnoid space form **cisterns.** It is in the subarachnoid space that cerebrospinal fluid circulates over the surfaces of the brain.

The innermost layer of the meninges is called the **pia mater.** The pia mater is rich in small blood vessels, which supply the brain with a large volume of blood. It is in direct contact with the external structure of the brain tissue.

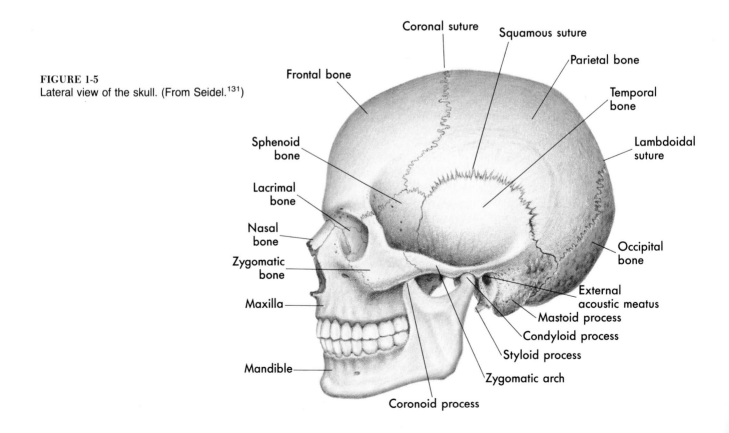

FIGURE 1-5
Lateral view of the skull. (From Seidel.[131])

Coronal suture

Squamous suture

Parietal bone

Frontal bone

Temporal bone

Sphenoid bone

Lambdoidal suture

Lacrimal bone

Nasal bone

Occipital bone

Zygomatic bone

External acoustic meatus

Maxilla

Mastoid process

Condyloid process

Styloid process

Mandible

Zygomatic arch

Coronoid process

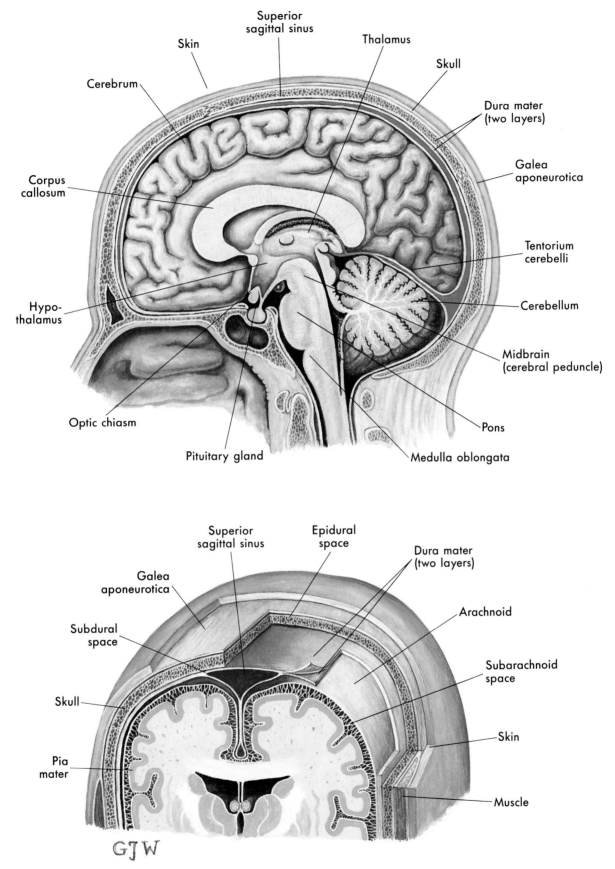

FIGURE 1-6
Meningeal layers of the brain.

CEREBRAL VENTRICULAR SYSTEM AND CEREBROSPINAL FLUID

The cerebral ventricular system consists of four interconnecting chambers that produce and circulate cerebrospinal fluid (Figure 1-7). The system is composed of two **lateral ventricles,** the **third ventricle,** and the **fourth ventricle.**

Cerebrospinal fluid is a colorless, odorless fluid that contains glucose, electrolytes, oxygen, water, carbon dioxide, small amounts of protein, and a few leukocytes. It is produced by the choroid plexus, which is located in the ventricular system. Cerebrospinal fluid cushions the central nervous system, removes metabolic wastes, provides nutrition, and maintains normal intracranial pressure.

BLOOD-BRAIN BARRIER

The neuronal tissues of the brain are extremely sensitive to any changes in the ionic concentration of their environment. Therefore the composition of the brain's internal environment must be delicately balanced to ensure normal functioning. The blood-brain barrier is a physiologic mechanism that helps maintain and protect this homeostatic balance by means of selective capillary permeability.

BLOOD SUPPLY TO THE BRAIN

Cerebral circulation is quite complex and uses 20% of the cardiac output. Because cerebral tissues have no oxygen and glucose reserves, inadequate blood supply to brain tissue results in irreversible damage.

The arterial blood supply to the brain is divided into two systems, the anterior circulation and the posterior circulation (Figure 1-8). The blood supply to the brain comes principally from two pairs of arteries: the internal carotid arteries, which supply the anterior circulation, and the vertebral arteries, which supply the posterior circulation (Figure 1-9 and Table 1-2). At the base of the brain the cerebral arteries are connected, by their communicating branches, into an arterial circle called the **circle of Willis.** The purpose of the circle of Willis is to ensure circulation if one of the four main blood vessels is interrupted. (See Figure 1-10.)

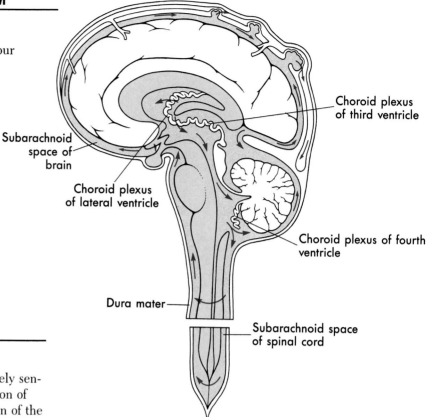

FIGURE 1-7
Cerebrospinal fluid (CSF) circulation. The arrows represent the route of flow. (From Seeley.[130])

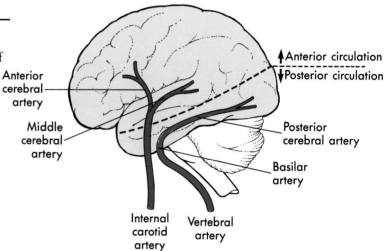

FIGURE 1-8
Arteries of anterior and posterior cerebral circulation. (From Thelan.[138])

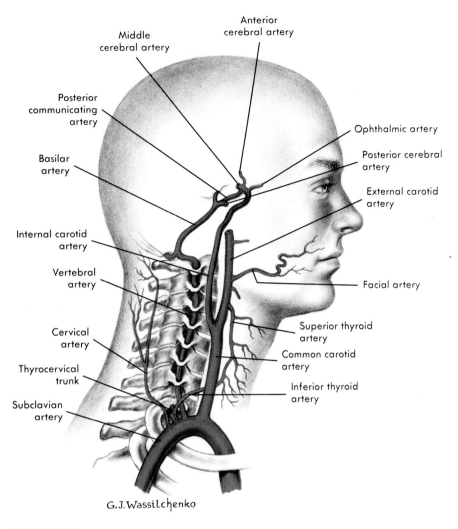

G.J.Wassilchenko

FIGURE 1-9
Feeder arteries to the brain. (From Thelan.[138])

Table 1-2

ARTERIAL SYSTEMS SUPPLYING THE BRAIN

Arterial origin	Structures served	Conditions caused by occlusion
Anterior cerebral artery	Basal ganglia; corpus callosum; medial surface of cerebral hemispheres; superior surface of frontal and parietal lobes	Hemiplegia on the contralateral side of the body, greater in the lower than in the upper extremities
Middle cerebral artery	Frontal lobe; parietal lobe; temporal lobe (primarily the cortical surfaces)	Aphasia in dominant hemisphere
Posterior cerebral artery	Part of the diencephalon and temporal lobe; occipital lobe	Contralateral hemiplegia, greater in the face and upper extremities than in the lower extremities; sensory loss; visual loss

From McCance.[98]

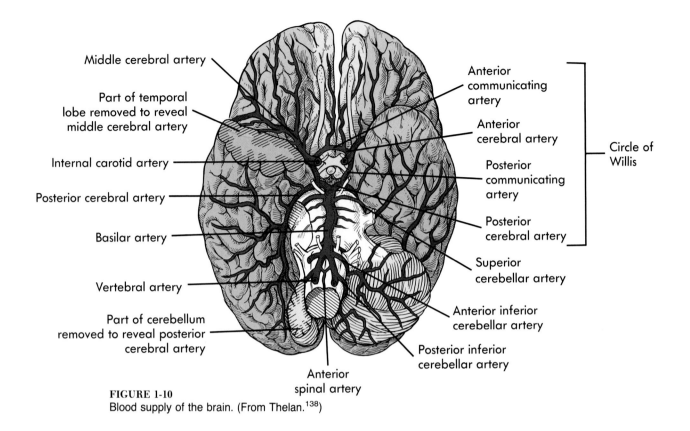

Middle cerebral artery

Part of temporal
lobe removed to reveal
middle cerebral artery

Internal carotid artery

Posterior cerebral artery

Basilar artery

Vertebral artery

Part of cerebellum
removed to reveal posterior
cerebral artery

Anterior
spinal artery

Anterior
communicating
artery

Anterior
cerebral artery

Posterior
communicating
artery

Posterior
cerebral artery

Superior
cerebellar artery

Anterior inferior
cerebellar artery

Posterior inferior
cerebellar artery

Circle of
Willis

FIGURE 1-10
Blood supply of the brain. (From Thelan.[138])

CEREBRAL STRUCTURES

CEREBRUM

The cerebrum is the largest anatomic portion of the
brain. It accounts for 80% of the brain's weight. The
cerebrum includes two cerebral hemispheres connected by a structure known as the **corpus callosum.**

Each cerebral hemisphere is divided into four
lobes (named for the overlying cranial bones): the frontal lobe, the parietal lobe, the temporal lobe, and the
occipital lobe (Figure 1-11, *A*). Each of the cerebral
hemispheres controls its respective functions for the
opposite (contralateral) side of the body.

The **frontal lobe** is responsible for functions related
to motor activity and contains the primary motor cortex. It also controls psychic and higher intellectual
functions. Broca's area, which controls the ability to
produce the spoken word, is located in the left frontal
lobe.

The **parietal lobe** contains the primary sensory cortex. One of its major functions is to process sensory
input such as position sense, touch, shape, and consistency of objects.

The **temporal lobe** contains the primary auditory
cortex. Wernicke's area, located in the left temporal
lobe, is responsible for comprehension of spoken and
written language. The temporal lobe contains the in-
terpretive area where auditory, visual, and somatic
input are integrated into thought and memory.

The **occipital lobe** contains the primary vision cortex and is responsible for receiving and interpreting
visual information.

DIENCEPHALON

The diencephalon lies on top of the brainstem and
comprises the thalamus, hypothalamus, epithalamus,
and subthalamus (Figure 1-11, *B*).

The **thalamus** functions as a relay and integration
station from the spinal cord to the cerebral cortex and
other parts of the brain.

The **hypothalamus** has a wide variety of functions
and plays an important role in maintaining homeosta-
sis. Among other functions, the hypothalamus regulates body temperature and hunger and thirst, gener-
ates autonomic nervous system responses, and controls
hormonal secretions of the pituitary gland.

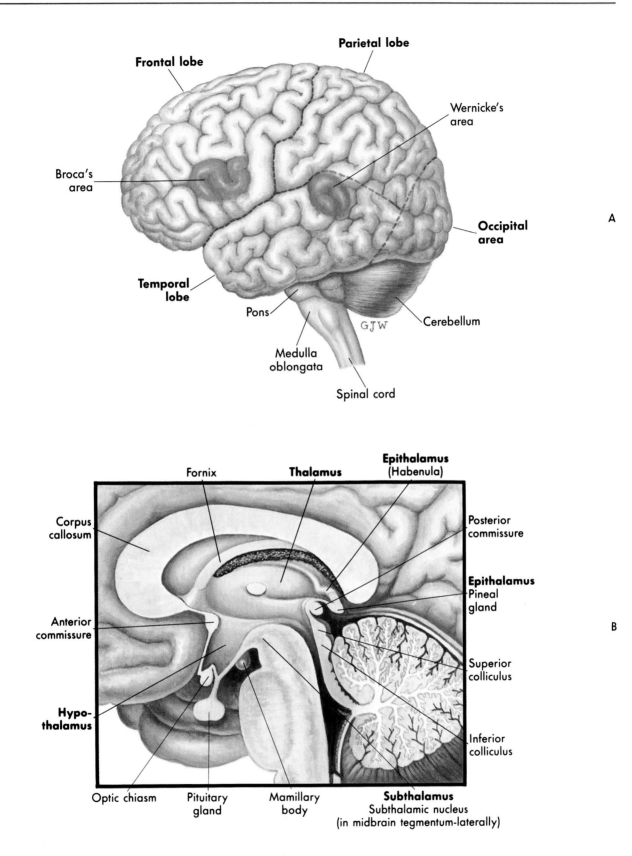

FIGURE 1-11
Lateral view of the brain. **A,** Cerebral hemispheres. **B,** Diencephalon.

The **epithalamus** contains the pineal gland, which is believed to play a role in physical growth and sexual development.

The **subthalamus** is part of the extrapyramidal systems of the autonomic nervous system and the basal ganglia.

BRAINSTEM

The brainstem consists of the midbrain (mesencephalon), the pons, and the medulla oblongata. The overall functions of the brainstem are to maintain involuntary reflexes for vital functioning of the body.

The major function of the **midbrain** is to relay stimuli concerning muscle movement to other brain structures. Arising from the midbrain are portions of motor tract pathways that control reflex motor movements in response to visual and auditory stimuli. Cranial nerves III and IV originate in the midbrain.

The **pons** connects the midbrain to the medulla oblongata and relays impulses to the brain centers and to the lower spinal centers. Cranial nerves V, VI, VII, and VIII originate in the pons.

The **medulla oblongata** contains the reflex centers for controlling involuntary functions such as breathing, sneezing, swallowing, coughing, salivation, vomiting, and vasoconstriction. Cranial nerves IX, X, XI, and XII originate in the medulla oblongata.

CEREBELLUM

The cerebellum is approximately one fifth the size of the cerebrum and consists of two lateral hemispheres and a medial portion, the vermis. It is separated from the cerebrum by the tentorium cerebelli. The cerebellum is involved primarily in coordinating movement, equilibrium, muscle tone, and proprioception. Each of the cerebellar hemispheres controls movement coordination for the same (ipsilateral) side of the body.

INTRACRANIAL PRESSURE: NORMAL DYNAMICS

Approximately 88% of the contents of the cranial cavity is brain tissue, 2% is intravascular blood, and the final 10% is cerebrospinal fluid. These three components are the essential elements of intracranial pressure (ICP) dynamics. Intracranial pressure equals the volume of brain tissue (BTV) plus the volume of blood (BV) plus the volume of cerebrospinal fluid (CSFV).

$$ICP = BTV + BV + CSFV$$

The normal intracranial pressure in the recumbent position is about 0 to 15 mm Hg (110 to 140 mm H_2O). Standing decreases intracranial pressure, whereas activities such as sneezing, coughing, isometric exercises, sexual intercourse, and the Valsalva maneuver cause a transient rise in intracranial pressure. Because the skull limits expansion of the brain, these activities normally are compensated for by redistribution of cerebrospinal fluid to the spinal subarachnoid space or by partial collapse of the cisterns and cerebral ventricles. (The skull of a young child is not rigid; thus expansion is not so severely limited.)

Another important determinant in the dynamics of intracranial pressure is the autoregulation of cerebral blood flow. The pressure of this blood flow generally is expressed as **cerebral perfusion pressure** (CPP) and is maintained by regulation of resistance vessel diameters. The cerebral perfusion pressure equals the **mean arterial blood pressure** (MABP) minus the **mean intracranial pressure** (MICP).

$$CPP = MABP - MICP$$

The normal range of cerebral perfusion pressure is 80 to 100 mm Hg. Cerebral perfusion pressure must be at least 50 mm Hg for the brain to receive an adequate blood supply. To maintain normal cerebral perfusion, the blood vessels constrict or dilate and therefore directly affect intracranial pressure.

The last component in intracranial pressure is the actual brain tissue. The compensatory mechanism of brain tissue displacement or shifting is not usually considered a part of normal dynamics.

Any activity or condition that causes a sustained increase in one of the three essential elements listed above must be compensated for by a decrease in one or both of the other two essential elements. This principle, known as the Monro-Kellie doctrine, must be understood as it affects both the normal dynamics of intracranial pressure and pathologic states that lead to increased pressure.

SPINAL VERTEBRAE AND SPINAL CORD

SPINAL VERTEBRAE

The vertebral column is made up of 33 vertebrae divided into five anatomic and functional regions: cervical, thoracic, lumbar, sacral, and coccygeal (Figure 1-12). There are seven cervical vertebrae (C1 to C7), 12 thoracic vertebrae (T1 to T12), five lumbar vertebrae (L1 to L5), five sacral vertebrae (S1 to S5), and four coccygeal vertebrae (fused as one). The vertebrae are connected by numerous ligaments and intervertebral disks, which provide strength and flexibility.

SPINAL CORD

The spinal cord originates at the foramen magnum and ends at the superior border of L2. It is a continuation from the medulla oblongata. The spinal cord consists of 31 segments, each giving rise to a pair of spinal nerves.

The spinal cord consists of white matter (**myelinated**) surrounding the butterfly-shaped gray matter (**unmyelinated**) (Figure 1-13). The paired gray-matter projections that form the front wings of the butterfly are the **anterior** (also called **ventral**) **horns.** The gray matter contains unmyelinated fibers and cell bodies. The anterior horns contain the motor efferent neurons of the spinal nerves. The pair of projections that form the back wings are called the **posterior** (also called **dorsal**) **horns.** The posterior horns contain axons from peripheral sensory neurons. In the thoracic and upper lumbar spinal regions, a lateral horn is found that contains cell bodies of the sympathetic nervous system.

The white matter contains mostly myelinated fibers, in which impulses are carried to and from the spinal cord and brain. These fibers compose the ascending (sensory) and descending (motor) tracts. The neurons in the ascending pathways transmit sensory information from

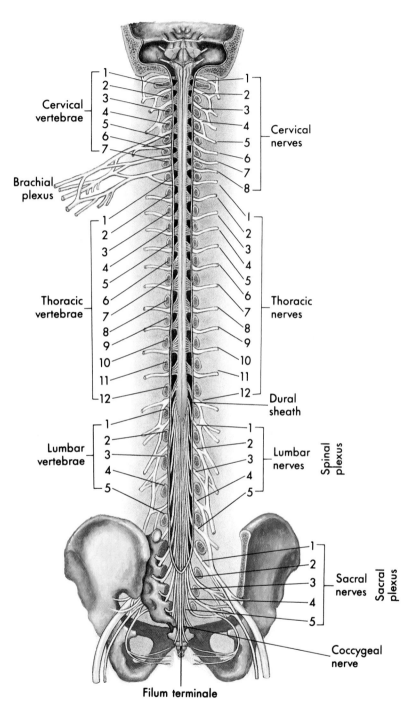

FIGURE 1-12
View of the spinal column showing vertebrae, spinal cord, and spinal nerves exiting.

peripheral receptors to the spinal cord and brain. The descending pathways transmit impulses from the brain to motor neurons in the anterior (ventral) horn of the spinal cord and to motor neurons in the cranial nerves (Table 1-3).

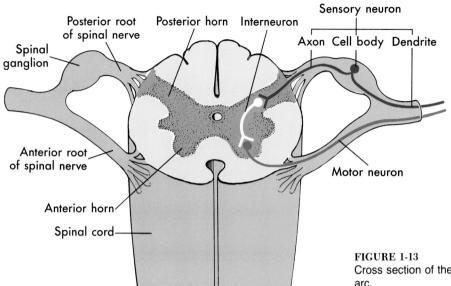

Spinal ganglion

Posterior root of spinal nerve

Posterior horn

Interneuron

Sensory neuron

Axon Cell body Dendrite

Anterior root of spinal nerve

Anterior horn

Spinal cord

Motor neuron

FIGURE 1-13
Cross section of the spinal cord showing three-neuron reflex arc.

Table 1-3

MAJOR ASCENDING AND DESCENDING SPINAL CORD TRACTS

Name	Function	Location	Origin*	Termination†
Ascending pathway				
Lateral spinothalamic	Pain, temperature, and crude touch opposite side	Lateral white columns	Posterior gray column opposite side	Thalamus
Ventral spinothalamic	Crude touch, pain, and temperature	Anterior white columns	Posterior gray column opposite side	Thalamus
Fasciculus gracilis and fasciculus cuneatus	Discriminating touch and pressure sensations, including vibration, stereognosis, and two-point discrimination; also conscious kinesthesia	Posterior white columns	Spinal ganglia same side	Medulla
Spinocerebellar	Unconscious kinesthesia	Lateral white columns	Posterior gray column	Cerebellum
Descending pathway				
Lateral corticospinal (or crossed pyramidal)	Voluntary movement, contraction of individual or small groups of muscles, particularly those moving hands, fingers, feet, and toes of opposite side	Lateral white columns	Motor areas of cerebral cortex (mainly areas 4 and 6) opposite side from tract location in cord	Intermediate or anterior gray columns
Ventral corticospinal (direct pyramidal)	Same as lateral corticospinal except mainly muscles of same side	Lateral white columns	Motor cortex but on same side as tract location in cord	Intermediate or anterior gray columns
Lateral reticulospinal	Mainly facilitatory influence on motor neurons to skeletal muscles	Lateral white columns	Reticular formation, midbrain, pons, and medulla	Intermediate or anterior gray columns
Medial reticulospinal	Mainly inhibitory influence on motor neurons to skeletal muscles	Anterior white columns	Reticular formation, medulla mainly	Intermediate or anterior gray columns

*Location of cell bodies of neurons from which axons of tract arise.
†Structure in which axons of tract terminate.

PERIPHERAL NERVOUS SYSTEM

CRANIAL NERVES

The 12 pairs of cranial nerves form the peripheral nerves of the brain. Some have only motor fibers (five pairs), some have only sensory fibers (three pairs), and the rest (four pairs) have both sensory and motor fibers. The cranial nerves are responsible for sensation, voluntary control of muscles, and autonomic functions; they also include the mechanism for the special senses of vision, hearing, smell, and taste (see box).

SPINAL NERVES

The 31 pairs of spinal nerves arise from different segments of the spinal cord (8 pairs of cervical nerves, 12 pairs of thoracic nerves, 5 pairs of lumbar nerves, 5 pairs of sacral nerves, and 1 pair of coccygeal nerves). Each pair of spinal nerves is formed by the union of anterior and posterior roots attached to the spinal cord. Each pair of spinal nerves and its corresponding part of the spinal cord constitute a spinal segment. Individual spinal segments in turn innervate specific body segments.

The first seven cervical nerves exit above their corresponding vertebrae. The remaining spinal nerves exit below the corresponding vertebrae.

DERMATOMES

Each spinal nerve root innervates a specific area, or dermatome, of the body surface for superficial or cutaneous sensation (Figure 1-14). Although areas innervated by the spinal nerves overlap considerably, knowledge of the distribution of dermatomes is useful for assessment and evaluation purposes.

CRANIAL NERVES AND THEIR FUNCTION

Cranial nerves	Function
Olfactory (I)	Sensory: smell reception and interpretation
Optic (II)	Sensory: visual acuity and visual fields
Oculomotor (III)	Motor: raise eyelids, most extraocular movements
	Parasympathetic: constrict pupils, change lens shape
Trochlear (IV)	Motor: downward, inward eye movement
Trigeminal (V)	Motor: jaw opening and clenching, chewing and mastication
	Sensory: sensation to cornea, iris, lacrimal glands, conjunctiva, eyelids, forehead, nose, nasal and oral mucosa, teeth, tongue, ear, facial skin
Abducens (VI)	Motor: lateral eye movement
Facial (VII)	Motor: movement of facial expression muscles except jaw, close eyes, labial speech sounds (b, m, w, and rounded vowels)
	Sensory: taste, anterior two thirds of tongue, sensation to pharynx
	Parasympathetic: secretion of saliva and tears
Acoustic (VIII)	Sensory: hearing and equilibrium
Glossopharyngeal (IX)	Motor: voluntary muscles for swallowing and phonation
	Sensory: sensation of nasopharynx, gag reflex, taste—posterior one third of tongue
	Parasympathetic: secretion of salivary glands, carotid reflex
Vagus (X)	Motor: voluntary muscles of phonation (guttural speech sounds) and swallowing
	Sensory: sensation behind ear and part of external ear canal
	Parasympathetic: secretion of digestive enzymes; peristalsis; carotid reflex; involuntary action of heart, lungs, and digestive tract
Spinal accessory (XI)	Motor: turn head, shrug shoulders, some actions for phonation
Hypoglossal (XII)	Motor: tongue movement for speech sound articulation (l, t, n) and swallowing

From Seidel.[131]

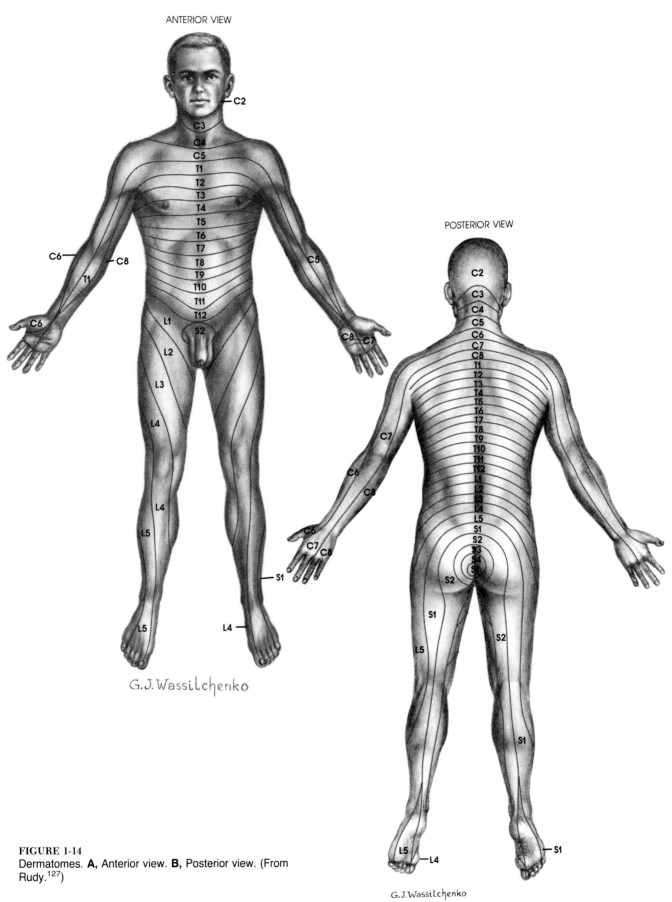

FIGURE 1-14
Dermatomes. **A,** Anterior view. **B,** Posterior view. (From
Rudy.[127])

AUTONOMIC NERVOUS SYSTEM

The autonomic nervous system (ANS) is considered part of the peripheral nervous system (Figure 1-15). It regulates the body's internal environment in close conjunction with the endocrine system. It is responsible for the unconscious, moment-to-moment functioning of all internal systems, including visceral organs (e.g., digestive and urogenital organs), involuntary muscle fibers (e.g., smooth muscle), and glandular functions (e.g., adrenal medulla and islets of Langerhans in the pancreas). The autonomic nervous system is activated by centers in the hypothalamus, brainstem, and spinal cord.

The autonomic nervous system has two components: the **sympathetic nervous system** and the **parasympathetic nervous system.** The sympathetic nervous system is activated during internal and external stress situations (the flight or fight response). Sympathetic responses to stressful situations include increased blood pressure and heart rate, vasoconstriction of peripheral blood vessels, inhibition of gastrointestinal peristalsis, and bronchodilation.

The parasympathetic nervous system controls vegetative functions. It is involved in those functions associated with conservation of energy. The functions of the parasympathetic nervous system include decreasing the rate and force of the heart's pumping action, decreasing blood pressure and respiration, and stimulating gastrointestinal peristalsis.

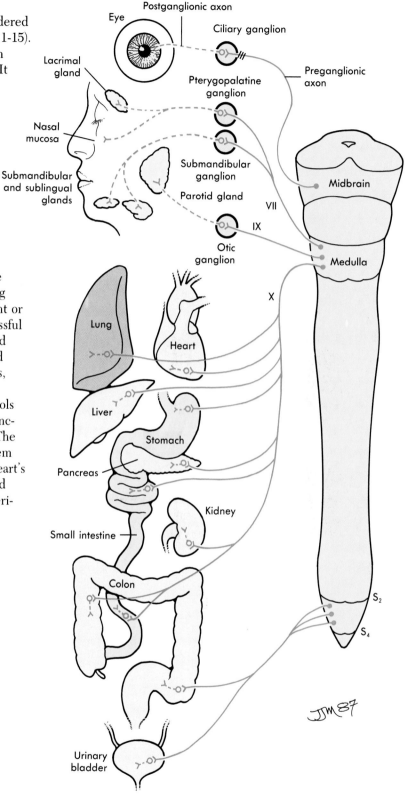

FIGURE 1-15
Autonomic nervous system. (From Rudy.[127])

Assessment

The neurologic evaluation is the cornerstone of care for a patient with a neurologic disorder. Assessment is the first phase of the nursing process, and all subsequent plans and interventions are based on accurate collection of data. Because the neurologic system is a major controlling mechanism for the body, a change in its function affects the functioning of other body systems. For example, a traumatic spinal cord injury affects the functioning not only of the neurologic system but also of the urinary, gastrointestinal, and respiratory systems. Therefore, although this chapter focuses on assessment of the neurologic system, it is always important to assess other body systems thoroughly when evaluating a patient.

ENVIRONMENT AND EQUIPMENT

The environment in which the neurologic examination is conducted usually is predetermined by the setting in which the patient is first encountered. This can range from a chaotic accident scene to a controlled setting in a neurologic clinic. The setting and purpose of the examination also determine the comprehensiveness of the assessment. In general, the examination should be done in a quiet room where the patient is comfortable, his privacy can be maintained, and appropriate instruments are available. Sufficient, uninterrupted time should be allotted for the assessment. The environment may need to be adapted to accommodate a patient's special needs or to eliminate distractions. Sufficient space and furniture should be available to assess the patient while walking, sitting in a chair, and lying on an examination table or bed.

EQUIPMENT

Penlight	Tongue blades	Sterile needles
Coin	Key	Paper clip
Cotton wisp	Reflex hammer	Cotton applicators
Cup of water	Emesis basin	Catheter-tip syringe
Snellen chart	Cup of ice water	Rubber catheter

Vials of aromatic substances: coffee, orange extract, peppermint extract, oil of cloves
Vials of solutions: glucose, salt, lemon, quinine
Tuning forks: 200-400 Hz and 500-1000 Hz
Test tubes of very warm and cold water

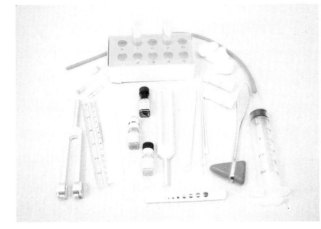

FIGURE 2-1
Equipment for neurologic assessment.

HISTORY

The patient's related history is obtained by interviewing the patient, reviewing data from medical records, discussing the patient's condition with other caregivers, and interviewing the patient's family. Each activity should be pursued separately, and the data should be compiled and compared with the assessment findings after the examination.

HEALTH HISTORY

General considerations

Demographic data: Age, sex, race, home address, religion

Occupation: Description of typical daily activities

Exposure to occupational and environmental hazards: Solvents, insecticides, pesticides, arsenic, lead, and other chemicals; use of heavy equipment; works with electricity, in or near water, or at heights

Intellectual level: Educational history, general communication pattern

Emotional status: Expression of emotion; feelings about self, family, and health care workers; perceived stresses; usual coping methods

Hand, eye, and foot dominance

Medication history: Current medications (note name, purpose, dosage, frequency, route, and time of last dose); significant past medications; recent changes in medications; use of over-the-counter drugs; drug and food allergies

Use of alcohol, tobacco products, mood-altering drugs

Source of health care: Family physician, nurse practitioner, clinic

Current problem

Trauma: Sequence of events, elapsed time, extent of known injury, care provided, medications administered, current status

Acute infection: Onset, symptoms, site of infection, source of infection, interventions done and related response

Seizures/convulsions: Sequence of events, character of symptoms, possible precipitating factors, history of previous seizures, use of anticonvulsants

Pain: Location, quality, intensity, duration (acute or chronic), constancy, related or precipitating activities or symptoms, interventions done and their effectiveness

Gait coordination: Balance, falling, related activities

Vertigo/dizziness: Onset, precipitating activity, sensation, nausea or vomiting, tinnitus, associated symptoms (loss of consciousness, numbness or tingling, cognitive changes, visual changes, chest pain, falling)

Weakness/numbness: Onset, duration, location, characteristics, precipitating activities, associated symptoms (pain, muscle spasms, shortness of breath)

Swallowing difficulties: Onset, drooling, presence of gagging or coughing, problems swallowing liquids or solids

Past medical history

Trauma: head, back, spinal cord, birth trauma, nerve injuries

Congenital anomalies, deformities

Cerebrovascular accident

Encephalitis, meningitis

Cardiovascular problems: hypertension, aneurysm, cardiac dysrhythmias or surgery, thrombophlebitis

Neurologic disorders

Psychiatric counseling

Family history

Epilepsy or seizures

Headaches

Mental retardation

Cerebrovascular accidents

Psychiatric disorders

Use of alcohol, tobacco products, or mood-altering drugs

Hereditary disorders: Huntington's chorea, muscular dystrophy, neurofibromatosis, Tay-Sachs disease

Neurologic diseases or disorders

ASSESSMENT OF MENTAL STATUS

Although there are specific assessment tools to use in evaluating a person's mental status (cerebral function), the assessment process continues throughout the physical examination. Note the person's physical appearance, behavior, orientation, speech patterns, logic, memory, and affect.

STATE OF CONSCIOUSNESS

A person's state of consciousness comprises the degree of arousal and the degree of awareness. Arousal is a measure of being awake, whereas awareness involves interpreting sensory input and giving an appropriate response. The truly comatose patient cannot be aroused, and she is neither aware of incoming sensory stimuli nor able to respond actively. A person in a persistent vegetative state arouses (episodically, not in response to external stimulation) but has no awareness. A person with locked-in syndrome can be aroused and is aware but cannot verbally communicate or purposefully move because the motor pathways in the brainstem have been damaged.[129]

GLASGOW COMA SCALE

The Glasgow Coma Scale is used to quickly determine the level of consciousness in a patient who cannot or will not participate in a more extensive cognitive examination (see inside front cover). When using the Glasgow Coma Scale, make sure to note if certain responses cannot be evaluated because the patient has been intubated or immobilized, is paralyzed, or the eyes are swollen shut. The painful stimulus can be a sternal rub or pressure applied to the nail bed or supraorbital notch.

THE RANCHO LOS AMIGOS LEVELS OF COGNITIVE FUNCTIONING

The Rancho Los Amigos Levels of Cognitive Functioning were developed to more descriptively categorize the cognitive functioning and behaviors of people with a brain injury. This scale is also useful in tracking the sequence of recovery from a coma (see inside front cover).

MINI-MENTAL STATE

The Mini-Mental State is a standardized examination tool that may be used to quantify cognitive function and document cognitive changes over time (Figure 2-2).

UNEXPECTED LEVELS OF CONSCIOUSNESS	
Confusion	Inappropriate response to question
	Decreased attention span and memory
Lethargy	Drowsy, falls asleep quickly
	Once aroused, responds appropriately
Delirium	Confusion with disordered perceptions and decreased attention span
	Marked anxiety with motor and sensory excitement
	Inappropriate reactions to stimuli
Stupor	Arousable for short periods to visual, verbal, or painful stimuli
	Simple motor or moaning responses to stimuli
	Slow responses
Coma	Neither awake nor aware
	Decerebrate posturing to painful stimuli

From Seidel.[131]

```
                                          Patient.................................
                                          Examiner...............................
                                          Date ...................................
                         "MINI-MENTAL STATE"
    Maximum
    Score    Score
                              ORIENTATION
      5      (  )   What is the (year) (season) (date) (day) (month)?
      5      (  )   Where are we: (state) (county) (town) (hospital) (floor).

                             REGISTRATION
      3      (  )   Name 3 objects: 1 second to say each. Then ask the patient all 3 after you have said them.
                          Give 1 point for each correct answer. Then repeat them until he learns all
                          3. Count trials and record.
                                         Trials

                     ATTENTION AND CALCULATION
      5      (  )   Serial 7's. 1 point for each correct. Stop after 5 answers. Alternatively spell "world"
                   backwards.

                                RECALL
      3      (  )   Ask for the 3 objects repeated above. Give 1 point for each correct.

                               LANGUAGE
      9      (  )   Name a pencil, and watch (2 points)
                   Repeat the following "No ifs, ands or buts." (1 point)
                   Follow a 3-stage command:
                          "Take a paper in your right hand, fold it in half, and put in on the floor"
                          (3 points)
                   Read and obey the following:
                          CLOSE YOUR EYES (1 point)
                   Write a sentence (1 point)
                   Copy design (1 point)
    _____     Total score
                   ASSESS level of consciousness along a continuum_____
                                          Alert   Drowsy   Stupor   Coma
```

INSTRUCTIONS FOR ADMINISTRATION OF MINI-MENTAL STATE EXAMINATION

ORIENTATION

(1) Ask for the date. Then ask specifically for parts omitted, e.g., "Can you also tell me what season it is?" One point for each correct.

(2) Ask in turn "Can you tell me the name of this hospital?" (town, county, etc.). One point for each correct.

REGISTRATION

Ask the patient if you may test his memory. Then say the name of 3 unrelated objects, clearly and slowly, about one second for each. After you have said 3, ask him to repeat them. The first repetition determines his score (0-3) but keep saying them until he can repeat all 3, up to 6 trials. If he does not eventually learn all 3, recall cannot be meaningfully tested.

ATTENTION AND CALCULATION

Ask the patient to begin with 100 and count backwards by 7. Stop after 5 subtracations (93,86,79,72,65). Score the total number of correct answers.

If the patient cannot or will not perform this task, ask him to spell the word "world" backwards. The score is the number of letters in correct order. E.g. dlrow = 5, dlorw = 3.

RECALL

Ask the patient if he can recall the 3 words you previously asked him to remember. Score 0-3.

LANGUAGE

Naming: Show the patient a wrist watch and ask him what it is. Repeat for pencil. Score 0-2.

Repetition: Ask the patient to repeat the sentence after you. Allow only one trial. Score 0 or 1.

3-Stage command: Give the patient a piece of plain blank paper and repeat the command. Score 1 point for each part correctly executed.

Reading: On a blank piece of paper print the sentence "Close your eyes", in letters large enough for the patient to see clearly. Ask him to read it and do what it says. Score 1 pcint only if he actually closes his eyes.

Writing: Give the patient a blank piece of paper and ask him to write a sentence for you. Do not dictate a sentence, it is to be written spontaneously. It must contain a subject and verb to be sensible. Correct grammer and puncuation are not necessary.

Copying: On a clean piece of paper, draw intersecting pentagons, each side about 1 in., and ask him to copy it exactly as it is. All 10 angles must be present and 2 must intersect to score 1 point. Tremor and rotation are ignored.

Estimate the patient's level of sensorium along a continuum, from alert on the left to coma on the right.

FIGURE 2-2

"Mini-mental state" examination tool. A score greater than 20 is acceptable. A score of 20 or less is found in patients with dementia, delirium, schizophrenia, or an affective disorder. (From Folstein et al.[53])

ASSESSMENT OF SPEECH AND LANGUAGE FUNCTIONS

A gross assessment of speech and language functions should be performed throughout the neurologic assessment. A more detailed evaluation is necessary if the patient demonstrates difficulty communicating. If significant problems are identified, the speech therapist should be consulted for a more thorough examination.

The patient's voice should be clear, with the ability to change volume and pitch. Speech should be fluent with expression of connected thoughts. Evaluate the pronunciation and rhythm of spontaneous speech. If the patient cannot communicate verbally, assess her ability to understand and use gestures. The patient's ability to read and write should always be assessed. This can be done by asking the patient to read several lines from a patient education brochure and to write down a list of past illnesses. Note if the patient normally wears glasses, contact lenses, hearing aids, or dentures. If the patient can communicate only by sign language, ask if a family member can help interpret during the interview and examination, or identify another member of the staff who can sign.

ASSESSMENT OF CRANIAL NERVE FUNCTION

Table 2-1 gives the procedures for testing cranial nerve functions.

Cranial Nerve I (Olfactory)

Have available several vials of familiar aromatic substances, such as fresh instant coffee, orange extract, peppermint extract, or oil of cloves. Do not let the patient see the vial labels. Before testing, ensure that the patient's nasal passages are open by asking her to occlude each naris, inhale, and then exhale. Have the patient close her eyes. Using the least irritating aroma first, occlude one naris and place the vial under the patient's nose (Figure 2-3). Ask the patient to inhale and identify the odor. Repeat the process, using a different vial and the opposite naris. Continue with other odors, alternating nares and allowing a minute or so between each test so the patient does not get confused. The patient should be sensitive to the odors in each naris and able to discriminate among them.

Cranial Nerve II (Optic)

Examination of the optic nerve involves testing visual acuity and the visual fields. Visual acuity is tested by positioning the patient 20 feet away from a well-lighted Snellen chart, having the patient cover one eye with an opaque card, and asking her to identify all the letters of any specific line. Determine the line with the smallest letters that the patient can read accurately and record the visual acuity designated by the line on the chart. Repeat the procedure for the opposite eye, asking the patient to read the letters from right to left to decrease the chance of the patient simply recalling the letters from memory. If the patient wears corrective lenses, test the vision without the lenses first, then with the

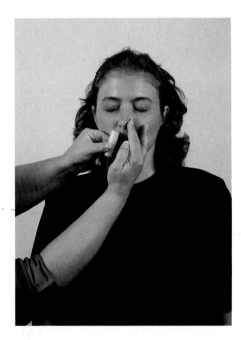

FIGURE 2-3
Examination of the olfactory cranial nerve (CN I).

lenses. Record both readings, designating which is with the corrective lenses.

Visual fields can be grossly measured by the confrontation test. Sit opposite the patient at eye level, about 2 feet away. Ask the patient to cover her left eye with an opaque card while you cover your right eye with a similar card. Have the patient look into your eye while you look into hers. Hold a small object such as a pencil in your left hand, and bring the object from the periphery into the patient's field of vision from direc-

Table 2-1

PROCEDURES FOR CRANIAL NERVE EXAMINATION

Cranial nerve (CN)	Procedure
CN I (olfactory)	Test ability to identify familiar aromatic odors, one naris at a time with eyes closed.
CN II (optic)	Test vision with Snellen chart and Rosenbaum near vision chart. Perform ophthalmoscopic examination of fundi. Test visual fields by confrontation and extinction of vision.
CN III, IV, and VI (oculomotor, trochlear, and abducens)	Inspect eyelids for drooping. Inspect pupils' size for equality and their direct and consensual response to light and accommodation. Assess cardinal fields of gaze.
CN V (trigeminal)	Inspect face for muscle atrophy and tremors. Palpate jaw muscles for tone and strength when patient clenches teeth. Test superficial pain and touch sensation in each branch. (Test temperature sensation if there are unexpected findings to pain or touch.) Test corneal reflex.
CN VII (facial)	Inspect symmetry of facial features with various expressions (smile, frown, puffed cheeks, wrinkled forehead, and so on). Test ability to identify sweet and salty tastes on each side of tongue.
CN VIII (acoustic)	Test sense of hearing with whisper screening tests or by audiometry. Compare bone and air conduction of sound. Test for lateralization of sound.
CN IX (glossopharyngeal)	Test ability to identify sour and bitter tastes. Test gag reflex and ability to swallow.
CN X (vagus)	Inspect palate and uvula for symmetry with speech sounds and gag reflex. Observe for swallowing difficulty. Evaluate quality of guttural speech sounds (presence of nasal or hoarse quality to voice).
CN XI (spinal accessory)	Test trapezius muscle strength (shrug shoulders against resistance). Test sternocleidomastoid muscle strength (turn head to each side against resistance).
CN XII (hypoglossal)	Inspect tongue in mouth and while protruded for symmetry, tremors, and atrophy. Inspect tongue movement toward nose and chin. Test tongue strength with index finger when tongue is pressed against cheek. Evaluate quality of lingual speech sounds (l, t, d, n).

From Seidel.[131]

tions shown in Figure 2-4. Keep the object equidistant between you and the patient, except when testing the temporal field (when the test object must be placed somewhat behind the patient). Move the object slowly, giving the patient time to respond; ask her to indicate when she first sees the object. Compare her response to your field (except temporal vision). Repeat with the other eye.

Cranial Nerves III, IV, and VI (Oculomotor, Trochlear, and Abducens)

Cranial nerves III, IV, and VI are examined as a group because they work together with the extraocular mus-

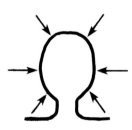

FIGURE 2-4
Field of vision.

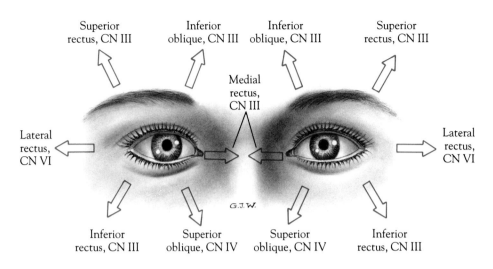

Superior rectus, CN III   Inferior oblique, CN III   Inferior oblique, CN III   Superior rectus, CN III

Medial rectus, CN III

Lateral rectus, CN VI

Lateral rectus, CN VI

G.J.W.

Inferior rectus, CN III   Superior oblique, CN IV   Superior oblique, CN IV   Inferior rectus, CN III

FIGURE 2-5
Testing the six cardinal fields of gaze. (From Seidel.[131])

cles to control eye movements. Inspect the eyelids for drooping. A drooping eyelid might indicate damage to the oculomotor nerve. Stabilize the patient's chin to prevent head movement, then have her watch your finger as you move it through the six cardinal fields of gaze (Figure 2-5). Movements should be smooth. Full movement indicates appropriate muscle strength and intact nerve function.

Next the pupils are tested for response to light both directly and consensually. Room lights should be dimmed so that the pupils dilate. First, shine a penlight directly into one eye. The pupil should constrict. There should be a consensual response in the opposite eye, causing that pupil to constrict simultaneously with the one being tested.

To test the pupils for constriction to accommodation, ask the patient to look at an object across the room and then at your finger, which is held about 4 inches in front of the bridge of the patient's nose. The pupils should constrict when the eyes focus on your finger after first looking at the distant object. Using a ruler or pupillary size chart (Figure 2-6), estimate resting pupil size and compare to see if the pupils are equal in size.

Cranial Nerve V (Trigeminal)

First, inspect the face for any tremors or muscle atrophy. Then palpate the jaw muscles for tone while the patient clenches her teeth (Figure 2-7, *A*). The sensory function of the trigeminal nerve is evaluated for sharp, dull, and light touch. Have the patient close her eyes, then randomly touch each side of the face on the forehead, cheek, and chin with a point, a rounded end of a paper clip, and then a wisp of cotton (Figure 2-7, *B*). Ask the patient to state where the stimulus is felt and

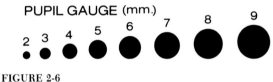

PUPIL GAUGE (mm.)

2 3 4 5 6 7 8 9

FIGURE 2-6
Pupillary size chart.

whether it is sharp or dull. Use a tongue blade to check sensation of the buccal mucosa. Temperature sensation over the face is tested by using capped test tubes filled with very warm and cold water. There should be symmetric sensory discrimination over the face to each stimulus.

The corneal reflex is tested by having the patient (with any contact lenses removed) look up and away from the examiner. Approaching from the side, lightly touch the cornea of one eye with a wisp of cotton. Repeat on the other eye with a clean wisp of cotton. A symmetric blink reflex should be present.

Cranial Nerve VII (Facial)

The motor function of the facial nerve is tested by having the patient raise her eyebrows and wrinkle the forehead, smile, puff out cheeks, purse lips and blow out, show her teeth, and squeeze her eyes shut while you try to open them. Movements should be smooth and symmetric (Figure 2-8).

The sensory functions of the facial nerve and the glossopharyngeal nerve are tested at the same time. The facial nerve is responsible for detecting sweet and salty tastes on each side of the anterior tongue, whereas the glossopharyngeal nerve detects sour and bitter

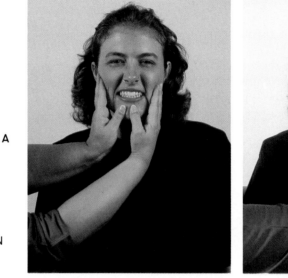
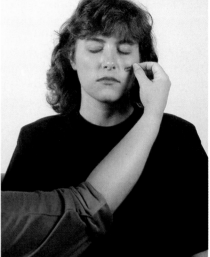

FIGURE 2-7
Examination of the trigeminal nerve (CN V) for motor function **(A)** and sensory function **(B)**.

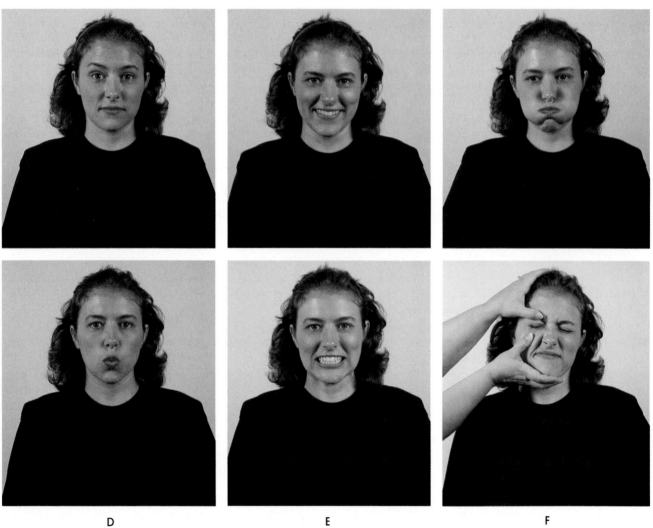

FIGURE 2-8
Examination of the facial nerve (CN VII). Ask the patient to **(A)** raise eyebrows and wrinkle forehead, **(B)** smile, **(C)** puff out cheeks, **(D)** purse lips and blow out, **(E)** show teeth, and **(F)** squeeze eyes shut while you try to open them.

tastes on each side of the posterior tongue (Figure 2-9). Place four vials of appropriate solutions (glucose, salt, lemon, and quinine) on a table with the labels facing away from the patient. Have the tastes written on a paper so the patient can point to the appropriate answer. Have the patient keep her tongue protruded while you apply one solution at a time to the appropriate region of the tongue. Using a clean swab, apply one taste at a time to one region, and ask the patient to point to the perceived taste on the sheet of paper. Have the patient rinse her mouth with water between tests. Apply tastes to each side of the tongue. The patient should be able to identify each taste bilaterally.

Cranial Nerve VIII (Acoustic)

Hearing initially can be screened at the beginning of the interview, when the patient states either that she understands or that she cannot hear your questions. Note whether the patient wears hearing aids, and if so, remove them while testing the acoustic nerve. First, see if the patient can hear one- and two-syllable words that you whisper 1 to 2 feet from each ear while the patient occludes the other ear. The patient should be able to repeat your spoken words with at least 50% accuracy. High-frequency hearing can be grossly tested by holding a ticking watch 10 inches from each ear while the other ear is occluded. Slowly bring the watch toward the ear until the patient hears the ticking. (Before using the watch, test the distance from the ear that the ticking can be heard by several co-workers.)

The tuning fork is used to compare hearing by bone conduction with that by air conduction. The tuning fork is set into vibration by holding the base with one hand and tapping the tines gently against the heel of the other hand. For the Weber test, the vibrating tuning fork is placed on the midline vertex of the patient's head. Ask if it is heard better in one ear or in both equally. If it is lateralized to one ear more than the other, have the patient identify which side. Test again, having the patient occlude one ear. Normally there should be no lateralization initially, but it will lateralize to the occluded ear. For the Rinne test, the base of the vibrating tuning fork is placed against the patient's mastoid bone. Begin timing with your watch. Have the patient tell you when the sound is no longer heard. Note the number of seconds. Quickly position the vibrating tines about ½ inch from the patient's auditory canal, and ask the patient to tell you when she can no longer hear the sound. Continue timing the interval to determine how long the sound is heard by air conduction. Compare the length of time the sound is heard by bone conduction versus air conduction. The ratio should be 2 to 1, since air conduction is heard twice as long as bone conduction. The Schwabach test involves placing the

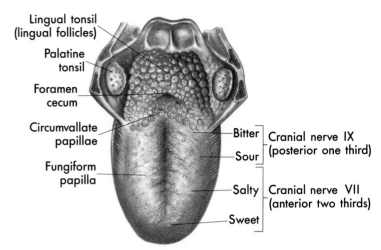

FIGURE 2-9
Location of taste bud regions tested for the sensory function of the facial and glossopharyngeal cranial nerves. (From Seidel.[131])

vibrating tuning fork alternately against the patient's mastoid bone and the examiner's mastoid bone. Normally, the patient should hear the vibration as long as the examiner.

To evaluate vestibular function, the caloric test is done. Place the patient in a supine position with her head elevated 30 degrees. Using a syringe and a soft rubber catheter, instill 5 to 10 ml of ice water into the ear under gentle pressure. This normally will cause vertigo, nystagmus, nausea, and possibly vomiting.

Cranial Nerve IX (Glossopharyngeal)

The taste function of the glossopharyngeal nerve is tested with the facial nerve as described on page 24. The glossopharyngeal sensation is tested with the vagus nerve by stimulating a gag reflex, and the motor function is tested with the vagus nerve by evaluating swallowing.

Cranial Nerve X (Vagus)

Nasopharyngeal sensation is tested by soliciting the gag reflex by touching the posterior wall of the pharynx with a tongue blade. The palate should move upward, and the pharyngeal muscles should contract. The uvula should remain midline.

Motor function is tested by having the patient say "ah" while observing the movement of the soft palate and uvula for symmetry. Also note whether the patient's voice has a nasal or hoarse quality when she speaks.

Swallowing can be grossly tested by having the patient take sips of water and swallow. The patient should swallow easily with no choking. If choking is noted,

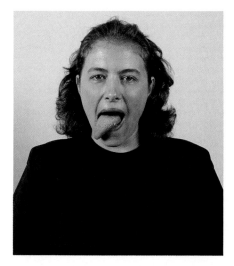

FIGURE 2-10
Examination of the hypoglossal nerve (CN XII).

consult the speech therapist to arrange for a thorough evaluation of swallowing by videofluoroscopy.

Cranial Nerve XI (Spinal Accessory)

The strength of the trapezius muscle is demonstrated by having the patient shrug her shoulders while the examiner applies manual resistance. The strength of the sternocleidomastoid muscle is tested by having the patient turn her head to each side against resistance.

Cranial Nerve XII (Hypoglossal)

First, inspect the tongue in the mouth and then protruded for symmetry, atrophy, and absence of tremors. Then ask the patient to move her tongue toward her nose, toward her chin, and side to side (Figure 2-10). The strength of the tongue can be tested by pressing against it with the index finger while it is pressed against the inside of the cheek. Have the person say the words "light" and "down" to evaluate the lingual sounds of l, t, d, and n.

ASSESSMENT OF PROPRIOCEPTION AND CEREBELLAR FUNCTION

COORDINATION AND FINE MOTOR SKILLS

The ability to do rhythmic, alternating movements quickly is tested by having the patient touch the thumb to each finger on the same hand sequentially back and forth with increasing speed (Figure 2-11). Test each hand separately. Movement should be smooth and rhythmic.

Movement accuracy is tested by having the patient touch her nose with her index finger and then touch your index finger, which is held about 18 inches from the patient (Figure 2-12). Change the location of your finger several times. Repeat the test with the patient using her other hand. Movements during the finger-to-finger test should be rapid, smooth, and accurate.

The second test of movement accuracy is the finger-to-nose test. Have the patient close her eyes, then touch her nose with the index finger of each hand. Repeat and increase speed. Movements should again be rapid, smooth, and accurate.

The third test of movement accuracy is the heel-to-shin test. It can be done while the patient is sitting, standing, or lying down. Ask the patient to lightly run the heel of one foot up and down the opposite shin (Figure 2-13). Repeat with the other heel. The patient should be able to do this in a smooth, straight line.

BALANCE: EQUILIBRIUM

A person's equilibrium is first tested by the Romberg test. Have the patient stand, feet together, arms at the sides, eyes open (Figure 2-14). Be prepared to steady the patient or catch him if he begins to fall. Slight swaying is normal, but a loss of balance (a positive Romberg sign) is abnormal. Repeat the test with the eyes closed. If the person has a positive Romberg sign, further balance tests may not be safe.

Balance is further evaluated by having the patient stand with her feet slightly apart. The examiner then pushes the shoulders to throw the patient off balance, being ready to catch the patient. The patient should recover balance quickly.

Balance is also tested by having the patient stand on one foot, eyes closed, and arms held straight at the sides. Repeat on the opposite foot. Slight swaying is normal, but balance should be maintained at least 5 seconds on each foot.

Finally, have the patient open his eyes and hop in place on one foot, then on the other (Figure 2-15). The patient should be able to balance and hop on each foot at least 5 seconds.

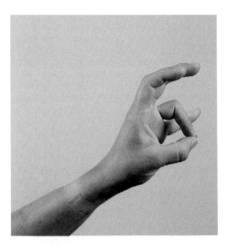

FIGURE 2-11

FIGURE 2-11
Examination of coordination with rapid alternating movements.

FIGURE 2-12
Examination of fine motor function. The patient touches her nose **(A)** and then the examiner's finger **(B).**

FIGURE 2-13
Examination of fine motor function. Ask the patient to run the heel of one foot up and down the opposite shin.

FIGURE 2-14
Evaluation of balance with the Romberg test. (From Seidel.[131])

FIGURE 2-15
Evaluation of balance with the patient hopping in place on one foot. (From Seidel.[131])

A
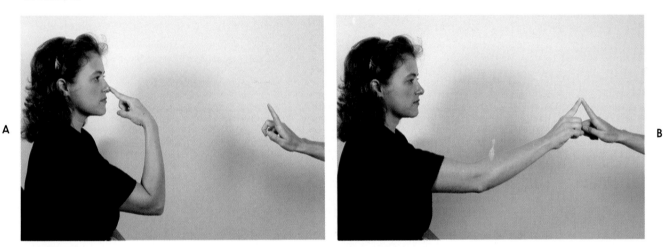
B

FIGURE 2-12

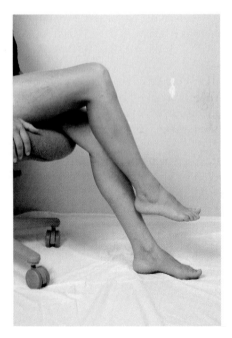

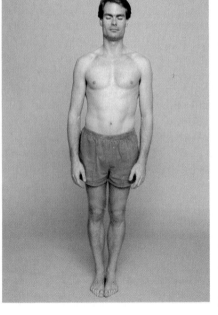

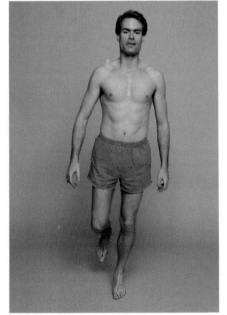

FIGURE 2-13   **FIGURE 2-14**   **FIGURE 2-15**

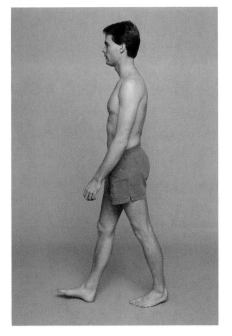

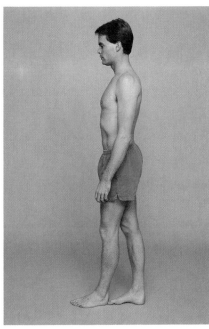

FIGURE 2-16
Evaluation of gait. (From Seidel.[131])

FIGURE 2-17
Evaluation of balance with
heel-toe walking on a straight
line.

FIGURE 2-16   **FIGURE 2-17**

BALANCE: GAIT

Observe the patient walk barefooted down the hallway, first with eyes open and then closed. Observe gait sequence, arm movements, and posture (Figure 2-16). Note any shuffling, toe walking, foot slapping, staggering, scissoring, widely placed feet, loss of arm swing, and hip hiking. The gait should be smooth and symmetric and have a regular rhythm. Posture should be a smooth sway with each step, and the arm swing should be smooth and symmetric.

Next, have the patient walk forward in a straight line heel to toe with eyes open (Figure 2-17). Then have the patient reverse and walk heel to toe backwards. Some swaying is normal, but the patient should be able to consistently touch heel to toe.

ASSESSMENT OF SENSORY FUNCTION

Complete assessment of peripheral nerve sensory function involves testing for superficial touch, superficial pain, temperature, deep pressure, vibration, and joint position in the distribution of each peripheral nerve. It routinely involves assessing the sensation of the hands, lower arms, abdomen, feet, and lower legs. Facial sensation is tested during the evaluation of cranial nerves.

Sensation is evaluated with the patient's eyes closed. The stimulation is presented minimally at first, then increased in intensity until the patient is aware of the stimulation. The patient should be asked to compare contralateral sides of the body's sensation. With each stimulus there should be minimal differences side to side, correct identification of the stimulus, and cor- rect location of the stimulus. Sensory impairments should be mapped on a body figure that has dermatomes noted (see Figure 1-14).

PERIPHERAL NERVE SENSORY FUNCTION

Superficial touch: Lightly stroke the skin with a wisp of cotton. Have the patient point to the area touched or say when the sensation is felt (Figure 2-18, *A*).

Superficial pain: Alternately use the point of a sterile needle and the rounded end of a paper clip to touch the patient's skin in a random pattern (Figure 2-18, *B*). Allow several seconds between stimuli. Have the patient identify if the sensation is sharp or dull and where it was felt.

SKULL X-RAYS

Skull x-rays visualize the bones, nasal sinuses, and any cerebral calcification of the cranium. These x-rays provide important diagnostic data in identifying fractures, cranial anomalies, vascular abnormalities, degenerative changes (i.e., bone erosion), unusual calcifications, and the position of the pineal body. Posteroanterior (PA), anteroposterior (AP), and lateral views commonly are ordered, but axial and half-axial views may also be requested. The procedure is painless but requires the patient's cooperation. The patient is placed on an x-ray table and asked to remain still for a few minutes (Figures 3-3 and 3-4). In the case of a head injury, the cervical spine should be treated as unstable. The neck should not be hyperextended or manipulated. Metal objects and dentures should be removed.

INDICATIONS

Head injury or fractures
Brain tumor
Vascular abnormalities
Degenerative changes

CONTRAINDICATIONS

None

NURSING CARE AND PATIENT TEACHING

Explain the purpose of the procedure, and assure the patient that it is painless. Instruct the patient to remove metal objects and dentures.

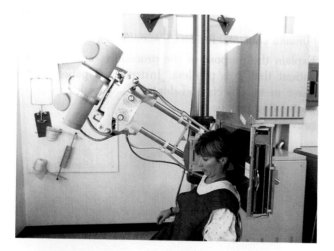

FIGURE 3-3
Patient positioned for a skull x-ray. (Towne view—AP projection with a posterior view.) A lead apron is placed on the patient to prevent unnecessary exposure to radiation.

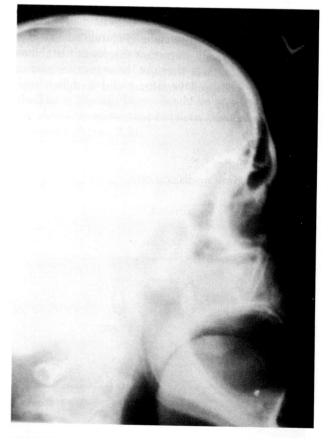

FIGURE 3-4
Lateral sinus view of head.

COMPUTED TOMOGRAPHY (CT)

Computed tomography (CT) scanning combines the technologies of radiologic imaging and computer analysis to provide detailed images of thin cross sections of the brain. CT scans use an x-ray beam to take several cross-sectional pictures of the brain. The computer then calculates the x-ray penetration of each tissue, creating a three-dimensional view. There are two methods of CT scanning, contrast and noncontrast. In contrast-enhanced scans, a special dye may be used to facilitate visualization of the vascular areas.

For a CT scan, the patient is placed supine on the x-ray table with the head placed inside the scanner (Figure 3-5). The head is immobilized in a device resembling a cap, and the patient is asked to remain still. If contrast dye is to be used, an intravenous line is initiated and dye is injected. The scanner takes a series of pictures by rotating around the head at 1-degree intervals until 180 degrees are completed (Figure 3-6).

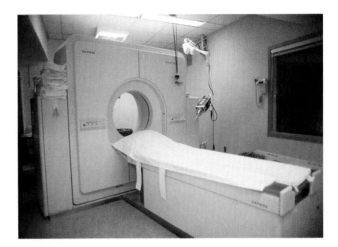

FIGURE 3-5
Clinical setting for CT. (Courtesy Doctors Hospital, Columbus, Ohio.)

INDICATIONS

Head trauma
Cerebrovascular disturbances
Identification of space-occupying lesions
Intracranial tumors
Brain abscesses
Intracranial hemorrhage
Hydrocephalus
Abnormal brain development

CONTRAINDICATIONS

Uncooperative patient
Allergy to iodine dye (only if contrast scan is needed)

COMPLICATIONS

Anaphylactic reaction following use of contrast dye.

NURSING CARE

All metal objects should be removed. A mild sedative may be given to anxious patients. If contrast dye is used, the patient should be NPO for 4 hours before the CT scan. The patient should be carefully questioned about any allergies he may have, particularly to iodine dyes, fish, or shellfish. After the procedure, if contrast dye was used, the patient should be monitored for any allergic reactions: tachycardia, increased respirations, flushing, urticaria, nausea, and vomiting. The patient should be encouraged to drink fluids, since the contrast dye causes a rapid diuresis. Furthermore, because the contrast dye is hypertonic, it may cause hypervolemia. Therefore patients with a known history of cardiac disease should be carefully monitored for the signs and symptoms of fluid overload.

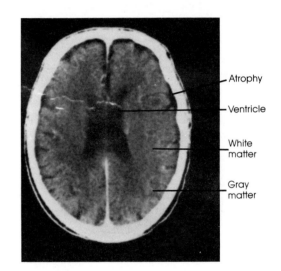

FIGURE 3-6
CT image of brain. (From Ballinger.[14])

Atrophy
Ventricle
White matter
Gray matter

PATIENT TEACHING

Explain the procedure, and describe the CT scan. Explain to the patient that he will be asked to lie still and that he will hear a clicking sound as the machine moves around his head. Explain the purpose of the intravenous line if contrast dye is to be used.

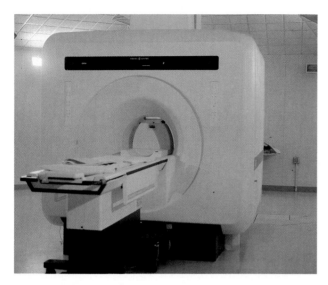

FIGURE 3-7
Clinical setting for magnetic resonance imaging. (From Mourad.[104])

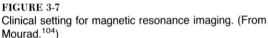
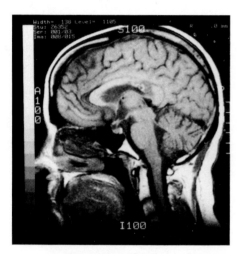

FIGURE 3-8
Midline sagittal brain (5 mm thick slice; T_1 weighted).

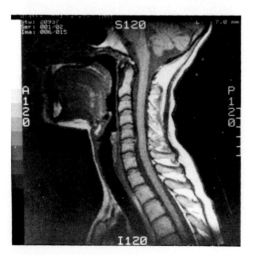

FIGURE 3-9
Midline sagittal cervical spine. Herniated disc at C5-C6.

MAGNETIC RESONANCE IMAGING (MRI)

Magnetic resonance imaging (MRI), also called nuclear magnetic resonance (NMR) imaging, is a technique of tomography based on the magnetic behavior of protons (hydrogen nuclei) in body tissues. The scanner produces images when protons are placed in a strong external magnetic field and then are subjected to short, computer-programmed pulses of additional energy in the form of radiofrequency waves (Figure 3-7). When placed in the magnetic field, positively charged nuclei and negatively charged electrons align uniformly. Short pulses of radiofrequency waves are then applied, which tip the atoms out of their magnetic alignment, causing uniform spinning (resonance) of the nuclei. When the radiofrequency wave is stopped, the atoms realign uniformly with the magnetic field and emit tissue-specific signals that are based on realignment time and the relative proton density (water content) of nuclei. These signals are then monitored, processed, and displayed as a high-resolution image by the MRI computer (Figures 3-8 and 3-9).

INDICATIONS

Central nervous system malignancies
Central nervous system disorders
Craniocerebral trauma
Spinal cord edema or lesions
Cerebral edema
Cerebral infarctions
Hemorrhagic areas of the central nervous system and spinal cord
Congenital anomalies

CONTRAINDICATIONS

Ferromagnetic implants (e.g., pacemakers, metallic orthopedic devices, metal aneurysm clips)
Pregnancy

NURSING CARE AND PATIENT TEACHING

Inform the patient that MRI is a painless procedure that does not require ionizing radiation and has no known risks. Describe the equipment and the procedure. Explain to the patient that she will lie flat on a narrow table inside the round opening of a large magnet and that she should lie still during the scan. Tell her that she will hear a soft humming sound and the on-off pulses of the radiofrequency waves.

CEREBRAL ANGIOGRAPHY

Cerebral angiography involves the infusion of a radiopaque substance into the cerebral arterial system (Figure 3-10). Cerebral angiography provides important diagnostic information about the patency, size, irregularities, or occlusion of the cerebral vessels.

The procedure can be performed via several injection sites: the femoral, carotid, or brachial artery, although the femoral artery is most commonly used. If the femoral artery is used, the catheter is threaded up into the aorta.

Catheter placement is verified by x-ray or fluoroscopy. After correct placement has been confirmed, the contrast medium is injected. Following the injection, a series of x-rays is taken for visualization of arterial and venous circulation (Figure 3-11). After the test, the catheter is removed and pressure is applied to the site.

INDICATIONS

Cerebral vascular anomalies
Aneurysms
Arteriovenous malformation
Visualization of cerebral arteries and veins

CONTRAINDICATIONS

Allergy to radiopaque dye
Anticoagulant therapy
Recent embolic or thrombotic occurrences
Severe liver, thyroid, or kidney disease

COMPLICATIONS

Anaphylactic reaction; seizures; cerebrovascular accident; visual disturbances; pulmonary emboli; hemorrhage from puncture site.

NURSING CARE

Obtain a careful history regarding any existing allergies (e.g., iodine, shellfish) and use of anticoagulants. The patient generally is made NPO after midnight on the night before the test. An IV line may be inserted to maintain hydration. Document baseline vital signs and neurologic status before the test. Check the procedure permission form to be sure it has been completed. Administer preprocedure drugs if prescribed.

After the procedure, bed rest is maintained for 12 to 24 hours, and the extremity in which the catheter was inserted is kept straight. Vital signs should be checked and neurologic assessment done every 15 minutes for the first hour, then every 30 minutes for the second hour, and then every hour for the next 4 hours.

The catheter insertion site should be assessed for bleeding, hematoma, and edema. If the brachial or femoral artery was used, check the appropriate extrem-

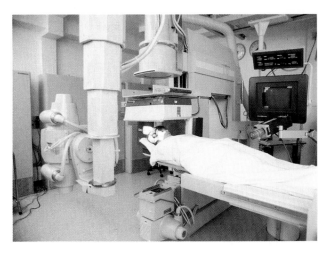

FIGURE 3-10
Positioning of patient for cerebral angiography. The equipment remains in position only while the pictures are being taken.

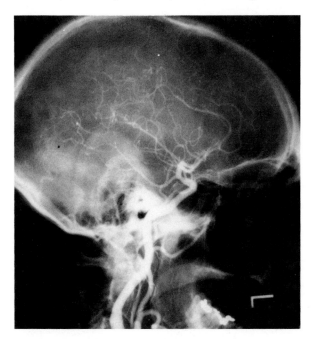

FIGURE 3-11
Left lateral common carotid angiogram.

ity for quality of pulse, color, temperature, paresthesias, or weakness. If the carotid artery was used, assess for signs of respiratory distress or dysphagia.

The patient should be encouraged to drink fluids, since this promotes excretion of the dye. A regular diet can be resumed.

PATIENT TEACHING

Explain the purpose of the procedure. Explain that if the femoral or carotid site is used, the area will be shaved. Explain that the patient will be asked to lie still on an x-ray table. Explain the reason for injecting the contrast medium, and tell the patient that he may experience a burning sensation, warm sensation, headache, or pressure. Explain the purpose of the pressure dressing. Stress the importance of bed rest and of keeping the extremity straight after the procedure. Also emphasize the need for increased fluid intake. Explain the nurse's role in monitoring the patient frequently after the test.

A

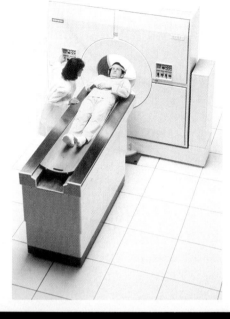

B

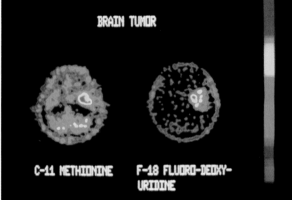

FIGURE 3-12
A, Clinical setting for positron emission tomography. Shown are the Siemens ECAT Scanner gantry and patient bed. **B,** Images received from a PET scan with different radioisotopes such as C-11 and F-18. This particular study positively indicates a brain tumor. (Courtesy Siemens Medical Systems, Inc., Hoffman Estates, Illinois.)

POSITRON EMISSION TOMOGRAPHY (PET)

Positron emission tomography (PET) is a relatively new and promising technique that uses the principles of CT scanning and radionuclide imaging. PET scanning provides important diagnostic information about cerebral function as well as cerebral structure. PET scanning uses radioactive materials that emit positrons (positive electrons), which can be combined with negatively charged electrons of biochemical substances in the brain (Figure 3-12, *A*). The positron emitters serve as chemical tags to evaluate the function of biochemical substances in the brain, such as glucose and neurotransmitters.

The patient either is injected with a substance that has been tagged with a radioactive material or is asked to inhale a radioactive gas. Once absorbed, the positron emitters react with a negative electron, releasing gamma rays. The scanner detects these gamma rays and codes them into a computer, which reconstructs the images. (Figure 3-12, *B*).

INDICATIONS

Cerebral injuries
Epilepsy
Alzheimer's disease
Cerebrovascular disease
Psychiatric disorders

CONTRAINDICATIONS

Uncooperative patient
Pregnancy

NURSING CARE

Obtain a careful history regarding any existing allergies. Encourage fluid intake after the test.

PATIENT TEACHING

Explain the procedure and that it is essentially painless. Reassure the patient that the radioactive material is excreted rapidly and poses no health hazard.

RADIONUCLIDE SCAN

Radionuclide scanning uses a gamma scintillation (Geiger) counter and the injection of a radioisotope (e.g., technetium-99) to detect pathologic conditions of the brain and to evaluate cerebral blood flow. The scintillation camera can detect areas of increased radioisotope uptake, which can then be displayed on the screen (Figures 3-13 and 3-14).

Under normal conditions radioisotopes cannot cross the blood-brain barrier. However, if this barrier has been disrupted, the radioisotope can become localized in an abnormal area. The precise nature of the pathologic process may not be specifically indicated.

After intravenous injection of the radioisotope, the head is scanned with a special sensing device to detect areas of concentrated radioisotope uptake. The procedure may last 35 to 45 minutes.

INDICATIONS

Brain tumors or masses
Cerebral infarction
Headaches
Seizure disorders
Other major neurologic disorders

CONTRAINDICATIONS

Uncooperative patient
Pregnancy

NURSING CARE

Obtain a careful history regarding any existing allergies, particularly to iodine. Encourage intake of fluids after the procedure.

PATIENT TEACHING

Explain the procedure and that it is essentially painless except for some mild burning that might be felt when the isotope is injected. Reassure the patient that the radioactive material is excreted rapidly and poses no health hazard.

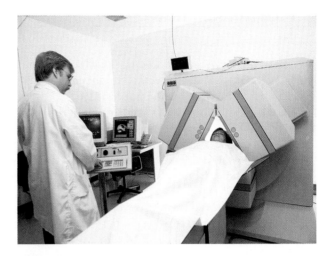

FIGURE 3-13
Patient positioned for a radionuclide scan of the brain. In this diagnostic study a small amount of radioactive material crosses the blood-brain barrier to produce an image. This study is known as SPECT—single photon emission computed tomography. (Courtesy Doctors Hospital, Columbus, Ohio.)

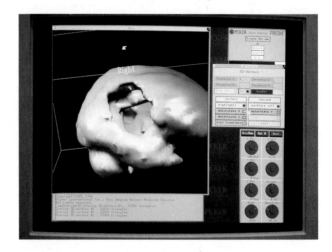

FIGURE 3-14
Image produced by radionuclide scan. This particular image demonstrates a deficit in cerebral blood flow caused by an arteriovenous malformation. (Courtesy Doctors Hospital, Columbus, Ohio.)

LUMBAR PUNCTURE

A lumbar puncture is a procedure in which the sub-arachnoid space is entered, either to obtain diagnostic information or as a therapeutic intervention.

For diagnostic purposes, a lumbar puncture is done to obtain samples of cerebrospinal fluid (CSF) and pressure readings (see Appendix, p. 311). It also may be performed to remove bloody or purulent CSF that may cause obstruction, to inject diagnostic agents, and to administer spinal anesthesia.

During the procedure the patient is positioned in the lateral recumbent position with the knees flexed and touching the chin (Figure 3-15). An 18- to 22-gauge needle is inserted into the subarachnoid space after a local anesthetic has been administered. The puncture usually is performed below the L2 at the L3-L4 space or the L2-L3 space. The stylet is removed from the needle, and CSF drips out. A sterile manometer is attached to the needle so that the pressure within the subarachnoid space can be measured. CSF specimens are collected, and the needle is removed. A Queckenstedt test may be performed if blockage of CSF is suspected; the jugular veins are occluded briefly (10 seconds). The CSF pressure should rapidly increase and then return to normal after release of the pressure. A sluggish rise of pressure indicates a partial block. No rise of pressure indicates a complete block. A cisternal puncture can be performed at the C1-C2 level if there is blockage along the spinal column, but this variation is associated with a much higher risk of complication.

INDICATIONS

To obtain CSF samples
To inject diagnostic agents
To obtain a pressure reading
To administer a spinal anesthetic
To remove purulent or bloody cerebrospinal fluid

CONTRAINDICATIONS

Elevated intracranial pressure
Uncooperative patient
Infection near the intended puncture site
Severe degenerative joint disease
Coagulation abnormalities

COMPLICATIONS

Meningitis; CSF leak; brain herniation; puncture of spinal cord; transient back pain or paresthesia in the legs.

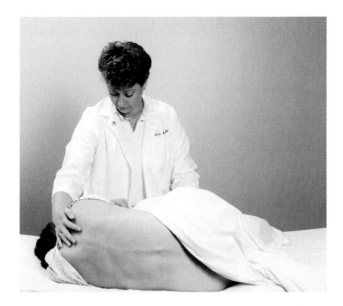

FIGURE 3-15
Patient positioned for a lumbar puncture. (From Grimes.[60])

NURSING CARE

Lumbar punctures frequently are performed in the patient's bed. Consent should be obtained. The patient is placed in the lateral recumbent position so that the back is curved outward and the spiny processes of the vertebrae are visible. After the needle has been removed, a small bandage is placed over the puncture site. Specimens should be collected and labeled. The patient should remain with the bed flat for at least 4 to 6 hours to prevent headaches. (The recommended number of hours of bed rest after a lumbar puncture may vary among institutions.) Fluids should be encouraged. The puncture site should be observed for drainage, edema, or hematoma. The patient should be observed for severe headache, any neurologic change, nuchal rigidity, and fever.

PATIENT TEACHING

Try to ease the patient's anxiety and fear by explaining the procedure and the care that follows it. Help the patient into the lateral recumbent position, and assure him that the nurse will be in the room during the procedure.

MYELOGRAPHY

Myelography uses the technologies of fluoroscopy and radiography to visualize the spinal subarachnoid space. To obtain a myelogram, a lumbar puncture is performed, and 2 to 6 ml of spinal fluid is removed. A radiopaque solution is injected and distributed to the various tissues and structures to be examined. The patient is placed in the prone position on a tilt table with the head tilted down while the study is performed (Figures 3-16 and 3-17).

Two types of contrast dye are available, a water-soluble radiopaque solution (metrizamide) and an oil-based solution (iophendylate). Metrizamide is absorbed into the cerebrospinal fluid rather quickly, but iophendylate must be removed by tilting the patient while observing the image monitor until the solution moves to the needle tip, through which it is withdrawn into a syringe. It is important that all or most of the iophendylate be removed, because even small amounts of retained solution may lead to persistent headaches and possibly adhesive arachnoiditis.

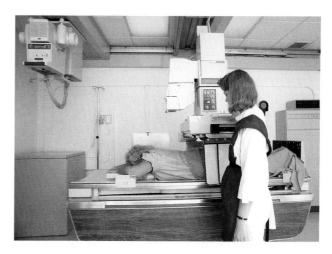

FIGURE 3-16
Positioning of patient for a myelogram. The procedure may last from 30 minutes to 1½ hours. (Courtesy Doctors Hospital, Columbus, Ohio.)

INDICATIONS

Spinal stenosis
Spinal obstruction
Ruptured or herniated intravertebral disks
Distortion of the spinal cord, spinal nerve roots, or subarachnoid space

CONTRAINDICATIONS

Increased intracranial pressure
Hypersensitivity to iodine or contrast medium
Infection near the intended puncture site

COMPLICATIONS

Complications vary, depending on whether metrizamide (water soluble) or iophendylate (oil based) is used. *With metrizamide:* nausea and vomiting, headache, seizures, chest pain, dysrhythmias, speech disorders. *With iophendylate:* headache; meningeal and nerve root irritation; adhesive arachnoiditis

NURSING CARE

Obtain a consent form, and question the patient about any allergies. The patient should be kept NPO for 4 hours before the procedure. A mild sedative may be given. Postprocedural care is dictated by the type of dye used. If oily iophendylate was used, the patient must lie flat in bed for 8 to 12 hours, and fluids are forced to replace the cerebrospinal fluid. If metriza-

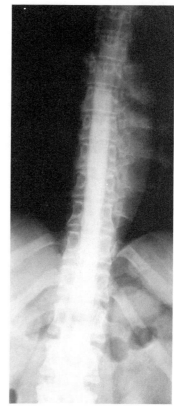

FIGURE 3-17
Posterior thoracic myelogram.

mide was used, the head of the bed should be raised and fluids forced. Vital signs, intake and output, and neurologic status should be monitored following administration of either dye. A mild analgesic may be ordered for persistent pain.

PATIENT TEACHING

Explain the procedure (i.e., the lumbar puncture, the use of dye, and the tilting of the table). Tell the patient that she may feel some discomfort. Explain the postprocedural care, emphasizing the importance of fluid intake and bed rest.

PNEUMOENCEPHALOGRAM

A pneumoencephalogram involves the injection of air, helium, or oxygen into the lumbar subarachnoid space after intermittent removal of cerebrospinal fluid by lumbar puncture. This procedure allows for x-ray visualization of the ventricular space, basal cisterns, and subarachnoid space overlying the cerebral hemispheres of the brain.

Before the procedure, the patient is mildly sedated and a local anesthetic is administered for the lumbar puncture. The patient is placed in the sitting position. After the lumbar puncture, a small amount of cerebrospinal fluid (about 5 ml) is withdrawn and replaced with an equal amount of air, helium, or oxygen. Serial x-rays are taken to visualize the ventricular system.

INDICATIONS

Localization of intracranial tumors
Visualization of the ventricular system and subarachnoid space
Detection of cerebral atrophy

CONTRAINDICATIONS

Infection at the puncture site
Increased intracranial pressure

COMPLICATIONS

Nausea and vomiting; headache; increased intracranial pressure; respiratory distress; seizures; air embolus; shock.

NURSING CARE

After the procedure, the patient should remain flat in bed for 12 to 24 hours. Fluids should be encouraged and intake and output carefully monitored. Vital signs and neurologic status should be monitored frequently (patients may be febrile for 36 to 48 hours after the procedure). Analgesics may be administered as prescribed.

PATIENT TEACHING

Explain the procedure. Explain to the patient that she may experience some discomfort, but sedatives and local anesthesia are used. Explain the importance of bed rest and increased fluid intake after the procedure.

ELECTROMYOGRAPHY (EMG)

Electromyography measures and records the electrical properties of skeletal muscle and nerve conduction. This electrical activity is recorded on a cathode-ray oscilloscope. An electromyogram (EMG) provides important diagnostic data about neuromuscular diseases and other pathologic conditions that affect neuromuscular transmission.

During the procedure a small needle is inserted into the muscle to be examined (Figure 3-18). Initially the patient is asked to keep the muscle still so that any unusual fasciculations or fibrillations can be noted. Gradually the patient is asked to increase movement of the muscle.

INDICATIONS

To diagnose: primary muscle disorders, other disorders affecting neuromuscular conduction

CONTRAINDICATIONS

Uncooperative patient
Anticoagulant therapy or a bleeding disorder
Extensive skin infection

NURSING CARE AND PATIENT TEACHING

The EMG may be done at the bedside but more often is performed in the EMG laboratory. After the proce-

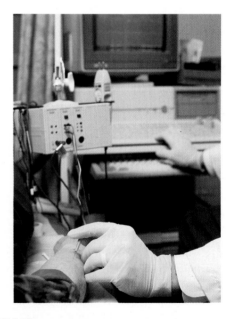

FIGURE 3-18
Electromyography. Small needle size makes the procedure virtually painless. (From Mourad.[104])

dure, check the needle site for hematoma or inflammation. Explain the procedure. Tell the patient that it takes about 20 minutes and that he may feel some discomfort.

ELECTROENCEPHALOGRAPHY

An electroencephalogram (EEG) is a graphic record of brain wave activity. It provides important diagnostic data about abnormal electrical activity in the brain. Generally, between 17 and 21 electrodes are attached with an adhesive called collodion to the patient's head at corresponding areas over the prefrontal, frontal, temporal, parietal, and occipital lobes (Figure 3-19). After the electrodes have been attached, the patient is instructed to remain quiet with the eyes closed and is informed of the need to refrain from talking or moving unless otherwise requested (the patient is asked to hyperventilate for a short period during the test to accentuate abnormalities).

The brain waves recorded during an EEG are called alpha, beta, delta, and theta rhythms (Figure 3-20). *Alpha* rhythms occur in the adult at 8 to 13 cycles per second and are most prominent in the occipital leads. Apprehension and anxiety can decrease the frequency of the alpha waves. *Beta* wave forms are prominent in the frontal and central areas and occur at a rate of 18 to 30 cycles per second. Beta rhythm indicates normal activity, when an individual is alert and attentive with the eyes open. *Delta* wave forms indicate serious brain dysfunction or deep sleep. This rhythm occurs at a rate of fewer than 4 cycles per second. *Theta* wave forms occur at a rate of 4 to 7 cycles per second and come primarily from the temporal and parietal areas. Theta rhythm indicates drowsiness or emotional stress in adults.

INDICATIONS

To diagnose: Epilepsy
           Cerebral death
To evaluate: Drug intoxication
           Cerebral blood flow

CONTRAINDICATIONS

None

NURSING CARE

The night before the EEG, the patient's hair should be shampooed. Stimulants such as coffee, tea, and cola are not permitted 8 hours before the procedure. After the procedure, the electrode paste should be removed completely and the hair should be shampooed again.

PATIENT TEACHING

Explain the procedure and its purpose. Reassure the patient that the procedure is painless and that he will not receive an electrical shock. Explain that during the procedure he will be asked to remain still with his eyes closed.

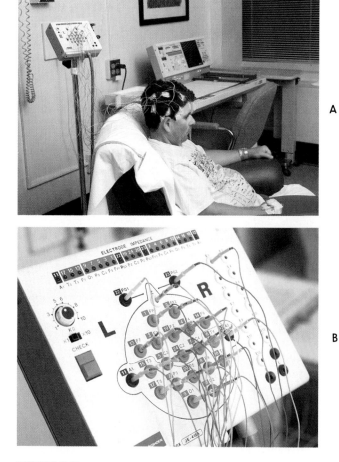

A

B

FIGURE 3-19
Electroencephalography. A routine EEG takes approximately 1¼ hours. The actual test lasts approximately 30 minutes. Electrodes are attached to the patient's head **(A)**, with the wires leading to corresponding areas on the equipment **(B)** for recording brain wave activity.

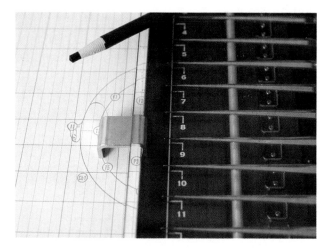

FIGURE 3-20
Equipment used to record brain waves during an EEG.

EVOKED POTENTIALS (EP)

Evoked potentials (EP) measure changes in brain electrical activity in response to sensory stimulation (Figure 3-21). In contrast to the EEG, which records spontaneous brain wave activity, the EP measures and records brain electrical activity after administration of selected visual, auditory, and somatosensory stimuli.

Visual evoked potentials measure the electrical response in the occipital lobe in response to a strobe light flash, reversible checkerboard pattern, or retinal stimuli. Auditory evoked potentials evaluate the central auditory pathways of the brainstem in response to clicking sounds. Somatosensory evoked potentials measure the length of time it takes for the stimulus to travel along the nerve to the cortex following somatosensory stimuli (e.g., an electrical stimulus).

INDICATIONS

Neuromuscular diseases
Cerebrovascular disease
Spinal cord injury
Head injury
Peripheral nerve disease
Intracranial or spinal tumors

CONTRAINDICATIONS

None

NURSING CARE

The patient's hair should be shampooed before and after the test.

PATIENT TEACHING

Explain the purpose of the procedure. Explain that the patient will be asked to perform a variety of activities, during which electrodes placed on the scalp will measure electrical activity.

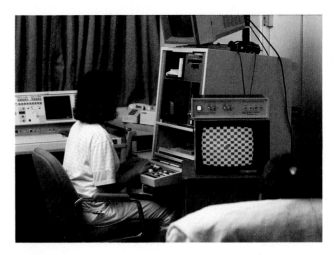

FIGURE 3-21
Patient undergoing evoked potentials diagnostic study. The patient is asked to concentrate on the yellow dot in the middle of the screen while the checkerboard pattern moves. Usually a patch is placed over one eye at a time. The room is darkened for the actual procedure.

CHAPTER 4

Central Nervous System Disorders

Craniocerebral Trauma

Craniocerebral trauma is severe physical injury to the brain or structures within the cranium.

Trauma is the leading cause of death for people between 1 and 44 years of age. Craniocerebral trauma is a major factor in half the deaths resulting from physical injuries and is the second most common cause of neurologic deficits. In addition to the 77,000 people who die each year in the United States from traumatic brain injury, 50,000 to 60,000 survive head injuries with varying levels of permanent deficit. There are no long-term studies documenting life expectancy after a moderate to severe head injury. Patients with a mild head injury need medical follow-up and therapy, but those with moderate to severe head injuries need intensive and often long-term rehabilitation. The leading causes of craniocerebral trauma are falls, industrial accidents, vehicular accidents (70% of victims sustain head injuries), assaults, sports accidents (e.g., football, boxing, diving), and intrauterine and birth injuries.[29]

The general physiologic effects of moderate to severe head injuries include cerebral edema, sensorimotor deficits, cognitive deficits, and increased intracranial pressure. After the initial brain injury, secondary damage can result from brain herniation, cerebral ischemia, and hypoxemia.

The effects of the physiological impairments can vary in intensity and duration, depending on the extent of brain damage and the quality of care after the injury.

Cognitive problems may include inconsistent responsiveness, impaired orientation, shortened attention span, impaired memory, impaired new learning, impaired problem solving, impaired organization, impaired judgment, impaired language, and impaired mathematical skills.

Sensory problems may include impaired vision and hearing, altered touch sensation, altered perception and body awareness, and unilateral neglect.

Motor problems may involve increased or decreased muscle tone, impaired motor control and strength, ataxia, apraxia, impaired coordination, impaired balance, impaired gait, and decreased endurance. The person also may have uncoordinated oral motor function, impaired swallowing, and dysarthria.

Behavioral problems may include agitation, resistance to treatment, lack of initiation, impulsivity, apathy, denial of deficits, disinhibition, sexually inappropriate behavior, depression, impaired social skills, confabulation, perseveration, and difficulty adjusting to a disability.

Functional problems arise from the interplay of all these deficits. The person usually is less able to complete activities of daily living (ADL); homemaking and driving skills are impaired, and sexual functioning is altered, as are leisure time skills, community integration skills, and vocational skills. Other issues that can arise include family education and social support, adapting the home with special equipment, arranging for adequate supervision of the person with the head injury, determining guardianship, and arranging for long-term rehabilitation and treatment.

PATHOPHYSIOLOGY

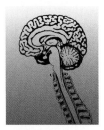 Craniocerebral injuries can result from primary or secondary injury to the head. Primary injury occurs when the head is subjected to traumatic forces. The mechanisms of primary injury are acceleration-deceleration force, rotation force and missile force. These forces can occur simultaneously or in succession and damage the brain by compression, shearing, or tension.

PRIMARY INJURY

Mechanism of Injury

Acceleration injuries result when the head is struck by a moving object and set in motion. Deceleration injuries occur when the moving head strikes a solid, immovable object. In either case, when the skull is hit by force, the brain tissue hits the skull, then reverses direction and hits the opposite side of the skull. Acceleration-deceleration injuries can result in contusion, laceration, and shearing, or tearing, of the brain tissue.[138]

Rotational injuries are caused by lateral flexion, hyperflexion, hyperextension, and turning movements of the head and neck. These movements cause the cerebrum to rotate about the brainstem and produce shearing, straining, and distortion of neural tissue. This rotational mechanism is a major cause of contrecoup lesions and may account for most of the contusions of brain tissue. The areas most frequently injured during rotation are the frontal and temporal lobes.[138]

Penetration injuries (missile injuries) involve direct cerebral tissue damage as a result of penetration of an object into or through brain tissue. These injuries often are associated with acts of violence and gunshot wounds (Figure 4-1). Further brain injury often results from the high energy released by the bullet.[138]

Open Head Injury

Head injuries can be classified as open or closed. Open head injuries result from skull fractures or penetrating wounds. The velocity, mass, and shape of the object, as well as the direction of impact, are the major determinants of the extent of brain injury. Open head injuries involve some type of skull fracture, be it linear, comminuted, depressed, or perforated.

A linear fracture is a simple break in bone continuity that produces an in-bending of the bone at the point

G.J.Wassilchenko

FIGURE 4-1
Penetrating bullet wound of the head. Bullet wound or other penetrating missile will cause an open (compound) skull fracture and damage to brain tissue. Shock wave effects are transmitted throughout the brain. (From Thelan.[138])

of impact and an out-bending of the skull in the surrounding area. A comminuted skull fracture occurs when two or more communicating breaks divide the bone into two or more fragments. Depressed fractures result when the bone is forced below the line of normal contour from collision with a moving object. Compound fractures may be linear, comminuted, or depressed.

A basilar fracture is a serious type of skull fracture involving disruption of the bones of the cranial vault particularly in the area of anterior and middle fossae. It can be linear, comminuted, or depressed. The structures most commonly damaged with this type of fracture are the internal carotid artery and cranial nerves I, II, VII, and VIII. Basilar skull fractures usually traverse the paranasal sinuses (frontal, maxillary, or ethmoid). The fragility of the bones and the close adherence of the dura account for the frequency of this type of fracture and the subsequent leakage of cerebrospinal fluid through the dural tear.[65]

Open head injuries can involve high-velocity or low-velocity impacts. The higher the velocity of impact, the greater the explosive effect within the cranium. For example, high-velocity impact, such as with gunshot wounds, causes laceration at the entry site, cerebral edema, hemorrhage into the destroyed area, and remote contusions (secondary to tissue displacement).[137] Low-velocity impact usually results in distortion and linear fractures of the skull.

Closed Head Injury

A closed, blunt head injury can produce the pathologic signs of cerebral concussion, contusion, or laceration. A concussion is a transient neurologic dysfunction or paralysis and is the least serious type of brain injury. A concussion may involve immediate and transitory disturbances in equilibrium, consciousness, and vision. Contusions result in bruising of brain tissue, usually accompanied by hemorrhage of surface vessels. Lacerations are the actual tearing of the cortical surface. Contusions and lacerations result in microscopic hemorrhages around blood vessels, with destruction of surrounding brain tissue.

A contusion or laceration directly beneath the site of impact is a coup lesion; those occurring opposite the site of impact are contrecoup lesions (Figure 4-2). The two major factors that determine the distribution of coup and contrecoup lesions are (1) the ability of cerebrospinal fluid to act as a shock absorber and (2) shifting of the intracranial contents. With a coup lesion, the impact causes greater displacement of the skull than the brain. At the site of impact the cerebrospinal fluid is squeezed out from between the brain and the skull, and the skull hits the brain at the point of impact.[84] Contrecoup lesions occur because of dissipation of the cerebrospinal fluid between the trailing edge of the brain and the trailing surface of the skull, and because of a compensatory increase in volume of cerebrospinal fluid between the leading edge of the brain and the leading surface of the skull.[84] The coup or contrecoup lesion may be accompanied by cavitation, which is the release of dissolved gases from cerebrospinal fluid, blood, or brain tissue. The release of these gases produces microscopic bubbles that extensively disrupt neural tissue, primarily in cerebrospinal pathways and near blood vessels.

SECONDARY HEAD INJURY

Primary trauma to the head may be followed by secondary injury that increases the morbidity and mortality of these patients. Secondary trauma to the head may result when tension strains and shearing forces are transmitted to the cranium by extreme torsion and stretching of the neck, as in a hard fall on the buttocks. Other factors, such as the development of a cerebral hemorrhage, sustained intracranial hypertension, sustained cerebral edema, hypercapnia, hypoxemia, systemic hypotension, infections, and respiratory trauma and its complications, may contribute to secondary injury to the brain.

Cerebral Hemorrhage

A head injury may be associated with the development of a hematoma (Figure 4-3). Hematomas result in a mass lesion effect that causes elevated intracranial pressure. Epidural and subdural hematomas occur outside the brain parenchyma, whereas intracerebral hematomas occur within the brain parenchyma.[138]

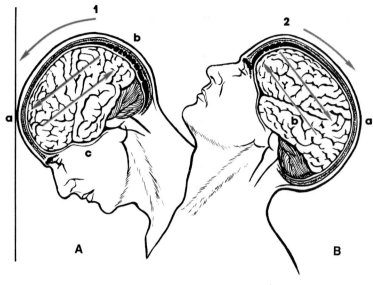

G.J. Wassilchenko

FIGURE 4-2
Coup and contrecoup head injury following blunt trauma. **A,** Coup injury: impact against object. a, Site of impact and direct trauma to brain. b, Shearing of subdural veins. c, Trauma to base of brain. **B,** Contrecoup injury: impact within skull. a, Site of impact from brain hitting opposite side of skull. b, Shearing forces through brain. These injuries occur in one continuous motion—the head strikes the wall (coup), then rebounds (contrecoup). (From Rudy.[127])

An epidural hematoma is a collection of blood between the inner periosteum of the skull and the dura mater. It occurs most often after a linear skull fracture that tears the middle meningeal artery. The patient usually has a brief period of unconsciousness followed by a lucid period that may last for a few hours to days. The lucid period is followed by rapid neurologic deterioration.[65]

A subdural hematoma results when blood accumulates between the dura mater and the subarachnoid layer. Because the subdural hematoma is venous, symptoms appear much later than with the arterial epidural hematoma; thus subdural hematomas can be classified as acute, subacute, or chronic. Acute subdural hematomas usually manifest symptoms within 24 to 48 hours after severe trauma. Symptoms of subacute subdural hematoma may develop anywhere from 48 hours to 2 weeks after severe head injury. Chronic subdural hematomas develop weeks, months, and possibly years after an apparently minor head injury. The chronic type of subdural hematoma is most common for individuals in the 60- to 70-year age group, since atrophy of the brain allows more room for expansion.[65]

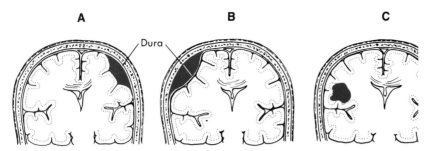

FIGURE 4-3
Different types of hematomas. **A,** Subdural. **B,** Epidural. **C,** Intracerebral. (From Thelan.[138])

An intracerebral hematoma is a collection of blood within the actual brain tissue that usually occurs in the temporal or frontal region. Intracerebral injuries often are associated with contusions.[65]

Cerebral Edema

Cerebral edema and expanding lesions (i.e., hematomas) are the major sources of increased intracranial pressure after craniocerebral trauma. Cerebral edema is an increase in tissue fluid content, either intracellular or extracellular, which results in increased brain volume.[133] It may be caused by the initial injury to the brain tissue or may be a secondary response to cerebral ischemia, hypoxia, and hypercapnia.[127] Cerebral edema after craniocerebral injury can occur around the injury (focal) and throughout the brain (generalized).

Cerebral edema that develops after a traumatic head injury is not a single clinical or pathologic entity, but rather exists in three forms: vasogenic, cytotoxic, and ischemic.[84] Vasogenic edema is extracellular and is caused by damage to the cerebral vasculature; capillary permeability is increased, and as a result plasma protein leaks out of the cerebral vessels into the extracellular space, followed by the influx of water into brain tissue.[127,133] Cytotoxic edema is intracellular and results from impairment or failure of the cation pump, allowing infiltration of water and sodium into the intracellular space. The mechanisms of ischemic cerebral edema are initiated by the infiltration of water and sodium into the intracellular space (cytotoxic edema). This intracellular edema affects the tight junctions of the endothelial cell, resulting in infiltration of plasma across the damaged capillaries into extracellular space (vasogenic edema).[84]

The mechanisms of traumatic cerebral edema are significant factors that affect both an individual's physiologic responses and survival after a severe head injury. If left untreated or uncontrolled, cerebral edema produces a cycle of intracranial hypertension, reduced cerebral perfusion, and increased cerebral hypoxia.

The peak of cerebral edema usually occurs about 72 hours after the traumatic injury. Responses to the cerebral edema include increased intracranial pressure and cerebral herniation.

Intracranial Pressure

Intracranial pressure (ICP) is the pressure exerted by the brain tissue, cerebrospinal fluid (CSF), and intravascular blood within the skull. Under normal conditions, intracranial pressure measures 0 to 15 mm Hg. Intracranial pressure is determined by the ratio of three components: brain tissue, cerebrospinal fluid, and intravascular blood. The exact amount of each component may vary, but the proportions generally are: brain tissue, 80%; cerebrospinal fluid, 10%; and intravascular blood, 10%.

Compensatory mechanisms maintain intracranial pressure within normal limits; an increase in any one of the intracranial components causes a decrease in volume in another component (Monro-Kellie hypothesis). Thus, the total intracranial volume remains the same. Intracranial volume can be adjusted to maintain normal intracranial pressure by (1) displacement of cerebrospinal fluid from the cranial cavity into the spinal subarachnoid space, (2) increased absorption of cerebrospinal fluid by arachnoid villi, and (3) reduction of intracranial blood volume. Intracranial pressure begins to rise when these compensation mechanisms can no longer maintain a state of equilibrium.

Brain Herniation

Brain herniation can occur after a head injury if increased intracranial pressure is not controlled. Brain herniation is the shifting of brain tissue from a compartment of high pressure to a compartment of low pressure.[120]

Brain herniation syndrome may be supratentorial or infratentorial (Figure 4-4). Supratentorial herniation syndromes include uncal (lateral), central (transtentorial), cingulate, and transcalvarial. Uncal (lateral) herniation involves displacement of the medial portion of the temporal lobe across the tentorium into the posterior fossa, compressing the midbrain and brainstem. Central (transtentorial) herniation involves downward displacement of the diencephalon through the tentorial notch. Cingulate herniation occurs when an expanding lesion from one hemisphere shifts laterally, forcing the cingulate gyrus under the falx cerebri. Transcalvarial herniation occurs when cerebral tissue expands through the cranium via an opening in the skull. Infratentorial herniation syndrome involves either downward displacement of the cerebellar tonsils through the foramen magnum or the upward movement of the cerebellar tonsils or the lower brainstem through the tentorial notch.[138]

COMPLICATIONS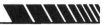

Focal neurologic deficits
Seizures
Neurogenic pulmonary edema
Pneumonia
Gastrointestinal hemorrhage
Cardiac dysrhythmias
Syndrome of inappropriate secretion of antidiuretic hormone (SIADH)
Diabetes insipidus
Disseminated intravascular coagulation
Pulmonary emboli
Heterotopic ossifications
Increased muscle tone
Contractures
Aspiration
Hydrocephalus
Hypertension
Disturbances of respiratory control
Hypopituitarism
Impaired nutritional status
Bladder incontinence
Bowel incontinence
Hyperphagia

FIGURE 4-4
Supratentorial herniation. **A,** Cingulate. **B,** Uncal. **C,** Central. **D,** Transcalvarial. (From Thelan.[138])

DIAGNOSTIC STUDIES AND FINDINGS

Diagnostic test	Findings
Skull x-ray	Calvarial fractures (simple, compound, depressed, or comminuted); bone fragments
Cervical x-ray	To confirm or rule out cervical spinal injury (assume neck injury until proven negative)
Chest x-ray	To check for aspiration, chest injuries, and atelectasis; to check placement of endotracheal tube
Computed tomography (CT) scan	May indicate subdural hematoma, intracerebral hematoma, or shift and distortion of cerebral ventricles
Magnetic resonance imaging (MRI) study	Same as with CT scan
Cerebrospinal fluid sampling (may be contraindicated with increased ICP)	Normal with cerebral edema and brain concussion; increased pressure and blood with laceration and contusion
Cerebral angiography	May indicate intracerebral or subdural hematoma by showing avascular areas with displacement of surrounding vessels
Electroencephalogram (EEG) (done serially)	Appearance or development of pathologic waves; determination of brain death
Echoencephalogram	To detect shifts in midline structures
Serum electrolytes	Hypernatremia; hyponatremia; elevated plasma cortisol; increased serum lactic dehydrogenase
Positron emission tomography (PET) study	Metabolically hypoactive but anatomically normal brain tissue can be identified
Serum alcohol	To detect alcohol ingested before injury
Serum drug screen	To detect drug use before injury
Urine drug screen	To detect drug use before injury
Gastric contents drug screen	To detect drug ingestion before injury
Serum human chorionic gonadotropin	To detect pregnancy
Urine osmolarity	Dilute and concentrated urine

MEDICAL MANAGEMENT

SURGERY

Suturing of head and scalp lacerations; Debridement of wounds; Insertion of ICP monitoring device; Ventriculostomy; Cranioplasty; Shunting procedures for hydrocephalus; Craniectomy; Craniotomy; Skull trephine (burr holes); Gastrostomy/jejunostomy; Tracheostomy.

DRUG THERAPY

Diuretics: Mannitol (osmotic diuretic); furosemide (Lasix) (loop diuretic).

Anticonvulsants: Phenytoin sodium (Dilantin); phenobarbital sodium; carbamazepine (Tegretol); valproic acid (Depakene); diazepam (Valium).

Corticosteroids (to control cerebral edema): Dexamethasone (Decadron).

Histamine antagonist: Cimetidine (Tagamet); ranitidine hydrochloride (Zantac).

Analgesic/antipyretics: Acetaminophen.

Antacids: Maalox.

Artificial tears: Prn.

Stool softeners: Docusate sodium (Colace).

Bulk laxatives: Psyllium (Metamucil).

Barbiturate coma therapy: Given by continuous IV infusion. Pentobarbital (Nembutal); thiopental (Pentothal).

Muscle relaxants and paralyzers: Pancuronium bromide (Pavulon); morphine sulfate.

Vitamins: Multiple vitamin.

Tricyclic antidepressants (for increasing neurotransmitters in the CNS): Amitriptyline hydrochloride (Elavil); doxepin hydrochloride (Sinequan).

Antihistamines (for sedative effect): Diphenhydramine hydrochloride (Benadryl).

Antianxiety agents (for severe agitation): Lorazepam (Ativan).

Antibiotics: Broad-spectrum agents used to prevent or control infections.

GENERAL MANAGEMENT—ACUTE PHASE

Respiratory: Controlled mechanical ventilation and hyperventilation are used to treat increased ICP. Carbon dioxide has a great effect on the cerebral vasculature, causing cerebral vasodilation. Hyperventilation is used to maintain the partial pressure of arterial carbon dioxide ($Paco_2$) between 25 and 30 mm Hg, such that mild vasoconstriction and reduction in cerebral blood volume occur.

ICP monitoring: May be used (see "Intracranial Pressure Monitoring," page 262).

Maintaining adequate cerebral perfusion pressure: Cerebral perfusion pressure (CPP) is the blood pressure gradient across the brain. Normal CPP is 80-100 mm Hg. A CPP of at least 60 mm Hg is necessary to provide perfusion to the brain. Cerebral perfusion pressure is found by subtracting the ICP from the mean arterial pressure (MAP) (MAP − ICP = CPP).

MEDICAL MANAGEMENT—cont'd

Cardiovascular/hemodynamic monitoring: Blood pressure is carefully monitored; a Swan-Ganz catheter may be inserted for hemodynamic monitoring.

Maintaining fluids and electrolytes: Fluids must be carefully administered; a state of mild dehydration may be maintained.

Temperature control: Hyperthermia increases cerebral blood flow and thus can increase ICP. Hyperthermia should be controlled with antipyretics. Shivering should be avoided, since this will increase ICP.

Preventing seizures: Seizure activity increases cerebral blood flow, thus increasing ICP. Anticonvulsants are prescribed.

Barbiturate coma therapy: May be used to treat ICP that has not responded to more conventional treatments. Barbiturates cause cerebral vasoconstriction and reduce cerebral blood volume. Large dosages of pentobarbital or thiopental are administered through a continuous-drip IV. This procedure requires that the patient be intubated and appropriately monitored.

Muscle relaxants and sedation: Used to decrease patient's response to noxious stimuli. Requires that the patient be intubated and appropriately monitored.

Facilitating venous drainage: Head of bed is kept at a 30- to 45-degree angle. The neck must be kept in proper alignment. Hip flexion is avoided.

Nutritional support: Above-normal caloric intake is needed initially. Parenteral or enteral therapy should be initiated as indicated.

Coma stimulation: The effectiveness of coma stimulation is still controversial. It involves periodic introduction of controlled stimuli to stimulate the brain's recovery from coma. One stimulus is introduced at a time. Common stimuli used include familiar strong odors (coffee, chocolate, orange, peppermint); familiar strong tastes (lemon, chocolate, sugar and salt solutions); familiar sounds (ringing of small bell, a favorite song, a family member's voice); tactile stimulation with different textures of fabric; and sometimes visual stimulation with large, colored cards.

GENERAL MANAGEMENT—REHABILITATION PHASE

Maintain skin integrity: Patient is at high risk of developing a pressure ulcer.

Maintain bowel elimination: Patient may or may not be able to control or be aware of bowel movements; establish regular bowel program.

Maintain urinary elimination: Patient initially may have an indwelling catheter to monitor urine output, but this should be removed as soon as medically indicated. Patient may or may not be able to control or be aware of urination; verify adequate bladder emptying by obtaining a postvoid residual.

Maintain body alignment and joint range of motion (ROM): Patient is at risk of developing contractures.

Facilitate orientation and memory: Patient may be disoriented and confused and may have posttraumatic amnesia.

Ensure patient's safety: Patient may have any combination of motor, sensory, and perceptual deficits and may be subject to agitation and wandering.

Address sexuality/sexual functioning issues: Patient may have altered inhibitions and may make socially inappropriate sexual comments or gestures. Impaired motor and sensory function and impaired communication may alter sexual functioning. The concerns of the patient, spouse or significant other, and family must be addressed early.

Maintain adequate nutrition: Evaluation of swallowing by videofluoroscopy often is necessary. Continued enteral feedings may be required. Changing activity levels necessitate changes in caloric needs. Memory and judgment impairments may cause patient to forget to eat or forget that she already has eaten.

MEDICAL MANAGEMENT—cont'd

Guide relearning of ADL: Impaired movement, sensation, perception, judgment, and memory will alter the patient's ability to independently perform her own bathing, grooming, dressing, feeding, and toileting.

Maintain mobility: Patient may have varying degrees of paralysis, lack of coordination, impaired judgment, decreased strength, and altered perception, all of which will influence bed mobility, transferring, and ambulation.

Support the family: Crisis reaction by family members. Patient may not perceive her own deficits. Counseling and social services are needed on an ongoing basis. Resources need to be identified, and the issue of competence may need to be addressed. Education sessions and support groups are important.

Discharge planning: Trajectory of patient care needs is identified as early as possible. Admission to an acute rehabilitation facility, day treatment program, extended care facility, or other type of program for the brain-injured person may need to be considered.

NEUROPSYCHOLOGIC ASSESSMENT

The physician often requests a neuropsychologic assessment of the patient who has had craniocerebral trauma. This assessment, performed by a specially trained clinician, assists in diagnosing brain damage and identifying the areas of abnormal brain function. It is extremely useful in describing the relationships between observed behavior and brain function. Neuropsychologists often use the results to help develop a program for remediation and rehabilitation. The different psychologic tests take varying lengths of time to complete, and administration of the tests may need to be adapted to accommodate the patient's physical impairments. Tests commonly included are the Halstead-Reitan Neuropsychological Battery, the Luria-Nebraska Neuropsychological Battery, the Minnesota Multiphasic Personality Inventory, and the Wechsler Adult Intelligence Scale (Revised).

BRAIN DEATH

The technologic advances in health care over the past few years have raised the issue of further defining the parameters of death. In the past, death was said to occur with the cessation of heart and respiratory function. Advances in emergency medicine and critical care have made this determination less clear, since some patients have irreversible loss of brain function but the heart and respiratory systems continue to function. The issue has been further complicated by the advances in organ transplantation, which identifies the comatose patient on life support as a potential ideal organ donor.

As the topic became a legal issue, as well as a medical and ethical issue, it became apparent that a more precise definition of death was needed. Brain death occurs when all brain function is irreversibly lost. The Harvard Medical School has defined brain death as meeting the following criteria: unresponsive coma, apnea, absent brainstem reflexes, absent spinal reflexes, two isoelectric electroencephalograms 24 hours apart, absence of drug intoxication, and absence of hypothermia.[138] The American Medical Association House of Delegates accepted the following definition in 1979:

An individual who has sustained either (a) irreversible cessation of circulatory and respiratory functions, or (b) irreversible cessation of all functions of the entire brain, should be considered dead. A determination of death shall be made in accordance with accepted medical standards.[138]

It is important that health care professionals know the current state law pertaining to brain death as well as the institutional guidelines where they practice. Review of individual cases by an institution's ethics committee is common practice.

1 ASSESS

ASSESSMENT	OBSERVATIONS
Skull fracture	Linear: No bone displacement; possible epidural hematoma Depressed: Focal neurologic deficits; cranial nerve injuries Basilar: Conjunctival hemorrhage; CSF rhinorrhea (drainage from nose); bilateral periorbital ecchymosis (raccoon eyes); CSF otorrhea (drainage from ear); mastoid bone ecchymosis (Battle's sign); hearing impairments; positive halo sign (drainage of blood encircled by CSF)
Closed head injury	Concussion: Transient period of unconsciousness with recovery in minutes to hours; residual amnesia; memory loss Contusion: Altered level of consciousness with signs of increasing ICP Laceration: Altered level of consciousness with signs of increasing ICP

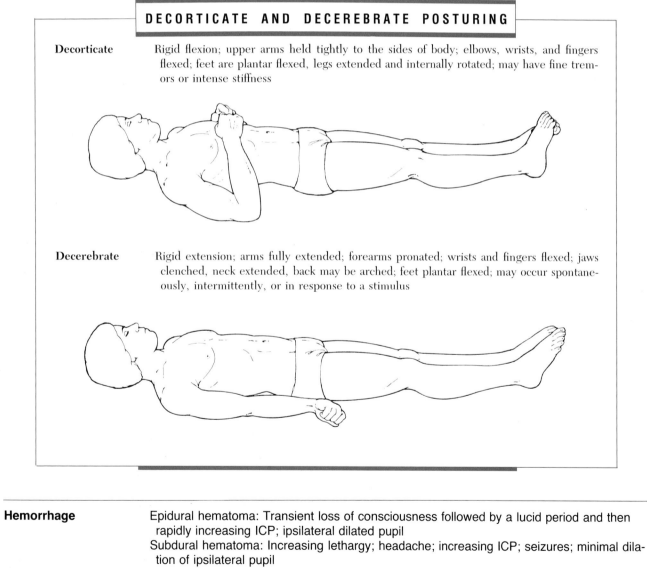

DECORTICATE AND DECEREBRATE POSTURING

Decorticate Rigid flexion; upper arms held tightly to the sides of body; elbows, wrists, and fingers flexed; feet are plantar flexed, legs extended and internally rotated; may have fine tremors or intense stiffness

Decerebrate Rigid extension; arms fully extended; forearms pronated; wrists and fingers flexed; jaws clenched, neck extended, back may be arched; feet plantar flexed; may occur spontaneously, intermittently, or in response to a stimulus

Hemorrhage	Epidural hematoma: Transient loss of consciousness followed by a lucid period and then rapidly increasing ICP; ipsilateral dilated pupil Subdural hematoma: Increasing lethargy; headache; increasing ICP; seizures; minimal dilation of ipsilateral pupil Intracerebral hematoma: Increasing ICP; contralateral hemiplegia; ipsilateral dilated pupil

➔ ❯ ❯

ASSESSMENT	OBSERVATIONS
Cranial nerve palsies	Bilateral anosmia; agnosia (less common); paralysis of ocular movements (diplopia, nystagmus); partial or complete blindness; vertigo; deafness; numbness, paresthesia, or neuralgia of areas supplied by trigeminal nerve; strabismus
Level of consciousness	Mental changes: irritability, restlessness, confusion, delirium, stupor, coma
Cognition	Posttraumatic amnesia (loss of day-to-day or minute-to-minute memory after the injury); disorientation, decreased focused attention Retrograde amnesia (loss of memory regarding events immediately preceding the injury) Impaired language and mathematical skills
Pain	Headache
Meningeal irritability	Nuchal rigidity; positive Kernig's sign (flex hip and knee; straighten knee; patient has pain in back and neck); positive Brudzinski's sign (passive flexion of neck produces neck pain and increased rigidity)
Cerebral edema/ICP	Changes in level of consciousness; slow, labored respirations; changes in arterial blood pressure and pulse pressure (later sign); bradycardia; anorexia; pupillary dysfunction; papilledema (late sign); changes in motor function (i.e., posturing); nausea and vomiting (may be projectile); positive Babinski's sign (usually contralateral to lesion); visual abnormalities (i.e., diplopia, visual blurring, decreased visual acuity); monoparesis or hemiparesis (usually contralateral)
Cardiac	Cardiac dysrhythmias
Respiratory	Rales, rhonchi, diminished breath sounds; shortness of breath; tachypnea; tracheal deviation; altered respiratory pattern

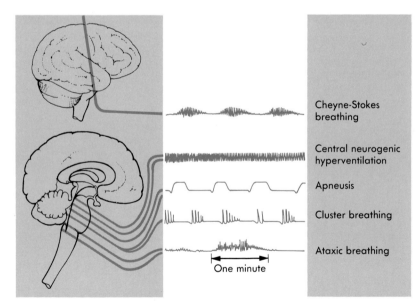

Abnormal respiratory patterns with corresponding level of central nervous system activity. (From Thelan.[138])

ASSESSMENT	OBSERVATIONS
Brain herniation	Uncal: Decreased level of consciousness with almost simultaneous rapid motor function changes; contralateral hemiplegia with progression to decerebrate or decorticate posturing; ipsilateral pupil dilation progressing to fixed dilated pupils; respiratory pattern changes; loss of oculocephalic reflex Central: Decreased level of consciousness; nuchal rigidity; headache; small reactive pupils that progress to fixed dilated pupils; Cheyne-Stokes respiration; cardiac dysrhythmias; decerebrate or decorticate posturing that progresses to flaccidity Infratentorial: Pupils constricted and nonreactive; decreased level of consciousness; apnea or ataxic respiration

OCULAR REFLEX TESTS

Oculocephalic (doll's eyes) reflex

To test: Hold the eyelids of the comatose patient open and briskly turn head to one side, then briskly turn head to the other side. Observe eye movements. Reflex is normal if eyes deviate to opposite direction when head is turned. (From Thelan.[138])

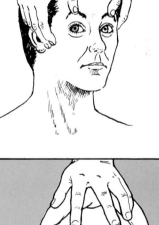

Oculovestibular reflex (cold caloric test)

To test: Physician injects 20-50 ml ice water into external ear canal. Reflex is normal if there is a quick, nystagmus-type deviation of both eyes toward the irrigated ear. (From Thelan.[138])

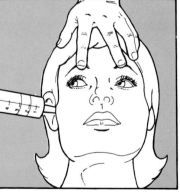

→ ＞ ＞

ASSESSMENT	OBSERVATIONS
Fluid balance	Decreased serum potassium; increased or decreased serum sodium; increased or decreased serum osmolarity; increased or decreased urine osmolarity; weight gain or loss; decreased skin turgor
Gastrointestinal	Abdominal distention; decreased pH of gastric secretions; bowel incontinence
Urinary	Bladder incontinence or retention
Swallowing	Coughing; choking; no gag reflex; no swallow reflex; uncoordinated oral movements
Sensory function	Visual field cuts; diplopia; impaired perception; neglect; impaired hearing; impaired tactile sensation; lack of body awareness
Behavior	Agitation; resistance to treatment; apathy; lack of initiation; denial of deficits; impulsivity; disinhibition; depression; sexually inappropriate behavior; perseveration; confabulation; lack of social skills; coping behavior (or lack of) related to the crisis or disability
ADL	Impaired ability to bathe, groom, dress, feed, and toilet
Patient/family knowledge and coping	Questioning (note depth and quantity); retention of information; repetitive questions; attentiveness; crying; anger; denial; conversing with other patients and families; attendance at educational and support group sessions; follow-up on tasks

2 DIAGNOSE

NURSING DIAGNOSIS	SUBJECTIVE FINDINGS	OBJECTIVE FINDINGS
Altered cerebral tissue perfusion related to disruption in cerebral blood flow secondary to cerebral edema	Complains of increasingly severe headache and anxiety	Restlessness; lethargy; change in level of consciousness (LOC); pupillary changes; focal neurologic deficits; change in respiratory pattern; widening pulse pressure; bradycardia; seizures; vomiting
Ineffective breathing pattern related to neuromuscular impairment, controlled mechanical ventilation, and/or pulmonary complications	Complains of shortness of breath (SOB)	Apnea; dyspnea; altered chest expansion; use of accessory muscles; rhonchi, rales, wheezing; diminished breath sounds; elevated arterial carbon dioxide pressure (Pa_{CO_2}); decreased arterial oxygen pressure (Pa_{O_2})
Potential fluid volume deficit related to osmotic diuretic therapy, fluid restriction, and/or onset of diabetes insipidus (DI)	Complains of thirst and dry mucous membranes, apprehensiveness	Apathy; weight loss; poor skin turgor; dry mucous membranes; increased or decreased urine output; increased or decreased specific gravity; decreased cardiac output (CO), pulmonary capillary wedge pressure (PCWP), central venous pressure (CVP); tachycardia; hypotension

NURSING DIAGNOSIS	SUBJECTIVE FINDINGS	OBJECTIVE FINDINGS
Potential fluid volume excess related to onset of syndrome of inappropriate secretion of antidiuretic hormone (SIADH)	Complains of fatigue, headache, muscle cramps, and anorexia	Change in LOC; weight gain; widespread generalized edema; seizures; decreased urine output; decreased serum sodium; increased urine osmolarity; increased urine sodium; decreased serum osmolarity
Sensory-perceptual alteration related to cognitive deficits, sensory alterations, and/or sensory overload	May report loss of memory, lack of concentration, confusion, disorientation, lack of motivation, decreased problem-solving ability	Impaired memory; short attention span; distractibility; illogical thinking; disorientation; impaired judgment; concreteness in thought; agitation; hostile or combative behavior; apathy; confabulation; impaired problem solving and decision making; disinhibition; egocentricity
Potential for injury related to altered sensory perception, agitation, poor judgment, impaired motor function, impaired communication, decreased endurance, seizure potential, and/or wandering	May report loss of memory, lack of concentration, confusion, disorientation, decreased problem-solving ability, difficulty with balance, problems moving arms or walking, problems with speech, having a seizure, or getting lost	Impaired memory; short attention span; distractibility; impaired judgment; agitation; hostile or combative behavior; impaired problem solving; unsteady gait; paralysis or paresis; sensory impairments; impaired speech; seizures; wandering and/or falling
Potential for aspiration related to reduced level of consciousness, seizures, depressed cough/gag reflexes, or impaired swallowing	Reports difficulty swallowing, history of aspiration, or seizures	Decreased or absent gag reflex; facial paralysis; reduced LOC; seizure activity; impaired perception and judgment; tracheostomy tube; hoarseness; aspiration; apraxia; dehydration; nasal regurgitation; residual food in oropharyngeal cavity; coughing immediately after swallowing; documented impaired swallowing by videofluoroscopy
Self-care deficit related to cognitive and sensory-perceptual impairment, memory loss, impaired balance and coordination, paralysis/paresis, spasticity, or increased muscle tone	May state that she cannot do specific ADL or needs help	Inability to independently bathe, brush teeth, comb hair, apply deodorant and makeup, feed and dress self, or do own toileting; cognitive and sensory-perceptual impairment; memory loss; impaired balance and coordination; paralysis or paresis; spasticity; or increased muscle tone

→ › ›

3 PLAN

Patient goals

1. The patient will demonstrate improved cerebral tissue perfusion.
2. The patient will demonstrate effective breathing patterns and improved ventilation and oxygenation.
3. The patient will maintain optimum fluid balance.
4. The patient will demonstrate improved cognitive functioning.
5. The patient will be free of injury.
6. The patient will not experience aspiration.
7. The patient will be able to accomplish activities of daily living on own.

4 IMPLEMENT

NURSING DIAGNOSIS	NURSING INTERVENTIONS	RATIONALE
Altered cerebral tissue perfusion related to disruption in cerebral blood flow secondary to cerebral edema	Assess LOC q 1 h/prn; evaluate and document patient's eye opening response, verbal response, and ability to follow simple commands.	LOC is the best indicator of neurologic change.
	Assess patient's pupils; note size, equality, response to light, and consensual response.	Pupillary function is controlled by cranial nerves (CN) II and III; as ICP rises, changes in pupillary size and reactivity occur, with the pupil dilating ipsilaterally and becoming sluggish in response to light.
	Assess position of patient's eyes; assess extraocular eye movements (EOM); note any abnormal gazes and loss of doll's eyes reflex (oculocephalic reflex).	EOM may be abnormal as ICP rises because of pressure on CN III, IV, and VI; loss of oculocephalic reflex indicates damage at the midbrain-pons level.
	Assess patient's corneal reflex and gag reflex.	Loss of corneal and gag reflexes indicates damage to the brainstem.
	Evaluate patient's motor and sensory function; observe spontaneous movements; evaluate the unconscious patient's motor response to painful stimuli; observe for any abnormal posturing (decorticate or decerebrate).	Motor dysfunction may develop because of pressure on pyramidal tract secondary to cerebral edema; late signs of increased ICP include decorticate, decerebrate, and flaccid postures.
	Monitor patient's BP, heart rate, and respiratory pattern q 1 h/prn.	Widening pulse pressure and bradycardia develop in later stages of increased ICP secondary to ischemia in the vasomotor center of the brainstem; changes in respiratory patterns correlate with level of brain dysfunction.
	Observe for any periorbital edema (raccoon eyes), ecchymosis on mastoid process (Battle's sign), or any scalp abrasions.	Raccoon eyes and Battle's sign indicate a basilar skull fracture.
	Observe for any clear or serosanguineous drainage from ears or nose; test drainage for glucose.	A tear in the dura mater can occur after some skull fractures, causing leakage of CSF.

NURSING DIAGNOSIS	NURSING INTERVENTIONS	RATIONALE
	Maintain head of bed between 30 and 45 degrees; maintain head and neck in mid-line position.	Facilitates venous drainage from cerebrum.
	Instruct patient to avoid flexion of hip, isometric exercise, coughing, and straining at stool.	These activities increase intrathoracic and intraabdominal pressure, which can contribute to increased ICP.
	Maintain normothermia.	Hyperthermia can increase cerebral blood flow, causing further cerebral edema; shivering can increase ICP.
	Monitor for seizure activity; maintain seizure precautions; give anticonvulsants as prescribed.	Seizures can occur from cerebral irritation caused by direct head injury or cerebral edema.
	Plan nursing care activities to minimize extraneous stimulation.	Even minimum stimulation can cause rapid elevation in ICP.
	Maintain patent airway and suction prn; hyperventilate with 100% oxygen before suctioning; suction for <15 sec.	To maintain adequate and continuous levels of oxygen; suctioning causes rapid increases in ICP.
	Monitor arterial blood gases (ABGs); maintain Pa_{CO_2} between 25 and 30 mm Hg and $Pa_{O_2} \geq 80$ mm Hg if controlled ventilation is used.	Carbon dioxide is a potent vasodilator; maintaining Pa_{CO_2} between 25 and 30 mm Hg produces mild cerebral vasoconstriction, reducing cerebral blood volume and ICP; adequate oxygenation is necessary to maintain cerebral metabolism; a reduction in Pa_{O_2} can increase cerebral blood volume.
	If intracranial monitoring system is used, monitor ICP; establish trend in pressure reading (see "ICP Monitoring," page 262).	ICP ≥ 15 mm Hg for longer than 15-30 min can increase cerebral ischemia.
	Administer IV fluids as prescribed.	IV fluids must be given with great caution so as not to exacerbate cerebral edema.
	Administer barbiturate coma therapy as prescribed; administer muscle relaxants and sedatives as prescribed.	High dose barbiturate therapy may be indicated to treat elevated ICP; muscle relaxants and sedatives are used to paralyze and sedate the patient; both therapies require intubation, ICP monitoring, hemodynamic monitoring, and intensive nursing care.
	Administer corticosteroids and osmotic diuretic therapy as prescribed.	Osmotic diuretic therapy draws water from the brain cells to reduce edema; corticosteroids, although controversial, are thought to reduce cerebral edema.

→ > >

NURSING DIAGNOSIS	NURSING INTERVENTIONS	RATIONALE
Ineffective breathing pattern related to neuromuscular impairment, controlled mechanical ventilation, and/or pulmonary complications	Assess patient's respiratory rate, depth, and rhythm q 1-2 h/prn.	Breathing irregularities such as apnea, dyspnea, SOB, rapid or shallow breathing, and altered chest expansion may reflect injury to the brain's respiratory centers.
	Auscultate breath sounds q 1-2 h/prn; note change in breath sounds.	Neurogenic pulmonary edema, adult respiratory distress syndrome (ARDS), pneumonia, and atelectasis are complications of head injury.
	Maintain patent airway and suction prn; hyperventilate with 100% oxygen before suctioning; suction for <15 sec.	To maintain adequate oxygenation; suctioning causes a rapid increase in ICP.
	Maintain oxygen at prescribed level; if controlled ventilation is used, maintain prescribed ventilator setting.	Pa_{O_2} must be maintained at $\geq$ 80 mm Hg.
	Monitor ABGs; report results to physician.	If controlled hyperventilation is used, Pa_{CO_2} is maintained between 25 and 30 mm Hg and Pa_{O_2} between 80 and 100 mm Hg.
Potential fluid volume deficit related to osmotic diuretic therapy, fluid restriction, and/or onset of diabetes insipidus (DI)	Monitor intake and output, specific gravity, and color of urine q 2 h.	DI, osmotic diuretic therapy, and fluid restriction may cause a severe volume depletion; early recognition makes treatment easier. Urine output > 200 ml/h, specific gravity < 1.005, and pale urine indicate onset of DI. Urine output < 30 ml/h with a specific gravity > 1.025 may indicate fluid volume deficit. Osmotic diuretic therapy (Mannitol) promotes diuresis, which can lead to dehydration.
	Monitor laboratory values: serum osmolarity, urine osmolarity, serum electrolytes, hematocrit.	DI occurs as a result of a lack of antidiuretic hormone (ADH); excessive water diuresis occurs because the renal tubules do not reabsorb water; DI is reflected in laboratory studies: urine osmolarity < 300 mOsm, serum osmolarity > 295 mOsm, serum sodium > 145 mEq/L, urine specific gravity < 1.005.
	Assess for signs of dehydration: polydipsia, dry skin, poor skin turgor, general weakness.	These signs are physiologic indicators of fluid volume depletion.
	Administer IV/PO fluid replacement as prescribed.	Fluid management after head injury is done with great caution; treatment of DI may involve replacement of urine output volume with IV fluid.
	Administer vasopressin for treatment of DI as prescribed.	Vasopressin is an exogenous form of ADH.

NURSING DIAGNOSIS	NURSING INTERVENTIONS	RATIONALE
Potential fluid volume excess related to onset of syndrome of inappropriate secretion of antidiuretic hormone (SIADH)	Monitor intake and output, specific gravity, and color of urine q 2 h.	SIADH can occur after head injury; it results from abnormally high levels of ADH secretion, which cause water to be continuously reabsorbed in the kidneys, resulting in water intoxication.
	Monitor laboratory values: serum osmolarity, urine sodium, urine osmolarity, serum electrolytes; serum sodium; blood urea nitrogen (BUN).	SIADH is associated with hyponatremia, increased urine sodium, hypoosmolar serum, and hyperosmolar urine.
	Monitor patient for signs of water intoxication: weight gain, generalized edema.	SIADH causes fluid retention over the total body.
	Monitor patient for CNS symptoms associated with hyponatremia: headache, lethargy, somnolence.	Hyponatremia can cause severe CNS depression.
	Maintain seizure precautions.	Hyponatremia can precipitate seizures.
	Maintain fluid restriction as prescribed.	Strict fluid restriction is maintained at approximately 500-1000 ml/day.
	Administer hypertonic saline intravenously as prescribed.	Hyponatremia can be treated with slow administration of 3% hypertonic saline.
Sensory-perceptual alteration related to cognitive deficits, sensory alterations, and/or sensory overload	**Memory** Develop and use memory aids.	Memory aids help patient remember.
	Post daily activity schedule.	Patient can review own schedule; helps relearn sequencing and passage of time.
	Encourage patient to make lists of things to do or to get.	Patient does not have to rely on memory.
	Post labeled photos of family, friends, home, pet; put patient's name on belongings.	Patient may not recognize own family and friends; labels help patient identify bed, closet, belongings, and clothing.
	Have visitors and staff members wear name tags.	Patient can identify people visiting or caring for her.
	Record visits from family and friends on calendar.	To help patient remember when family last visited and when they will return.
	Do simple memory exercises.	Memory exercises may help patient relearn information and associations.
	Cue patient to use memory aids.	Initially, patient often will need cues to use memory aid.
	Document observations of patient's memory skills.	Memory improves after clearing of post-traumatic amnesia.

→ ❯ ❯

NURSING DIAGNOSIS	NURSING INTERVENTIONS	RATIONALE
	Orientation	
	Assess orientation and reorient patient frequently; prompt patient if needed.	Memory problems interfere with orientation.
	Call patient by preferred name.	To aid in self-recognition.
	Introduce yourself before each new interaction with patient.	Patient may not remember you and may be afraid.
	Assign consistent caregivers.	Patient eventually may remember caregiver; keeps routine more consistent.
	Maintain simple, consistent daily routine.	To help patient remember and anticipate activities.
	Tell patient what you are doing and going to do.	To decrease anxiety and increase understanding.
	Post large calendar where patient can see it; cross off days as they pass.	To help time orientation and to mark the passage of time.
	Have clock in patient's view; refer to times of activities.	To aid in time orientation and to mark the passage of time.
	Maintain appropriate day/night, light/dark schedule.	To assist in day/night orientation and sleep patterns.
	Evaluate positive or negative effect of radio and television on orientation.	Radio and television may help orient patient or may cause confusion.
	Agitation	
	Maintain simple, nonconfusing environment. Decrease amount and complexity of stimuli if patient shows signs of frustration and agitation.	Internal confusion results in frustration and agitation.
	Keep window and cubicle curtains closed when working with patient. Keep radio and television off.	To decrease stimuli and help patient focus attention.
	Evaluate positive or negative effect of roommate.	Patient may be distracted by activities of roommate.
	Speak slowly in a calm voice.	Patient can detect anxiety in your voice; may have difficulty following conversation.
	Provide care at unhurried pace.	To avoid confusing patient.
	Observe and document any factors that cause agitation; eliminate or modify such factors.	Preventive and early intervention may decrease incidence and severity of agitation.
	Provide therapy/meals in quiet environment.	To help patient focus on task at hand.

NURSING DIAGNOSIS	NURSING INTERVENTIONS	RATIONALE
Potential for injury related to altered sensory perception, agitation, poor judgment, impaired motor function, impaired communication, decreased endurance, seizure potential, and/or wandering	Maintain seizure precautions: side rails up and padded, suction apparatus available.	Seizure activity may cause injury.
	Keep environment simple, free of clutter.	Too much stimulation increases patient's frustration.
	Keep area free of sharp objects and potentially harmful substances: glass (cups, mirrors, pictures), razor blades, matches, lighters, antiseptic solutions.	Patient may not recognize hazard these objects pose.
	Consider applying shatter-resistant film to windows.	To decrease risk of shattering glass if window is hit.
	Consider using a securing bed belt if patient tries to climb out of bed (belt fastens around waist and to bed frame).	Allows full arm and leg movement, patient can sit or lie in bed.
	Use secure seat belt when patient is up in chair.	To prevent patient from getting up without assistance.
	Keep call light within reach, and reinforce its use; assess patient's understanding.	Patient should always have a way to call for assistance, but impaired memory may prevent her from using it.
	Have staff available to assist with ADL and transfers as needed.	Patient's poor judgment, impulsiveness, and impaired balance influence safety.
	Consider need for checks q 15 min, trained sitter, or video camera to monitor patient activities.	To detect hazardous activities, and properly cue and monitor patient; necessary if patient cannot call for assistance or use call light.
	Keep identification band on patient and name in clothes.	To help identify person as a patient.
	Consider fire code-approved code locks on unit exit doors and facility security system for wandering patients.	To prevent patient from leaving unit and building undetected.
Potential for aspiration related to reduced level of consciousness, seizures, depressed cough/gag reflexes, or impaired swallowing	Provide a quiet, supervised, nondistracting environment at meals.	To allow patient to focus on task of eating.
	Check for presence of gag reflex, and evaluate patient's alertness.	Do not feed patient if gag reflex is absent; presence of gag reflex does not necessarily mean effective swallowing.
	Keep suction equipment readily available.	To use if patient needs suctioning.
	Work with trained speech therapist to evaluate swallowing before providing meals for patient.	May discuss use of videofluoroscopy to test effectiveness of swallowing foods of different consistencies.

→ › ›

NURSING DIAGNOSIS	NURSING INTERVENTIONS	RATIONALE
	Sit patient at 90° angle or leaning slightly forward for meals, unless contraindicated.	This is the proper body position to facilitate adequate swallowing.
	Begin with small amounts of semisolid food; thicken liquids if necessary.	Patient probably will have the most difficulty with thin liquids.
	Remind patient to chew food well before swallowing. Remind patient to eat slowly, swallowing each bite before taking another.	Impulsiveness may cause patient to attempt swallowing before food has been chewed thoroughly and to put several bites of food into her mouth before swallowing.
	Remind patient to keep head tilted slightly downward.	To help keep airway closed during swallowing.
	Tell patient to think "swallow."	Sometimes a conscious thought helps trigger swallow reflex.
	Stroke neck lightly.	May trigger swallowing.
	Observe for coughing, gagging, nasal regurgitation, or holding of food in mouth.	These are signs of potential aspiration.
	Encourage patient to be as independent with her own feeding as possible.	Increased independence helps build self-confidence.
	Keep patient in upright position or head of bed elevated 30 to 45 degrees for at least 1 h after eating, longer if prescribed.	Food could reflux from stomach, causing patient to aspirate.
	Teach family members how to perform Heimlich maneuver.	To use in case patient chokes.
Self-care deficit related to cognitive and sensory-perceptual impairment, memory loss, impaired balance and coordination, paralysis/paresis, spasticity, or increased muscle tone	Allow sufficient time to have patient do as much of her own care as possible.	Patient will be less confused if ADL is done in unhurried manner.
	Provide quiet, nondistracting environment with privacy.	Fewer distractions allow patient to focus on task at hand.
	Work with occupational and physical therapists to determine method for doing activity.	Teamwork will give thorough evaluation of patient's skills and adaptive techniques.
	Have patient involved in selecting clothing, food, and so forth as much as possible.	To acknowledge preferences and allow patient to determine own self-care.
	Give patient simple verbal or visual cues. Increase use of simple gestures.	To remind patient of next step. To help patient understand.
	Develop a routine for ADL. Assign consistent caregivers.	To help patient remember steps of ADL. To provide a more consistent routine.

NURSING DIAGNOSIS	NURSING INTERVENTIONS	RATIONALE
	Allow patient to do as much of her own care as possible.	To increase self-esteem and improve endurance.
	Encourage patient, and acknowledge progress.	To motivate patient to keep trying.
Knowledge deficit	See Patient Teaching.	

5 EVALUATE

PATIENT OUTCOME	DATA INDICATING THAT OUTCOME IS REACHED
Patient demonstrates improved cerebral tissue perfusion.	LOC has improved; there is no neurologic deficit or seizure activity.
Patient demonstrates effective breathing patterns and improved ventilation and oxygenation.	Airway is patent; chest excursion is symmetric; breath sounds are normal; ABG are within normal limits or prescribed parameters; there are no subjective or objective findings of SOB, air hunger, or dyspnea.
Patient maintains optimum fluid balance.	Intake and output are balanced; specific gravity is between 1.010 and 1.023; skin turgor and mucous membranes are normal; serum osmolarity, urine osmolarity, serum and urine electrolytes, Hgb, and Hct are within normal limits; BP and heart rate are normal.
Patient shows improved cognitive functioning.	Patient demonstrates improved memory and orientation and little or no agitation.
Patient remains free of injury.	Patient uses safety measures to prevent injury.
Patient does not experience aspiration.	There is no evidence of aspiration.
Patient can independently do own ADL.	Patient completes ADL independently or as independently as possible within physical limitations.

PATIENT TEACHING

1. Instruct the patient to avoid flexion of the hip, isometric exercise, coughing, and straining at stool as long as increased ICP is a potential problem.
2. Keep the patient and family informed about progress and what care is being done, test results, etc.
3. Teach the patient and family about traumatic brain injury, its effects, and the treatment plan. Adjust patient teaching to the patient's comprehension level.
4. Involve the family in the patient's care, based on their readiness to learn.
5. Teach the patient how to adapt to residual impairments.

Cerebrovascular Accident

A **cerebrovascular accident (CVA),** otherwise known as a stroke or apoplexy, occurs when a cerebral blood vessel is occluded by a thrombus or embolus, or when cerebrovascular hemorrhage occurs. Both mechanisms result in ischemia of the brain tissue normally perfused by the damaged vessel.

Stroke is the third leading cause of death in the United States, accounting for approximately 150,300 deaths annually, 60.6% of whom are women. It has been estimated that 500,000 strokes occur each year, and that almost 3 million living Americans have had a stroke. Although a stroke can occur at any age, 72% occur in people over 65 years of age.[3]

Stroke is the second leading cause of chronic disability and illness. Since the sequelae of a stroke depend on the extent and location of the ischemia, the degree of disability varies greatly.

Certain risk factors may predispose an individual to a stroke; hypertension is the major risk factor. Risk factors showing some familial tendencies include diabetes mellitus, hypertension, cardiac disease, subclavian steal syndrome, and a high serum cholesterol level. Obesity, a sedentary life-style, cigarette smoking, stress, and high serum levels of cholesterol, lipoprotein, and tri-

glycerides make an individual a high-risk candidate for stroke. In women, use of oral contraceptives and cigarette smoking increase the risk of stroke. Combinations of risk factors put an individual at even greater risk.[39]

PATHOPHYSIOLOGY

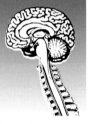

The pathologic mechanisms of stroke are commonly listed as hemorrhagic, thrombotic, and embolic in the most recent vascular literature. Hemorrhage may be subarachnoid from rupture of the subarachnoid artery, or intraparenchymal from rupture of an intraparenchymal artery. Embolic occlusion stems from tumors, valvular cardiac diseases, and, most commonly, plaques released from cerebral vessels that produce infarction. Thrombotic arterial occlusion produces various ischemic or hypoxic insults.[84] Table 4-1 compares seven types of strokes.

Cerebral Hemorrhage

The pathogenesis of hypertensive cerebral hemorrhage is not completely understood. However, several facts are known: the hemorrhage usually occurs in relation to

Table 4-1

COMPARISON OF SEVEN TYPES OF STROKES

	Intracerebral hemorrhage	Subarachnoid hemorrhage	Subdural hemorrhage
Onset	Rapid; minutes to 1-2 h	Sudden; varied progression	Insidious; occasionally acute
Duration	Permanent if lesion is large; small lesions are potentially reversible	Variable; complete clearing may occur in days or weeks	Hours to months
Relation to activity	Usually occurs during activity	Most commonly related to head trauma	Usually related to head trauma
Contributing or associated factors	Hypertensive cardiovascular disease; coagulation defects	Intracerebral arterial aneurysm; trauma; vascular malformations	Chronic alcoholism
Sensorium	Coma common	Coma common	Generally clouded
Nuchal (neck) rigidity	Frequently present	Present	Rare
Location of cerebral deficit	Focal; arterial syndrome not common	Diffuse aneurysm may give focal sign before and after	Frontal lobe signs; ipsilateral pupil may dilate
Convulsions	Common	Common	Infrequent
Cerebrospinal fluid	Bloody unless hemorrhage entirely intracerebral	Grossly bloody; increased pressure	Normal to slightly elevated protein
Skull x-rays	Pineal shift, edema, hemorrhage, or hematoma	Normal or calcified aneurysm	Frequent contralateral shift of pineal gland

some mild exertion, and it occurs in individuals who have experienced significant increases in systolic-diastolic pressures for several years. Some researchers theorize that microaneurysms, known as *Charcot-Bouchard aneurysms,* in small arteries or arteriolar necrosis may precipitate the bleeding. The major sites of bleeding in hypertensive cerebral hemorrhage include the putamen (55%), cortex and subcortex (15%), thalamus (10%), pons (10%), and cerebellar hemisphere (10%).[29,123]

Hypertensive vascular disorders primarily affect the smaller arteries and arterioles, causing thickening of vessel walls, increase in cellularity of some vessels, and hyalinization, possibly with necrosis.[29,123]

Resolution of the hemorrhage occurs through resorption and begins when macrophages and reactive fibrillary astrocytes appear. After the tissue has been cleared of blood by the macrophages, there is a cavity surrounded by dense, fibrillary gliosis and hemosiderin-laden macrophages.[29,123]

Cerebral Infarction

Cerebral infarction occurs when a local area of brain tissue is deprived of blood supply because of vascular occlusion. Several hypotheses regarding the pathogenesis of cerebral infarcts include: abrupt vessel occlusion (e.g., embolus) that results in tissue infarction in the distribution supply of the occluded vessel; gradual ves-

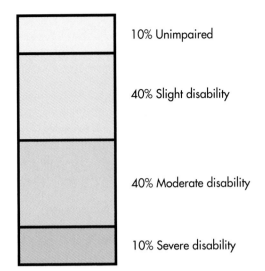

10% Unimpaired

40% Slight disability

40% Moderate disability

10% Severe disability

Degree of disability in survivors of stroke.[3]

sel occlusion (e.g., atheroma), which may not result in an infarction if collateral blood supply is sufficient; and vessels that are stenosed but not completely occluded. This may precipitate an infarction if the collateral blood supply to the hypoxic area becomes comprised.[29,123]

Cerebral thrombi and cerebral emboli are common causes of vascular occlusion. Thrombi usually occur in larger vessels (e.g., internal carotid arteries) and are associated with localized damage to the vessel wall at the

Epidural hemorrhage	Focal cerebral ischemia	Cerebral thrombosis	Cerebral embolism
Rapid; minutes to hours	Rapid; seconds to minutes	Minutes to hours	Sudden
Initially fluctuating; then steadily progressive	Seconds to minutes	Permanent if lesion is large; potentially reversible if lesion is small	Rapid improvement may occur, depending on collateral flow
Almost always related to head trauma	Occurs during activity if related to decreased cardiac output	Usually occurs at rest	Unrelated to activity
Any condition that predisposes to trauma	Peripheral and coronary atherosclerosis; hypertension	Peripheral and coronary atherosclerosis; hypertension	Atrial fibrillation; aortic and mitral valve disease; myocardial infarct; atherosclerotic plaque
Rapidly advancing coma	Usually conscious	Usually conscious	Usually conscious
Rare	Absent	Absent	Absent
Temporal lobe signs; ipsilateral pupil may dilate; high intracranial pressure (ICP)	Focal; or arterial syndrome	Focal; or arterial syndrome	Focal; or arterial syndrome
Common	Rare	Rare	Rare
Increased pressure; color and cells usually normal	Usually normal	Usually normal	Usually normal
Frequently fracture across middle meningeal artery groove	May show calcification of intracranial arteries	Possible arterial calcification and pineal shift from edema	Usually normal

point of occlusion. Atherosclerosis and hypotension are important underlying processes, but other types of vascular injury (e.g., arteritis) can initiate thrombosis. Emboli usually affect smaller vessels and are commonly found at points of narrowed vessel lumen and bifurcation. The sources of cerebral emboli vary, but the most common is a mural thrombus in the left atrium or ventricle. Septic emboli may originate from bacterial endocarditis. Cerebral infarcts from embolic occlusions frequently are hemorrhagic, whereas thrombotic infarcts are bland or ischemic. Emboli occur most frequently in the middle cerebral artery.

A cerebral infarction may be ischemic or hemorrhagic. *Ischemic* infarctions usually are not demonstrable on gross examination for 6 to 12 hours. The initial change of the affected area is a slight discoloration and softening, with the gray matter taking on a muddy color and the white matter losing its normal fine-grained appearance.[123] After 48 to 72 hours, infarction, necrosis, circumlesional swelling, and mushy disintegration of the affected area are evident. Eventually there is liquefaction and formation of a cyst surrounded by firm glial tissue.

Histologic changes after an infarction include cell body changes, interruption and disintegration of the myelin sheath and axis cylinder, and loss of oligodendroglia and astrocytes. Polymorphonuclear leukocytes begin to appear 48 hours after infarct. At 78 to 96 hours, macrophages appear around blood vessels.[29]

Hemorrhagic infarctions usually occur in the cerebral cortex and result from a reflow of blood into the infarcted area. This reperfusion is caused by a fragmentation, or lysis, of the embolus or a reduction of vascular compression and reestablishment of blood flow.[123] Hemorrhagic infarcts therefore are ischemic in origin.

Lacunar Strokes

Lacunar strokes are less than 1 cubic centimeter in size and occur only where small perforating arterioles branch off large vessels, as in the basal ganglia, internal capsule, and brainstem. The small arterioles are damaged over time by hypertension, resulting in small infarcts. This often is a chronic process. Because a lacunar stroke has a subcortical location, the results usually are pure motor or pure sensory deficits.[42]

ONSET OF SYMPTOMS

The classic warning signals of a stroke are minor numbness, temporary speech difficulties, blurred vision, headache, dizziness, loss of consciousness, and/or paralysis. If the person experiences a transient ischemic attack (TIA), complete clinical recovery occurs in 24 hours or less. A TIA often is thought to be caused by a vessel spasm or by a small piece of

plaque that breaks off and blocks a vessel, mimicking an embolus. Patients may report TIAs as blackouts, spells, or fainting. A report of TIAs by a patient should be investigated further, since they may be a precursor to an actual stroke. A reversible ischemic neurologic deficit (RIND) is similar to a TIA, but the symptoms can last 24 to 48 hours.[25]

A progressive stroke, also known as a stroke in evolution, manifests some evidence of neurologic deficit, and the condition worsens. A progressive stroke frequently is caused by the formation of a thrombus, by trauma, or by a slow hemorrhage. A tumor can cause a similar effect as it slowly occludes a blood vessel. A completed stroke is said to have occurred when the maximum deficit has been acquired and the patient's condition stabilizes. A completed stroke can occur rapidly, as with an aneurysm rupture, or more slowly, as with the stroke in evolution.

PATIENT OUTCOME AND REHABILITATION

The patient outcome after a completed stroke is determined by the cause of the stroke, its severity, and its location. Other factors include the specific neurologic deficits, the patient's age, his motivation, and the family and its resources. Function returns proximal to distal, meaning that hip and knee flexion may return but not ankle dorsiflexion. The muscles of affected extremities usually are flaccid at first, and deep tendon reflexes are absent. Reflexes usually return within the first 2 days. The flaccid tone progresses to spasticity, then to normal tone. The extent of return of function cannot be accurately predicted, but it is known that the most progress is made within the first month after the stroke. Slow progress may continue for 1 to 2 years, but it sometimes is difficult to discern when neurologic healing stops and learned compensatory function begins.[42]

Stroke rehabilitation focuses on facilitating return of function, teaching compensatory techniques, and helping the patient and family cope with the effects of the stroke. Conventional stroke rehabilitation includes maintaining range of motion, exercising to strengthen muscles, doing activities to increase mobilization, and learning compensatory techniques for activities of daily living. Bobath techniques focus on using specific posturing for positioning and activities, and controlling synergies with sensory input and motor feedback. Proprioceptive neuromuscular facilitation (PNF) focuses on using reflexes and patterning techniques. Many stroke rehabilitation programs currently use a combination of these techniques, based on the individual patient's needs and responses.[42]

COMPLICATIONS

Hypertension/hypotension
Seizures
Increased intracranial pressure (ICP)
Subsequent cerebrovascular accidents
Contractures
Abnormal muscle tone
Deep vein thrombosis
Pulmonary embolism
Malnutrition

Aspiration
Urinary incontinence
Bowel incontinence
Shoulder subluxation
Brachial plexus injury
Shoulder-hand syndrome
Heterotopic ossification
Depression

DIAGNOSTIC STUDIES AND FINDINGS

Diagnostic Test	Findings
Computed tomography (CT) scan	Infarct: appears initially (24 h) as area of decreased density surrounded by area of intermediate density; shifts in midline structures and ventricular system Older infarct: area of low density extending toward cortex or shift in ventricular system toward lesion
Magnetic resonance imaging (MRI) study	Same as CT scan; hemorrhage: rounded shape and uniformly high density
Lumbar puncture NOTE: Perform with caution in presence of elevated ICP	Increased pressure; bloody spinal fluid
Electroencephalography (EEG)	May show focal slowing around area of lesion
Brain scan	Diminished perfusion; detection of infarction, encapsulated hemorrhage, hematoma, and arteriovenous malformations
Cerebral angiography	Shows occlusion or narrowing of large vessels, particularly carotid artery occlusions
B mode ultrasonography	Outlines with ultrasound the flow of blood through large neck vessels
Skull x-ray	Pineal body position; intracranial calcifications
Echoencephalography	Shifts in midline structures; displaced ventricles
Doppler ultrasonography	Direction and velocity of blood flow through vessels
Electrocardiogram (ECG)	Myocardial infarction; dysrhythmias

MEDICAL MANAGEMENT

GENERAL MANAGEMENT – ACUTE PHASE

Mechanical ventilation: Controlled mechanical ventilation and hyperventilation are used to treat increased ICP.

ICP monitoring: See "Intracranial Pressure Monitoring," page 262.

Hypothermia blanket: Used to control hyperthermia and/or to lower body temperature to reduce metabolic demands of body tissues.

Cardiac monitoring: Pathologic cardiac conditions commonly exist in this population since risk factors are similar; embolic stroke may have cardiac origin.

Serial ABG analysis: Monitors the changing respiratory and metabolic body functions.

Aneurysm precautions: Used if patient has had an aneurysm rupture. (See "Cerebral Aneurysm," p. 88.)

Bed positioning: Head of bed is kept flat if increased cerebral perfusion is desired (thrombotic or embolic stroke); head of bed is elevated if decreased cerebral perfusion is desired (hemorrhagic stroke or increased ICP). Bed rest is desired initially.

Continued.

MEDICAL MANAGEMENT—cont'd

Seizure control: Anticonvulsants and seizure precautions are necessary, since risk of seizures is greatest in first weeks after the stroke.

Nasogastric tube: Initially used for gastric decompression, then may be used for enteral feeding until swallowing status has been evaluated.

Preventing pulmonary embolism and thrombophlebitis: Anticoagulants, elastic stockings, or sequential leg circulation pumps may be used.

Monitoring fluid and electrolyte balance: Indwelling urethral catheter may be used initially to monitor output accurately.

Use of thrombolytic enzymes: Still somewhat controversial; enzymes cause lysis of thrombi obstructing cerebral arteries in an acute stroke.

GENERAL MANAGEMENT–REHABILITATION PHASE

Maintain adequate nutrition: Difficulty swallowing and decreased level of consciousness (LOC) may necessitate enteral tube feeding.

Establish bladder management program: Initially patient may have flaccid bladder, followed by spastic bladder. Thorough urologic workup may be necessary for urinary incontinence.

Establish bowel management program: Bowel control is affected by amount of fluids and bulk in diet, decrease in activity, impaired mobility, and/or impaired communication.

Maintain body alignment and joint range of motion (ROM): Proper positioning and exercise are necessary; patient is at risk of developing contractures.

Prevent aspiration: Ineffective swallowing is common; swallowing evaluation is necessary, because the risk of aspiration is high.

Maintain skin integrity: Decreased mobility and sensation, incontinence, impaired nutrition, and age increase patient's risk of developing pressure ulcers.

Establish effective communication: Aphasia, dysarthria, apraxia, diplopia, and/or impaired arm function can cause significant communication deficits.

Establish and maintain safe ambulation: Paralysis, perceptual problems, impaired sensation, and impaired balance can affect safe ambulation; patient may need to learn bed mobility, transfer, and wheelchair skills. Use of a quad-cane or regular cane and ankle-foot orthosis is common.

Prevention and treatment of shoulder-hand syndrome (reflex sympathetic dystrophy): Usually develops 2-4 mo after stroke; may cause rapid, painful loss of ROM in affected arm. Treatment addresses pain control, passive stretching of the arm, and decreasing hand and arm edema.

Address sexuality and sexual functioning issues: Impaired motor/sensory function, impaired communication, and perceptual disturbances may alter sexual functioning. Emotional lability may also affect self-esteem. The concerns of the patient, spouse or significant other, and family must be addressed early.

Guide relearning of ADL: Impaired movement, sensation, perception, judgment, and memory will alter the patient's ability to independently perform own bathing, grooming, dressing, feeding, and toileting.

Ensure patient's safety from injury: Patient may have a combination of motor, sensory, and/or perceptual deficits that put him at high risk for falls, burns, accidental poisoning, and so forth.

Support the family: Crisis reaction by family members. Patient may not perceive his own deficits. Counseling and social services may be needed on an ongoing basis. Resources need to be identified. Guardianship may need to be addressed. Education sessions and support groups are important.

MEDICAL MANAGEMENT—cont'd

Discharge planning: Trajectory of patient care needs is identified as early as possible. Admission to acute rehabilitation facility, day treatment program, or extended care facility, or adapting the home for wheelchair accessibility may need to be considered.

SURGERY

Carotid endarterectomy (see "Carotid Endarterectomy," page 258); ICP monitoring (see "ICP Monitoring," p. 262)

DRUG THERAPY

Anticoagulants: Warfarin sodium (Coumadin); heparin sodium.

Antihypertensives: Diazoxide (Hyperstat).

Diuretics: Mannitol; furosemide (Lasix).

Corticosteroids: Dexamethasone (Decadron).

Anticonvulsants: Phenytoin (Dilantin); carbamazepine (Tegretol).

Narcotic analgesic: Codeine sulfate.

Analgesic/antipyretic: Acetaminophen.

Antiplatelet agents: Aspirin; dipyridamole (Persantine).

Antiulcer agents: Ranitidine hydrochloride (Zantac).

Stool softener: Docusate sodium (Colace).

Vasodilators: Papaverine hydrochloride (Pavabid).

Dilutional or hypoviscosity agents: Used to maintain cerebral perfusion.

Calcium channel blockers: Used in the treatment of vasospasm following subarachnoid hemorrhage.

1 ASSESS

ASSESSMENT	OBSERVATIONS
Motor paralysis/ paresis	Hemiplegia/hemiparesis: Paralysis or weakness of side of face, arm, and leg on side of body opposite brain lesion Monoplegia: Usually paralysis of arm on side opposite brain lesion Triplegia: Paralysis of three limbs, usually both arms and one leg Bilateral hemiplegia: Paralysis of all four limbs and facial muscles
Sensory alterations	Hemianesthesia: Loss of sensation on side of face, arm, and leg on side of body opposite brain lesion Hyperesthesia/pain: Enhanced sensitivity and/or pain, usually in paralyzed arm and shoulder

→ 〉 〉

ASSESSMENT	OBSERVATIONS
Dysphagia	Difficulty swallowing because of paralysis of tongue and larynx
Visual alterations	Diplopia: Double vision Homonymous hemianopia: Visual field cut on side opposite brain lesion
Anosognosia	Physiologic denial of current condition and resulting deficits; unable to realize something has happened to him
Agnosia	Unable to recognize previously familiar objects; however, once an object has been identified, can use it appropriately Visual: Unable to recognize an object by sight Auditory: Able to hear sounds but does not understand what they mean Tactile: Unable to recognize shapes or objects by touch, even though sensation is intact
Apraxia	Unable to physically perform a task, even though motor and sensory functions are intact Ideomotor: Able to understand a task but cannot do it when asked; however, may be able to do the task spontaneously Ideational: Unable to comprehend a task and thus cannot do it either when asked or spontaneously Constructional: Unable to produce designs by drawing, copying, or building Dressing: Unable to dress self
Communication disorders	Impaired ability to communicate; dominant hemisphere lesion (left in most people) Wernicke's aphasia (receptive or sensory aphasia): (Affects auditory comprehension); able to speak but may use nonexistent words; unable to understand or monitor own speech Broca's aphasia (expressive or motor aphasia): Able to hear and comprehend but cannot express own thoughts Global aphasia (sensory-motor, receptive-expressive, or mixed aphasia): Makes communication extremely difficult Anomia: Has difficulty mentally finding appropriate words Syntactical aphasia: Transposes first letters of words or uses words in wrong syntax Jargon: Able to make word sounds, but words are unknown Agraphia: Unable to write Alexia: Unable to read Automatic speech: Retains use of automatic words and phrases such as "yes" and "no," "hello," "good-bye," cursing, and words and phrases in native language, even though normal speech has been severely impaired; word and phrase usage is not always accurate or appropriate
Dysarthria	Unable to articulate words because of facial paralysis (also affects tongue, palate, pharynx, and lips)
Perseveration	Repeats a word, phrase, or motor action
Spatial perception deficit	Has difficulty perceiving verticals and horizontals, right and left, in and out, and up and down
Inability to revisualize	Gets lost easily; wanders
Emotional lability	Has easily triggered, dramatic mood swings; laughs or cries excessively; expression may not indicate true emotions; expression stops or changes with distraction
Impaired judgment	Is influenced greatly by sensation and perceptual deficits (creates increased risk for injury, especially falls)

ASSESSMENT	OBSERVATIONS
Impulsiveness	(Related to impaired judgment); is aware of safety measures but acts quickly without considering consequences
Short-term memory deficit	(Often labeled as stubbornness, noncompliance, and lack of motivation); has minimum day-to-day learning
Unilateral neglect	Neglects side of body and environmental space on contralateral side from lesion
Level of consciousness	Has varying levels of consciousness (assess and document changes over time)
Bladder functioning	May have urinary retention and/or incontinence (also evaluate prestroke urinary problems, urinalysis, urine culture, urodynamic studies as prescribed); may have functional incontinence
Bowel functioning	May have bowel incontinence or constipation/impaction (also evaluate prestroke bowel problems, fluid and dietary bulk intake, and functional incontinence)
Sexuality/sexual functioning	May be concerned and apprehensive (convey willingness to address issues, and identify functional deficits that may need to be addressed)

2 DIAGNOSE

NURSING DIAGNOSIS	SUBJECTIVE FINDINGS	OBJECTIVE FINDINGS
Altered cerebral tissue perfusion related to impaired cerebral blood flow, increased ICP, and hypoxia	Complains of increasingly severe headache and anxiety	Restlessness; lethargy; change in LOC; pupillary changes; focal neurologic deficits; change in respiratory pattern; widening pulse pressure; seizures; vomiting
Impaired physical mobility related to hemiplegia/hemiparesis, decreased LOC, sensory/perceptual deficits	Complains of inability to move arm and/or leg and to turn and position self in bed; cannot get out of bed; unable to walk or do ADL	Hemiplegia/hemiparesis; impaired ability to turn and position self in bed, get out of bed, and ambulate
Self-care deficit related to hemiplegia/hemiparesis, sensory/perceptual deficit	Complains of inability to do own ADL	Impaired ability to bathe, dress, groom, feed, and toilet self
Impaired communication related to aphasia, dysarthria, visual deficits, alexia, and/or agraphia	Complains of difficulty reading, writing, and speaking	Inappropriate responses to questions; words slurred and speech unintelligible; unable to read or write

NURSING DIAGNOSIS	SUBJECTIVE FINDINGS	OBJECTIVE FINDINGS
Functional urinary incontinence related to decreased sensation, cognitive dysfunction, impaired mobility, and/or impaired communication	Complains of urinary incontinence, inability to get to the bathroom quickly enough	Urinary incontinence; unaware of incontinence or full bladder; no communication of need to toilet
Bowel incontinence related to decreased sensation, cognitive dysfunction, impaired mobility, impaired communication, and/or lack of sufficient fluids and/or bulk in diet	Complains of soiling clothes, sheets, etc., constipation, diarrhea, inability to get to the bathroom quickly enough	Bowel incontinence; unaware of need to defecate or of incontinence; no communication of need to toilet; impaction, constipation, and diarrhea

Other Related Nursing Diagnoses: Impaired swallowing related to decreased/absent gag reflex, weakness, paralysis, and/or lack of coordination of swallowing musculature and/or reflex; **Potential/actual impaired skin integrity** related to decreased sensation, impaired mobility, urinary and/or bowel incontinence; **Potential for injury** related to paralysis/paresis, sensory-perceptual alterations, impaired judgment, impulsiveness, visual disturbances, apraxia, agnosia, impaired communication, and/or anosognosia; **Potential for aspiration** related to decreased/absent gag reflex, weakness, paralysis, and/or lack of coordination of swallowing musculature and reflex; **Ineffective airway clearance, impaired gas exchange, and ineffective breathing pattern** related to impaired cough, impaired ability to swallow secretions, decreased LOC, and/or impaired mobility; **Altered sexuality patterns or sexual dysfunction** related to impaired communication, decreased sensation, impaired perception, impaired mobility, and/or body image disturbance; **Body image disturbance** related to deficits of the CVA.

3   PLAN

Patient goals

1. The patient will demonstrate improved cerebral tissue perfusion.
2. The patient will be able to independently turn and position self in bed, get out of bed, ambulate or propel wheelchair.
3. The patient will be able to do activities of daily living on his own.
4. The patient will demonstrate improved ability to express self and relate decreased frustration with communication efforts.
5. The patient will be continent of urine.
6. The patient will be continent of stool.

4   IMPLEMENT

NURSING DIAGNOSIS	IMPLEMENTATION	RATIONALE
Altered cerebral tissue perfusion related to impaired cerebral blood flow, increased ICP, and hypoxia	(See implementation guidelines and rationale for altered cerebral tissue perfusion, page 266.)	

NURSING DIAGNOSIS	IMPLEMENTATION	RATIONALE
Impaired physical mobility related to hemiplegia/ hemiparesis, decreased LOC, sensory/perceptual deficits	Consult physical therapist.	Therapist will assist in developing a plan.
	Perform ROM exercises qd with active patient participation.	To prevent contractures and decrease risk of shoulder-hand syndrome.
	Properly position patient in bed.	Support affected arm on pillow to prevent edema; use pillow or trochanter roll to prevent severe external rotation of leg; use of footboard to prevent plantar flexion is controversial, since it has been found to stimulate reflex plantar flexion; use hard, cone-shaped device in paralyzed hand to prevent finger contractures; turn patient q 2 h; discuss positioning of affected side with therapist.
	Have trapeze placed on bed and instruct patient in its use.	To aid in patient's bed mobility; ensure patient does not do Valsalva maneuver when using trapeze.
	Keep bed side rails up on paralyzed side; both rails up if patient is impulsive.	To help patient use good arm to turn self and to prevent patient from falling out of bed or getting up without assistance.
	Teach or reinforce bed mobility skills.	Includes turning and positioning himself and bridging hips by flexing knee and placing feet flat on bed, then raising hips up off of mattress.
	Teach or reinforce technique for coming to a sitting position.	Includes getting feet off bed, rolling onto good arm, and pushing up on arm until in sitting position.
	Help patient regain sitting balance.	Begin on stable surface before bed mattress; gently push against patient, and teach him how to regain his balance.
	Teach patient how to stand up from a sitting position safely.	Use nonslip shoes; have him keep feet flat on floor and back near center of gravity; have him lean forward and push self up with unaffected arm on mattress or chair.
	Teach use of hemi-wheelchair; use seat belt.	Hemi-wheelchair has seat closer to the floor; remove footrest on unaffected side, and have patient propel wheelchair with foot; a brake extension handle is needed on affected side.
	Consider use of arm trough or clear lapboard on wheelchair.	Arm trough holds arm and hand in position to prevent hand edema, shoulder in place to prevent subluxation, and arm up and away from spokes of wheels; clear lapboard allows patient to see in front of wheelchair and provides arm support and work surface.

NURSING DIAGNOSIS	IMPLEMENTATION	RATIONALE
	Teach or reinforce technique for transferring safely into chair or wheelchair; if patient cannot do own transfer, do stand-pivot transfer. Properly position wheelchair and lock brakes.	Develop a consistent technique with physical therapist; adaptive approach is to transfer toward patient's unaffected side; if Bobath method is used, transfer toward patient's affected side.
	Remind patient to call for assistance before transfers.	Patient is at high risk for falls when transferring.
	Reinforce proper use of ambulation aids.	Patients commonly use quad-cane or regular cane on side opposite weak leg.
	Teach patient how to properly don any prescribed orthosis.	Patients commonly need an ankle-foot orthosis to hold ankle in neutral or slight dorsiflexion.
Self-care deficit related to hemiplegia/hemiparesis, sensory/perceptual deficit	Consult occupational therapist to assist in teaching one-handed self-care skills.	Most occupational therapists are trained in evaluation of ADL skills and teaching one-handed ADL techniques; assures a consistent approach between therapist and nurse.
	Develop consistent routine for self-care activities. Assign consistent caregivers.	To facilitate learning of new skills and to minimize frustration. To facilitate consistent approach.
	If patient has aphasia, increase use of gestures and demonstrations in teaching; if patient has perceptual problems without aphasia, increase use of verbal cues.	Nonverbal communication helps patients with aphasia; however, nonverbal cues can be confusing to patient with perceptual problems.
	Allow patient to do as much of his own care as possible.	To facilitate learning, independence, and self-esteem.
	Allow adequate time for patient to complete ADL skills.	Patient is more likely to do more on his own and to feel less frustrated if not hurried.
	Position objects within visual field; cue patient to scan environment on side of visual field cut; patch one eye if patient has diplopia.	Visual field cut and unilateral neglect can cause safety hazards and confusion; patching eliminates one visual image, thereby eliminating diplopia—alternate patched eye daily.
	Report to occupational therapist on patient follow-through on learned techniques.	To evaluate effectiveness of teaching, patient follow-through, and need for modifying techniques or reteaching.
	Evaluate home environment for safety and accessibility.	Home environment may need to be adapted for accessibility, and ADL techniques may need to be modified.

NURSING DIAGNOSIS	IMPLEMENTATION	RATIONALE
Impaired communication related to aphasia, dysarthria, visual deficits, alexia, and/or agraphia	Consult speech therapist to aid in developing effective communication with patient.	Early consultation with and intervention by speech therapist increases patient's safety and decreases frustration for both patient and nurse.
	Allow patient sufficient time to communicate.	Patients with dysarthria need time to articulate words; patients with aphasia need time to formulate thoughts and to try to communicate.
	Do not finish patient's sentences for him.	This discourages and frustrates patient.
	Treat patient in age-appropriate manner.	Do not talk to patient with speech difficulty as if he were a child.
	Slow and simplify your speech; increase redundancy.	To make it easier for patient to understand.
	Speak in normal tone of voice.	Do not talk louder if patient cannot communicate well unless patient has hearing loss.
	Encourage patient to increase use of gestures.	To aid in understanding communication.
	Be sure patient can use call light or bell.	To ensure patient's safety.
	Assess reliability of yes and no answers; use yes and no questions to simplify urgent communication.	To simplify learning patient's needs in urgent situations.
	Evaluate patient's ability to use communication board.	May facilitate communication in urgent situations.
	If you are unable to understand the patient, assure him that you will try again in a few minutes if the message is not urgent.	Patient's frustration with communication difficulties may increase inability to understand or to express thoughts.
Functional urinary incontinence related to decreased sensation, cognitive dysfunction, impaired mobility, and/or impaired communication	Develop a reliable method for patient to communicate need to void; keep call light within reach.	Patient with dysarthria or aphasia must be able to indicate need to go to bathroom.
	Remove potential obstacles between bed and bathroom.	To decrease risk of falls and discourage use of bedpan.
	Consider need for sturdy bedside commode.	Bathroom may be too far away when patient has urgent need to urinate.
	Evaluate patient's pattern of fluid intake, activity, and incontinence.	To identify patterns of heavy fluid intake and times/amounts of incontinence.
	Develop or modify fluid intake pattern to distribute fluid intake evenly throughout day, minimizing fluid intake after 7 PM.	Fluids evenly consumed during day prevent rapid filling of bladder at unexpected times; minimizing intake after 7 PM allows patient to void before retiring for night and minimizes need to get up during night.

NURSING DIAGNOSIS	IMPLEMENTATION	RATIONALE
	Develop or modify toileting schedule to establish a routine. Adjust to patient's voiding pattern.	Assures patient of being assisted to bathroom before and after activities. Common schedule is q 2-3 h during day, once during night.
	Observe for any signs of urinary tract infection or other urinary problems.	Incontinence can have numerous causative factors, including UTI and retention.
	Use adult diapers or condom catheters and leg-bags only when incontinence interferes with other therapy or skin problems exist.	To maintain patient's dignity and help break incontinence habit; small absorbent pads can absorb dribbling.
	Evaluate patient's safety and balance on commode.	Patient may be at high risk for falls during transfers, when cleansing self, and when pulling up pants and underwear.
	Provide privacy.	To protect patient's dignity and to help him focus on toileting.
	Praise patient's successes; never scold him for incontinence.	Process may take several weeks; encouragement reinforces success.
	Cleanse skin well after any incontinence.	To decrease risk of skin breakdown.
Bowel incontinence related to decreased sensation, cognitive dysfunction, impaired mobility, impaired communication, and/ or lack of sufficient fluids and bulk in diet	Develop reliable method for patient to communicate need to defecate; keep call light within reach.	Person with dysarthria or aphasia must be able to indicate need to go to bathroom.
	Remove barriers between bed and bathroom.	To decrease risk of falls and discourage use of bedpan.
	Consider need for sturdy bedside commode.	Distance to bathroom may be too far when patient has urgent need to defecate.
	Evaluate patient's pattern of stool incontinence, regularity of bowel movements, daily fluid intake, amount of bulk in diet, and prestroke pattern of bowel evacuation.	To help identify timing of bowel program, dietary factors that need to be modified, and past bowel habits.
	Establish or modify bowel program.	Consistent implementation is the key to establishing continence.
	Ensure that patient does not have an impaction or other cause for incontinence.	Impaction may cause oozing of stool; infection may cause diarrhea.
	Use adult diapers only when bowel incontinence may interfere with therapy.	To maintain patient's dignity and to assist in breaking incontinence habit.

NURSING DIAGNOSIS	IMPLEMENTATION	RATIONALE
	Evaluate patient's safety and balance on commode.	Patient may be at high risk for falls during transfers, while cleansing, or while pulling up pants and underwear.
	Provide privacy.	To maintain patient's dignity and to help patient focus on bowel elimination.
	Encourage patient; never scold when patient soils himself.	Process may take several weeks; encouragement reinforces success.
	Cleanse skin well after bowel incontinence.	To decrease risk of skin breakdown.
Knowledge deficit	See Patient Teaching.	

5 EVALUATE

PATIENT OUTCOME	DATA INDICATING THAT OUTCOME IS REACHED
Patient demonstrates improved cerebral tissue perfusion.	(See evaluation guidelines for altered cerebral tissue perfusion, page 268.)
Patient can independently turn and position self in bed, get out of bed, ambulate or propel wheelchair.	Patient can do his own bed mobility skills and transfers and ambulates safely or safely uses a wheelchair.
Patient can independently do own ADL.	Patient can do his own bathing, grooming, dressing, feeding, and toileting.
Patient has improved ability to express himself and relates decreased frustration with communication efforts.	Patient demonstrates increased skill at understanding others and expressing his own needs and thoughts; he shows less frustration when trying to communicate.
Patient is continent of urine.	Patient has no episodes of urinary incontinence.
Patient is continent of stool.	Patient has no episodes of bowel incontinence.

PATIENT TEACHING

1. Involve family members in the patient's care when appropriate and when they are ready.
2. Teach the patient and family members about a stroke, its effects, and how to compensate for and adapt to residual impairments.
3. Encourage the patient and family to attend educa-

tional sessions and support group meetings, both separately and as a family.

4. Stress the importance of continuing activities after discharge and of following up with outpatient therapy as prescribed.

5. Stress the need for a regular exercise program.

6. Encourage independent activities within the limits of safety.

7. Teach the patient how to do activities of daily living one-handed.

8. Teach the patient to eat slowly, to follow food consistency instructions, and to check the affected side of the mouth for pocketing of food.

9. Teach the patient and family how to do the Heimlich maneuver.

10. Teach the patient mobility skills, and teach the family how to assist safely.

11. Teach family members how to use good body mechanics and protect their backs.

12. Teach the patient and family how to adapt the home for accessibility.

13. Instruct the patient and family about medications: their purpose, dosage, route and frequency of administration, and side effects; also caution the patient not to use over-the-counter medications without consulting the physician.

14. Stress the importance of communication; encourage the patient to socialize with friends and family.

15. Teach the patient and family about seizures and first aid for seizures.

16. Refer the patient for driving evaluation; caution the family that the patient may not be able to drive vehicles safely.

Cerebral Aneurysm

A cerebral **aneurysm** is a localized dilation that develops secondary to a weakness of the arterial wall.

Cerebral aneurysm is the fourth most frequent cerebrovascular disorder, with an incidence of 9.6 cases per 100,000 in the general population. The peak incidence occurs between 35 and 60 years of age, and women are affected slightly more often than men. Cerebral aneurysms rarely occur in children and adolescents. Hypertension is found more frequently in people who have aneurysms than in the average population; however, aneurysms also occur in normotensive individuals.

A ruptured cerebral aneurysm is the most common cause of nontraumatic subarachnoid hemorrhage. At least 28% of individuals who have a ruptured cerebral aneurysm die immediately. Of individuals who survive the initial hemorrhage but are not treated, approximately 50% experience rebleeding within a year. Approximately one third of individuals who survive a ruptured cerebral aneurysm have some residual paralysis, headaches and mental changes, or epilepsy. Rupture of an aneurysm often is associated with physical exertion (e.g., sports or coitus), intense emotional excitement, and a sudden rise in blood pressure, but it also can occur during sleep.

PATHOPHYSIOLOGY

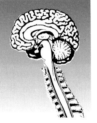

No single mechanism has been identified in the pathogenesis of an intracranial aneurysm. Possible causes are congenital structural defects in the media and elastica of the vessel wall, incomplete involution of embryonic vessels, and secondary factors such as arterial hypertension, atherosclerotic changes, hemodynamic disturbances, and polycystic disease. Intracranial aneurysms also may be caused by shearing forces during craniocerebral trauma. These shearing forces may weaken the arterial wall, which expands or dilates with each arterial pulsation until bleeding or symptoms occur.

Cerebral aneurysms normally vary in size from 2 to 6 mm in diameter, but they can be as large as 6 cm. Single aneurysms are common, but multiple aneurysms occur in 20% to 25% of the cases.[138]

Cerebral aneurysms are classified according to their predominant characteristics. Saccular aneurysms (also called berry aneurysms) account for 95% of all ruptured aneurysms (Figure 4-5). They look like small, thin-walled berries protruding from arteries, primarily at the points of bifurcation of the circle of Willis.

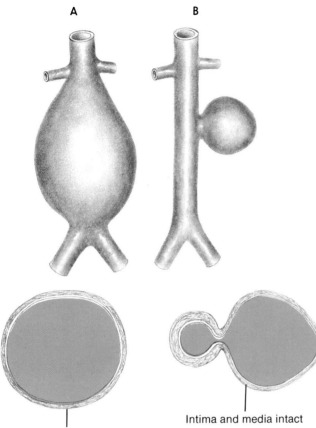

A   B

Stretched intima and media

Intima and media intact

FIGURE 4-5
A, Fusiform aneurysm. **B,** Saccular aneurysm. (From Canobbio.[31])

Fusiform (giant) aneurysms are spindle-shaped dilations of the entire circumference of an artery for several centimeters. They are characterized by diffuse arteriosclerotic changes. These aneurysms occur most commonly along the trunk of the basilar artery. Although they rupture only infrequently, they act as space-occupying lesions. When rupture does occur, it often is fatal.

Mycotic aneurysms are rare and result when a septic embolus from another infection causes arterial necrosis that leads to formation of aneurysms. Several mycotic aneurysms usually form, and they characteristically are found along the distal branches of the middle and anterior cerebral arteries.[149]

Traumatic aneurysms result from a weakened arterial wall secondary to direct damage by shearing forces or fracture of the skull. These aneurysms have been reported after such neurosurgical procedures as tumor removal, hematoma evacuation, and clipping of aneurysms.[96]

Cerebral aneurysms most often occur on the circle of Willis; 30% occur on the anterior communicating artery, 25% on the posterior communicating artery, 13% at the branching of the middle cerebral artery, and 32% in other locations.[138]

A cerebral aneurysm ruptures when the vessel wall becomes so thin that it can no longer withstand the surrounding arterial pressure. This causes direct hemorrhage of arterial blood into the subarachnoid space, resulting in a subarachnoid hemorrhage. Such a hemorrhage spreads rapidly, producing localized changes in the underlying cortex and focal irritation of the cranial nerves and arteries.

Immediately after rupture, intracranial pressure (ICP) rises, approaching the mean arterial pressure, with a resultant fall in cerebral perfusion pressure. Furthermore, the expanding hematoma acts as a space-occupying lesion, compressing or displacing brain tissue. Blood in the basal cisterns and subarachnoid space may impede the flow and resorption of cerebrospinal fluid, resulting in hydrocephalus.

The bleeding ceases with the formation of a fibrin-platelet plug at the point of rupture and by tissue compression. Within approximately 3 weeks, the hemorrhage undergoes resorption. Resorption occurs by the arachnoidal villi after leukocytes and macrophages have begun their scavenging.

Rebleeding is a major complication following the rupture of a cerebral aneurysm. It may occur anytime, but the risk is highest in the first 24 to 48 hours after the initial hemorrhage and again 7 to 10 days after the first episode. The mortality rate with rebleeding may be as high as 70%.[138]

Cerebral vasospasms are a common complication of subarachnoid hemorrhage, occurring in 35% to 40% of individuals. Cerebral vasospasm, defined as narrowing of the vessel lumen, may be caused by actual constriction or by inflammation of the vessel wall.[138] Cerebral vasospasms usually appear 4 to 10 days after the hemorrhage.[48] They decrease cerebral blood flow, producing further neurologic deterioration, cerebral ischemia, and cerebral infarction.

The pathophysiology of vasospasms is not clearly understood, but it is believed that they are precipitated by certain vasoactive substances (i.e., prostaglandins, serotonin, catecholamines, and methemoglobin) released by the blood into the subarachnoid space. Edema, media necrosis, and proliferation of the intima have been described as sequelae to the initial vasospasms.

CLINICAL MANIFESTATIONS

Cerebral aneurysms generally are asymptomatic until they rupture. However, some patients may experience a headache, lethargy, neck discomfort, and other neurologic deficits attributed to the location of the aneurysm. A bruit may be evident upon examination.

The signs and symptoms of a ruptured aneurysm are related to the effects of a subarachnoid hemorrhage. Initially, symptoms may range from reports of sudden onset of "the worst headache of my life" to immediate death.

A severe headache and vomiting are symptoms commonly reported. Physical examination may reveal decreasing level of consciousness, hemiplegia, and other focal neurologic deficits. Meningeal signs may be evident because of contact of blood with the meninges.

Subarachnoid hemorrhages are graded according to their severity (see box below). This grading system is useful in determining the medical interventions and clinical outcome.

COMPLICATIONS

Increased intracranial pressure
Rebleeding
Cerebral vasospasm
Hydrocephalus

CLASSIFICATION OF CEREBRAL ANEURYSM RUPTURE

Grade		Criteria
I	(minimal bleed)	Asymptomatic; alert; minimal headache and minimal nuchal rigidity; no neurologic deficits
II	(mild bleed)	Mild to severe headache; alert; nuchal rigidity; minimal neurologic deficits
III	(moderate bleed)	Lethargic or confused; severe headache; nuchal rigidity; mild focal neurologic deficits
IV	(moderate to severe bleed)	Stuporous; nuchal rigidity; mild to severe hemiparesis; may exhibit decerebrate posturing
V	(severe bleed)	Comatose; decerebrate posturing

DIAGNOSTIC STUDIES AND FINDINGS

Diagnostic test	Findings
Lumbar puncture (*Note:* Should be done with caution)	Increased opening pressures; elevated protein content (80-130 mg/dl); increased white blood count (WBC); slightly decreased glucose; bloody cerebrospinal fluid (CSF) with xanthochromia (hemolyzed red blood cells)
Computed tomography (CT) scan (serial)	Blood in subarachnoid space; displaced midline structures; localized blood clots (may show location)
Magnetic resonance imaging	Same as with CT scan
Cerebral angiogram	Locates site of aneurysm; identifies local or general vasospasm; outlines cerebral vasculature
Skull x-rays	May reveal calcified wall of aneurysm and areas of bone erosion
Echoencephalogram	Shifts in midline structure
Brain scan	May indicate local diminution of flow
Regional cerebral blood flow (rCBF)	Mean flow values for both hemispheres and determination of status of cerebral vasospasm
Electrocardiogram (ECG)	Q waves, elevated ST segments, ST and T wave changes
Serum tests	Electrolyte imbalances; changes in bleeding parameters (i.e., prothrombin time, partial thromboplastin time, and platelet count)

MEDICAL MANAGEMENT

The major goal of medical management is to repair the aneurysm and prevent rebleeding and vasospasm.

GENERAL MANAGEMENT

Aneurysm precautions: Initiated to prevent rebleeding (see Nursing Interventions).

Activity: Complete bed rest.

Diet: Soft, high fiber to prevent straining.

Fluids: Induced hypertensive-hypervolemic therapy is used to treat vasospasm; cardiac output and blood pressure are elevated with volume expanders and fluid; the hypervolemic state forces blood through the vasospastic vessels.

Hemodynamic monitoring: Careful monitoring of pulmonary capillary wedge pressure (PCWP), cardiac output (CO), blood pressure (BP), and heart rate during hypertensive-hypervolemic therapy.

Respiratory: Mechanical ventilation may be indicated because of clinical condition or need to hyperventilate to control ICP; chest x-rays should be carefully monitored because of risk of pulmonary edema with induced hypertensive-hypervolemic therapy.

SURGERY

Craniotomy for aneurysm repair: The timing of aneurysm surgery is the subject of much debate because of the risk of rebleeding and vasospasm. Historically, surgical repair of aneurysm was done 10-14 days after the initial hemorrhage. Recent studies have advocated surgical intervention within the first 48 h for grades I-III aneurysm ruptures (Figure 4-6). This is believed to reduce the risk of rebleeding and vasospasm.[90,138]

The goal of surgery is to repair the aneurysm and prevent rebleeding; this requires a craniotomy. Several techniques are available: clipping, which involves placing a clip on the neck of the aneurysm; wrapping, which involves reinforcement of the weakened arterial wall with substances such as muscle fasciae and muslin; and ligation of the neck of the aneurysm (Figure 4-6).[128]

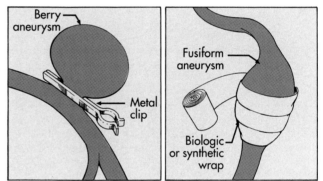

FIGURE 4-6
Clipping and wrapping of aneurysms.

Ventriculostomy: Temporary catheter is placed into the lateral ventricles used to drain CSF; procedure is used to treat elevated ICP and hydrocephalus.

DRUG THERAPY

Anticonvulsants: Phenytoin (Dilantin); phenobarbital.

Antihypertensive agents: Hydralazine (Apresoline); methyldopa (Aldomet).

Antifibrinolytic agents (given to prevent lysis of fibrin clot and reduce potential for rebleeding): Aminocaproic acid (Amicar). Use is controversial.[90]

Corticosteroids: Dexamethasone (Decadron).

Analgesics/antipyretics: Acetaminophen (Tylenol).

Pituitary hormone: Vasopressin injection (Pitressin) (treatment of diabetes insipidus).

Continued.

MEDICAL MANAGEMENT—cont'd

Narcotic analgesics: Acetaminophen with codeine.

Stool softeners: Docusate sodium (Colace).

Psychotherapeutic agents: Chlorpromazine (Thorazine) (for shivering).

Agents to control vasospasms (experimental): methysergide maleate (Sansert); phenoxybenzamine (Dibenzyline); reserpine (Serpasil); kanamycin sulfate (Kantrex); Nifedipine (Adalat, Procardia); nimodipine (Nimotop).

1 ASSESS

ASSESSMENT	OBSERVATIONS
LOC	Varies from brief loss of consciousness to persistent coma
Pain	Sudden onset of severe headache, usually beginning as localized frontally or temporally and then generalizing to involve entire head
Meningeal irritation	Nuchal rigidity; photophobia; positive Kernig's sign; positive Brudzinski's sign; fever; irritability; restlessness; later stages: seizures and blurred vision
Visual disturbances	Blurred vision; double vision; visual field defect: unilateral blindness
Cranial nerve involvement	Ptosis and dilation of pupil; inability to move eye upward or inward; papilledema
Motor function	Onset and worsening of hemiparesis; aphasia; dysphagia; hemiplegia; unilateral or bilateral transient paresis of lower extremities
Increased ICP	Restlessness and lethargy; changes in LOC; changes in vital signs (i.e., Cushing's response with increased systolic BP, wide pulse pressure, and decreased pulse rate [late symptom]); pupillary changes; papilledema (late symptom); vomiting; fluctuations in temperature; seizures; worsening of focal neurologic signs; changes in respiratory patterns
Vasospasms	Drowsiness and worsening headache followed by hemiplegia or hemiparesis; aphasia; focal neurologic deficits; seizures, rise in BP
Autonomic function	Diaphoresis; chills; changes in heart rate and BP; slight temperature elevation (37.8°-38.9° C; 100°-102° F); altered respiratory rhythm

2 DIAGNOSE

NURSING DIAGNOSIS	SUBJECTIVE FINDINGS	OBJECTIVE FINDINGS
Altered cerebral tissue perfusion related to increasing ICP secondary to subarachnoid hemorrhage	Complains of worsening headache, blurry vision, and photophobia	Decreasing LOC; restlessness; pupillary changes; focal neurologic deficits; speech deficits; widening pulse pressure; bradycardia; change in respiratory pattern
Fluid volume excess related to induced hypervolemic-hypertensive therapy	Complains of shortness of breath (SOB)	Increasing PCWP, PAS, PAD, central venous pressure (CVP), SVR, BP; rales on lung auscultation; distended jugular veins; peripheral edema; S_3 murmur
Pain related to severe headache, nuchal rigidity, and photophobia	Complains of severe headache	Restlessness; grimacing; increased BP, heart rate

Other related nursing diagnoses: Social isolation related to reduced environmental stimuli; **Impaired gas exchange** related to alveolar hypoventilation secondary to altered level of consciousness; **Altered family processes** related to situational crisis.

3 PLAN

Patient goals

1. The patient will demonstrate improved cerebral tissue perfusion.
2. The patient will demonstrate no complications secondary to induced fluid volume excess.
3. The patient will demonstrate relief of discomfort.

4 IMPLEMENT

NURSING DIAGNOSIS	NURSING INTERVENTIONS	RATIONALE
Altered cerebral tissue perfusion related to increasing ICP secondary to subarachnoid hemorrhage	Assess neurologic status and ICP q 1 h/prn.	Further neurologic deterioration may indicate rebleeding or onset of vasospasm; sustained ICP >15 mm Hg can cause severe neurologic deterioration.
	Monitor for signs of brain herniation: change in LOC; worsening hemiplegia or change in response to painful stimuli; change in pupil size or shape; widening pulse pressure; change in respiratory pattern; bradycardia	Indicates shifting of brain tissues; can be reversed if noted early.
	Carefully monitor BP and heart rate.	Sudden rise in BP can cause rebleeding; a decrease in BP can cause cerebral ischemia.

NURSING DIAGNOSIS	NURSING INTERVENTIONS	RATIONALE
	Elevate head of bed 30 to 45 degrees; maintain head and neck in neutral position.	To facilitate venous drainage from cranial vessels.
	Avoid hip flexion and isometric exercises.	These impede venous drainage.
	Maintain normothermia.	Hyperthermia increases cerebral blood flow.
	Provide adequate ventilation and oxygenation: arterial oxygen pressure (Pao_2) > 80 mm Hg; arterial carbon dioxide pressure ($Paco_2$) between 25 and 30 mm Hg if intubated.	Hyperventilation is prescribed to maintain partial pressure of carbon dioxide ($Paco_2$) between 25 and 30 mm Hg; increases in $Paco_2$ cause vasodilation, which increases ICP.
	Hyperoxygenate and hyperventilate before suctioning; suction for < 15 sec.	Suctioning causes hypoxia and hypercapnia, which increase ICP.
	Plan nursing care to minimize elevations in ICP.	Even minimum stimulation can markedly elevate ICP.
	Monitor for seizure activity.	Seizures increase cerebral blood flow.
	Administer antifibrinolytic agent as prescribed and monitor for deep vein thrombosis, pulmonary embolus, and ischemic complication.	Use is controversial; prevents lysis of clot around aneurysm and may minimize rebleeding; these are potential side effects of antifibrinolytic agents.
	Administer calcium channel blockers as prescribed.	To treat vasospasm; these drugs are believed to reduce the influx of calcium ions into muscle layers of cerebral vessels.
	Maintain aneurysm precautions: maintain bed rest in quiet environment; darken room; restrict visitors; administer mild sedatives and analgesic; provide soft, high-fiber diet; give stool softeners (no enemas); perform ADL for patient.	To prevent rebleeding; extent of aneurysm precautions may vary, depending on patient's clinical condition and physician's philosophy.
Fluid volume excess related to induced hypervolemic-hypertensive therapy	Monitor BP and heart rate.	Systolic BP usually is maintained between 150 and 160 mm Hg to increase perfusion through the vasospastic cerebral vessels.
	Monitor PAS, PAD, PCWP and SVR, and CO.	PCWP is increased to 16-20 mm Hg; CO is increased to 6.5-8 L/min.
	Administer fluids as prescribed.	Hypervolemia increases blood flow through vasospastic cerebral vessels.
	Maintain strict intake and output.	Fluid balances must be carefully monitored.
	Monitor lung sounds and chest x-rays.	Pulmonary edema is a complication of hypervolemic-hypertensive therapy.

NURSING DIAGNOSIS	NURSING INTERVENTIONS	RATIONALE
	Monitor for signs of congestive heart failure: jugular vein distention, peripheral edema, S_3 murmur.	Congestive heart failure is a complication of hypervolemic-hypertensive therapy.
	Monitor electrolytes.	Electrolyte balance may reflect volume status.
	Continuously assess neurologic status and report any changes to the physician	Elevated ICP and rebleeding are common complications of SAH.
Pain related to severe headache, nuchal rigidity, and photophobia	Monitor headache, nuchal rigidity, and photophobia.	Severe headache, nuchal rigidity, and photophobia are common complaints caused by meningeal irritation.
	Reduce environmental stimuli, and dim lighting; administer analgesics as prescribed; reposition patient q 2 h.	To help reduce discomfort.
	Investigate alternative relaxation techniques.	To reduce muscle tension and facilitate relaxation.
Knowledge deficit	See Patient Teaching.	

5 EVALUATE

PATIENT OUTCOME	DATA INDICATING THAT OUTCOME IS REACHED
Patient maintains adequate cerebral tissue perfusion.	LOC is unchanged; there is no evidence of neurologic deficits; ICP remains ≤15 mm Hg.
Patient demonstrates minimal complications of fluid volume excess.	Lung sounds and chest x-ray remain clear; electrolytes are within normal limits; there are no signs of peripheral edema or jugular vein distension.
Patient demonstrates minimum discomfort.	Patient has no headache, nuchal rigidity, or photophobia; there are no signs of grimacing.

PATIENT TEACHING

1. Involve the family in the patient's care, as possible; teach them the essential aspects of care.
2. Emphasize the importance of minimizing external stimuli and of maintaining aneurysm precautions.
3. Reinforce the physician's explanation of medical management.
4. Stress the importance of ongoing outpatient care and follow-up visits.

Intracranial Tumors

Intracranial tumors include both benign space-occupying and malignant lesions. Intracranial tumors can occur in any structural area of the brain and in all age groups. Growth rates range from the rapid growth of glioblastomas to the almost imperceptible changes of some meningiomas.

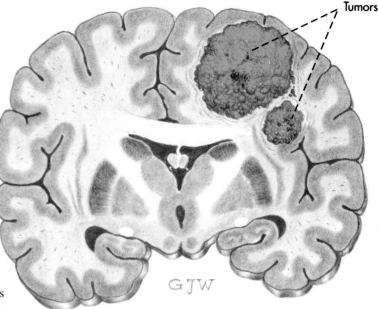

BRAIN TUMOR

About 10,000 people develop intracranial tumors in the United States each year. The peak incidence occurs in childhood (3 to 12 years of age) and in older adults (50 to 70 years of age).[138] Seventy percent of intracranial tumors in children occur infratentorially, whereas 70% of intracranial tumors in adults occur supratentorially.

Brain tumors are named according to the tissues from which they arise. Primary intracerebral brain tumors are those whose cells originate from brain substances; these tumors include oligodendrogliomas, ependymomas, astrocytomas, glioblastomas, and medulloblastomas. Primary extracerebral tumors are those that originate outside the substance of the brain, such as meningiomas, acoustic neuromas, and pituitary tumors (see Table 4-2). Secondary or metastatic tumors arise from metastatic carcinoma or sarcoma.[98]

PRIMARY INTRACEREBRAL TUMORS

The gliomas are tumors within brain tissue that arise from glial cells. They include oligodendroglioma, ependymoma, astrocytoma, and medulloblastoma.

Oligodendrogliomas form in the oligodendroglial cells that are responsible for forming the central nervous system (CNS) myelin sheaths. These tumors evolve slowly and may be detected on a routine skull x-ray because of intracranial calcification. The most common site of oligodendrogliomas is the frontal lobe.[98] This type of tumor makes up only 5%-7% of all intracranial tumors. There is a high incidence of this tumor among young adults who have a childhood history of temporal lobe epilepsy.[84]

Ependymomas are fairly rare in the general adult population and make up only 5% of all intracranial tumors. They are more commonly found in young children and adolescents and account for 20% of brain tumors in this age group. Ependymomas form in the ependymal cells and astrocytes that line the walls of the cerebral ventricular system and most commonly affect the fourth ventricle.[98]

Astrocytomas form in astrocyte cells at any level of the central nervous system. In adults they usually are lateral and supratentorial, whereas astrocytes in children are in or near the midline.[84] Cerebellar astrocytomas, which constitute 30% of all pediatric brain tumors, usually are located just lateral to the midline in the cerebellar hemisphere. Simple surgical excision of these tumors can achieve long-term survival. Brainstem astrocytomas primarily affect school-aged children, who have a high mortality rate because of destruction of the local cranial nerve nuclei and the long tracts.

Cerebral astrocytomas are classified by grade (Table 4-3). They are common between 30 and 50 years of age, making up 30% of the brain tumors for this age group. The growth rate for these tumors reflects their grade; for example, a grade I or grade II tumor grows slowly, whereas a grade III or grade IV tumor grows rapidly, advancing to a more malignant tumor, called a glioblastoma multiforme.

Medulloblastomas constitute 20% of brain tumors in children and occur most frequently in children under 10 years of age. The tumor eventually obstructs the flow of cerebrospinal fluid from the aqueduct, resulting in hydrocephalus and cerebellar signs. Without irradiation, the tumor is fatal; with irradiation, there is a 30% survival rate.

PRIMARY EXTRACEREBRAL TUMORS

Meningiomas, which occur in adults, arise from the cells of vessels, pia-arachnoid, and surrounding fibro-

Table 4-2

TYPES OF BRAIN TUMORS

Tumor	Location	Characteristics	Cell of origin
Gliomas			
Astrocytoma	Anywhere in the brain	Slow growing, invasive	Astrocytes
Glioblastoma multiforme	Predominantly in cerebral hemispheres	Highly invasive and malignant	Thought to arise from mature astrocytes
Oligodendroglioma	Most common in frontal lobes deep in white matter; may arise in brainstem, cerebellum, and spinal cord	Relatively avascular; tends to be encapsulated	Oligodendrites
Ependymoma	Wall of ventricle; may arise in caudal tail of spinal cord	Most common in children; variable growth rate; may extend into ventricle or invade brain tissue	Ependymal cells
Neuronal cell tumor			
Medulloblastoma	Posterior cerebellar vermis, roof of fourth ventricle	Well demarcated, rapid growing, fills fourth ventricle	Embryonic cells
Mesodermal tissue tumor			
Meningioma	Parasagittal falx of frontal and parietal lobes, sylvian fissure region, olfactory groove wing of sphenoid bone; superior surface of cerebellum; cerebellopontine angle, spinal cord	Slow growing, circumscribed, encapsulated, demarcated from normal tissue, compressive in nature	Arachnoid cells; may be from fibroblasts
Cranial nerve and spinal nerve root tumors			
Neurilemmoma	Cranial nerves (most commonly vestibular division or cranial nerve VIII)	Slow growing	Schwann cells
Pituitary tumors	Pituitary gland; may extend to invade floor of third ventricle	Age linked; several types; slow growing	Pituitary cells
Blood vessel tumors			
Angioma	Predominantly in posterior cerebral hemispheres	Slow growing	Arises from congenitally malformed arteriovenous connections
Hemangioblastoma	Predominantly in cerebellum	Slow growing	Embryonic vascular tissue
Congenital tumors			
Craniopharyngioma	Predominantly around the sella turcica; tends to grow upward and invade third ventricle	Slow growing	Arises from remnants of the hypophyseal pouch

Adapted from McCance.[98]

Table 4-3

GRADES OF ASTROCYTOMA

Grade	Growth rate	Prognosis
Astrocytoma		
Grade I	Slow	Good; 15-20 yr survival after surgery
Grade II	Slow	Good; 10-15 yr survival after surgery
Glioblastoma		
Grade III	Rapid, invasive	Poor; less than 2 yr survival without therapy
Grade IV (glioblastoma multiforme)	Rapid, invasive	Very poor; 6-9 mo survival without surgery

blasts. Meningiomas make up 15% of all adult tumors of the central nervous system and its coverings.[67,126] They occur more frequently in women and are found in approximately 40% to 50% of patients with von Recklinghausen's disease (neurofibromatosis). The symptoms of a meningioma are manifested as the tumor indents a local area of the brain and raises the intracranial pressure.

Acoustic neuromas (acoustic neurofibromas) arise from the Schwann cells of the vestibular portion of the eighth cranial nerve. Acoustic neuromas represent 5% to 10% of all intracranial tumors. Acoustic neuromas are slow-growing tumors that often grow quite large before becoming symptomatic. The symptoms of an acoustic neuroma are manifested as the tumor invades the cerebellopontine angle, compressing cranial nerves V, VII, VIII, IX, and X. Large tumors may cause symptoms attributed to disturbances in the cerebellum.[126]

Pituitary tumors account for 7% of all intracranial lesions. Pituitary tumors were previously identified by cell type: acidophil, basophil, or chromophobe. However, they are now described in terms of their ability to secrete hormones and are identified as nonfunctioning (nonsecreting) or functioning (secreting). Most pituitary tumors are benign and arise in the anterior lobe. However, benign tumors occupy space in the sella turcica, exerting pressure on the surrounding structures.[35]

METASTATIC TUMORS

It is estimated that 25% of patients with cancer develop metastases to the brain. Metastases can occur to the dura, meninges, or brain parenchyma.

Metastatic tumors may originate in the lungs, breasts, gastrointestinal tract, kidneys, gallbladder, liver, thyroid, testes, uterus, ovaries, and pancreas. The tumor cells are disseminated through the bloodstream.[98]

PATHOPHYSIOLOGY

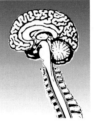

Primary tumors arise from tissue within the intracranial vault. These tumors rarely metastasize outside the brain. Classification of brain tumors is the subject of much controversy. However, classification is based on cell histology, cell features, and grade of malignancy. The prognosis depends on the tumor's classification and its intracranial location. Benign tumors in a surgically inaccessible part of the brain may offer a poorer prognosis than a malignant tumor that is surgically accessible. There is evidence that benign tumors can undergo anaplasia and become malignant.[67]

CLINICAL MANIFESTATIONS

Regardless of the pathologic type of intracranial tumor, the signs and symptoms reflect progressive neurologic deficits caused by focal disturbances and increased intracranial pressure. Focal disturbances are caused by increasing compression of brain tissue and the infiltration or direct invasion of brain parenchyma, resulting in destruction of neural tissue.[119] The cerebral blood supply may be diminished as the tumor compresses blood vessels, resulting in necrotic cerebral tissue or seizures. Approximately 30% of adults with intracranial tumors develop focal or generalized seizure activity. Increased intracranial pressure may result from regional edema, changes in cerebrospinal fluid circulation, and an increase in tissue within the skull. Hydrocephalus results from disruption in the circulation of cerebrospinal fluid from the cerebral ventricles to the subarachnoid spaces.

The size and location of the specific tumor can cause shifts of brain tissue, with associated brain herniation syndromes. If left untreated, herniation can lead to infarction, hemorrhage, and cerebral death.

Table 4-4

CLINICAL MANIFESTATIONS OF BRAIN TUMORS ASSOCIATED WITH PARTICULAR BRAIN REGIONS

Tumor location	Symptoms
Frontal lobe	
Anterior portion	Disturbances in mental function
Posterior portion	Motor system dysfunction; seizures; aphasia (dominant hemisphere)
Parietal lobe	Sensory deficits (contralateral)—paresthesia, hyperesthesia, astereognosis, loss of two-point discrimination, finger agnosia; seizures; visual field deficits; defects in integration
Temporal lobe	Psychomotor seizures; visual field deficits; auditory disturbances; Wernicke's aphasia (dominant hemisphere)
Occipital lobe	Headache; seizures with visual aura; visual field deficit
Pituitary	Headaches; visual problems; endocrine problems
Cerebellum	Nystagmus; ataxia; unsteady gait; intention tumors; dysmetria; problems with rapid alternating movements
Brainstem and cranial nerve	Hemiparesis; nystagmus; extraocular nerve palsies; facial paralysis; depressed corneal reflex; hearing loss, tinnitus; difficulty swallowing; drooling; vertigo and dizziness; ataxia; vomiting

Adapted from Rudy.[127]

COMPLICATIONS

Cerebral edema
Increased intracranial pressure
Brain herniation
Hydrocephalus
Seizures
Metastasis to other sites

DIAGNOSTIC STUDIES AND FINDINGS

Diagnostic test	Findings	Diagnostic test	Findings
Brain scan	Increased uptake of isotope in the tumor	**Computed tomography (CT) scan/ magnetic resonance imaging (MRI) study**	Identification of vascular tumors; shifts in midline structures; changes in cerebral ventricular size
Pneumoencephalogram (Contraindicated if increased ICP is suspected)	Tumor localization		
		Electroencephalogram (EEG)	Marked focal slowing (with rapidly developing tumors); rhythmic, periodic, and high-voltage slowing (with increased ICP)
Cerebral angiography	Cerebral vascularity; blood vessel deviations		
Positron emission tomography (PET) scan	Same as CT scan (see below) but also details sites of glucose metabolism in the brain under various conditions	**Dural sinus venography**	May indicate narrowed sinuses and interference with cranial drainage
		Echoencephalogram	Shifts in midline structures
Skull x-rays	Erosion of posterior clinoid process or presence of intracranial calcifications	**Stereotactic biopsy**	Identifies histologic cell type
		Ophthalmoscopic examination	Papilledema
Chest x-rays	Detection of primary lung tumor or metastatic disease		

MEDICAL MANAGEMENT

Treatment of brain tumors may involve surgery, chemotherapy, radiation, or any combination of the three.

GENERAL MANAGEMENT

Radiation therapy:[147]   May be the mainstay treatment for tumors that are not surgically accessible.

   External beam radiation therapy: May be performed postoperatively to destroy remaining tumor cells.

   Brachytherapy (interstitial radiation therapy):   Radioactive seeds are implanted by stereotactic techniques directly into tumor bed.

Nutrition: Adequate caloric intake.

SURGERY

Craniotomy: For excision of supratentorial tumors (see Cranial Surgery, page 236).

Craniectomy: For excision of infratentorial tumors (see Cranial Surgery, page 236).

Transsphenoidal procedure: For excision of pituitary tumors (see Transsphenoidal Surgery, page 253).

Shunting procedures: To treat the secondary complications of hydrocephalus (see Hydrocephalus, page 98).

Ommaya reservoir: Inserted for intraventricular chemotherapy.

DRUG THERAPY

Corticosteroids: Dexamethasone (Decadron).

Anticonvulsants: Phenytoin (Dilantin).

Analgesics/antipyretics: Acetaminophen.

Laxatives: Docusate sodium (Colace).

Histamine receptor antagonist: Cimetidine (Tagamet); Ranitidine (Zantac).

Antacids: Magnesium hydroxide (Maalox).

Systemic chemotherapy: Choice of pharmaceutic agents depends on tumor type and protocol; drugs selected must be able to cross blood-brain barrier.[88,147]

1   ASSESS

ASSESSMENT	OBSERVATIONS
Focal neurologic disturbance	Symptoms depend on tumor location (See Table 4-4)
Increased ICP	Restlessness, lethargy; changes in level of consciousness (LOC); changes in vital signs: widening pulse pressure, decreased heart rate; pupillary changes (i.e., mydriasis); papilledema (70%-75% of patients); vomiting (may be projectile); fluctuations in temperature; seizures; worsening of focal neurologic signs; changes in respiratory patterns

ASSESSMENT	OBSERVATIONS
Mentation	Personality changes (i.e., loss of emotional restraints); insidious decrease in mentation; depression; memory and judgment deficits
Pituitary dysfunction	Cushing's syndrome; acromegaly; giantism; hypopituitarism
Pain	Headaches with steady, persistent, or intractable dull pain; changes in character of headaches; stress-induced headaches
Seizure activity	Initial symptom in 15% of patients
Fluid status	Nausea and vomiting; decreased urine output; increased urine specific gravity; dry mucous membranes; decreased skin turgor; elevated serum sodium, blood urea nitrogen (BUN), hemoglobin and hematocrit; hypotension; tachycardia; weight loss
Psychosocial	Grief; anger; hostility; fear

2 DIAGNOSE

NURSING DIAGNOSIS	SUBJECTIVE FINDINGS	OBJECTIVE FINDINGS
Potential fluid volume deficit related to side effects of chemotherapeutic agents and radiation therapy	Complains of generalized weakness and thirst	Change in urine output; increased urine specific gravity; increased serum sodium, BUN, hemoglobin and hematocrit; decreased skin turgor; dry mucous membranes; hypotension; tachycardia; weight loss
Body image disturbance related to hair loss and change in body structure and function	Expresses fear of rejection, negative self-image, feeling of hopelessness	Hair loss; change in sensory/motor function; social withdrawal
Impaired skin integrity related to effects of chemotherapy and radiation therapy	Complains of dry, itchy, red, sore skin	Red, dry skin
Anticipatory grieving related to actual or perceived death	Expresses feelings of grief, depression, and hopelessness	Weight loss; lack of appetite; social withdrawal; changes in sleep pattern; decreased interest in activities and participation in self-care

Other related nursing diagnoses: Altered cerebral tissue perfusion related to surgical excision of tumor, brain tissue compression, and cerebral edema (see Cranial Surgery, page 236); **Altered nutrition: less than body requirements** related to persistent nausea and vomiting; **Pain** related to severe headaches and side effects of treatment; **Potential sensory-perceptual alteration** related to brain tissue compression.

PLAN

Patient goals

1. The patient will demonstrate adequate fluid volume.
2. The patient will come to accept changes in body image.
3. The patient's skin integrity will be maintained.
4. The patient will be able to express feelings of fear and depression.

4   IMPLEMENT

NURSING DIAGNOSIS	NURSING INTERVENTIONS	RATIONALE
Potential fluid volume deficit related to side effects of chemotherapeutic agents and radiation therapy	Assess physiologic signs of fluid deficit: skin turgor, mucous membranes, thirst, BP, and heart rate; monitor serum electrolytes, serum albumin, and CBC.	These parameters reflect state of hydration.
	Monitor intake and output.	Excessive vomiting may occur with chemotherapy and radiation therapy.
	Encourage adequate fluid intake. Administer IV fluids as prescribed.	To help maintain adequate hydration.
	Administer antiemetics as prescribed.	May reduce nausea and vomiting, which impede oral fluid intake.
Body image disturbance related to hair loss and change in body structure and function	Assess patient's awareness of and reaction to body changes.	To determine patient's reaction to change in body image.
	Observe patient's social interactions.	Social withdrawal may occur because of embarrassment or fear of rejection.
	Establish a therapeutic relationship with patient.	To facilitate an open, trusting relationship.
	Encourage friends and family to promote positive self-image for patient.	To bolster patient's self-esteem.
	Encourage patient to communicate openly with health care personnel and significant others.	Openly expressing fears and concerns can reduce anxiety.
	Help patient devise realistic strategies in coping with change in body image.	Helping patient discover coping strategies can reduce anxiety and fear.
Impaired skin integrity related to effects of chemotherapy and radiation therapy	Assess skin integrity q 4 h.	A reddened, dry, sore area can develop in the area of radiation; chemotherapy may cause rashes, hyperpigmentation, and hair loss.
	Keep skin clean and dry; use mild soap and water to bathe patient.	To maintain clean, dry skin and to prevent skin breakdown.
	Use foam egg-crate pad, water mattress, or other pressure-reducing devices.	To reduce pressure on tender skin.

NURSING DIAGNOSIS	NURSING INTERVENTIONS	RATIONALE
	Reposition patient q 2 h.	To increase circulation and prevent pressure ulcers.
	Encourage adequate fluid and nutrition intake.	Dehydration and malnutrition can increase risk of pressure ulcer development.
Anticipatory grieving related to actual or perceived death	Assess patient's and family's reaction to diagnosis.	To determine grieving process and coping strategies of patient and family.
	Encourage patient to be open in expressing feelings.	To reduce anxiety and fear.
	Anticipate patient's feelings of anger and fear.	Mood swings are common after initial shock of diagnosis.
	Assist patient in reviewing past life experiences.	To help patient recognize previous coping mechanisms.
	Encourage patient to participate in ADL.	To reduce feelings of powerlessness.
	Help patient and family make preparatory plans for death.	To allow opportunity to discuss family business and to prepare for death.
	Refer patient and family to support groups and hospice counseling services.	Community agencies can provide financial, physical, and emotional support.
Knowledge deficit	See Patient Teaching.	

5 EVALUATE

PATIENT OUTCOME	DATA INDICATING THAT OUTCOME IS REACHED
Adequate fluid balance is maintained.	Intake and output are equal; specific gravity is within normal limits; skin turgor is within normal limits; mucous membranes are moist; vital signs within normal limits; serum electrolytes, hemoglobin, and hematocrit are within normal limits.
Patient expresses a positive self-image.	Patient has expressed her acceptance of changes in her body image.
Patient's skin integrity is maintained.	Skin remains intact with no signs of redness or breakdown.
Patient/family are able to express grief.	Patient's and family's feelings of grief are appropriately expressed.

→ > >

PATIENT TEACHING

1. Involve the family in the patient's care, as possible; teach them the essential aspects of care.
2. Reinforce the physician's explanation of medical management.
3. Stress the importance of ongoing outpatient care and follow-up visits.
4. Encourage independent activities, as possible:
   a. Alert the patient to limitations.
   b. Avoid overprotection.
   c. Stress the need for supportive devices as indicated.
5. Stress the need for a regular exercise program; teach the family range-of-motion exercises.
6. Stress the importance of diet as ordered:
   a. Offer supplemental feedings.
   b. Offer small portions, and instruct the patient to chew slowly.
7. Stress the importance of safety measures: side rails, ramps, shower chairs, and walkers and canes.
8. Teach the patient about medications: name, dosage, time of administration, and toxic or side effects.
9. Instruct the patient not to take over-the-counter medications without first consulting physician.
10. Encourage the patient to socialize with friends and family.
11. Stress the importance of expressing feelings of anxiety, fear, and concern about body image changes.
12. Teach the patient and family about seizures: safety measures and whom to contact.
13. Refer the patient and family to appropriate community agencies.

Hydrocephalus

Hydrocephalus is characterized by an abnormal accumulation of cerebrospinal fluid within the cranial vault, with subsequent dilation of the cerebral ventricles.[119]

Hydrocephalus has an incidence of 4 cases per 1,000 infants from birth through 3 months of age, but it can occur at any age. In infants it is considered a primary disease, whereas in later life it occurs as a complication of other diseases.

Hydrocephalus has several known causes, which can be categorized as congenital or acquired. Congenital abnormalities obstruct the flow of cerebrospinal fluid (CSF); 70% of these obstructions result from stenosis of the aqueduct of Sylvius. Other anomalies causing or associated with congenital hydrocephalus are Arnold-Chiari deformity, Dandy-Walker syndrome, and spina bifida cystica.[113] Acquired hydrocephalus may be caused by hemorrhage, infection, trauma, or neoplasm.[59]

There are two types of hydrocephalus, communicating and noncommunicating. Communicating (extraventricular) hydrocephalus results when the obstruction is outside the ventricular system. In these cases there is no blockage of CSF flow between the ventricles, but either CSF is overproduced or its absorption is diminished. Communicating hydrocephalus may result from subarachnoid hemorrhage, head injury, or a choroid plexus papilloma, which causes increased production of CSF. Noncommu-

nicating (intraventricular) hydrocephalus results when CSF accumulates because the normal flow of CSF has been blocked at some point in the ventricular system; this causes the cerebral ventricles proximal to the block to dilate. Noncommunicating hydrocephalus is associated with congenital abnormalities or tumors near or within the ventricular system.[11,59]

PATHOPHYSIOLOGY

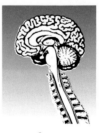

The causative mechanism of hydrocephalus may be related to excessive production of CSF or, more commonly, impaired absorption of CSF because of blockage of the ventricles or subarachnoid space. Impaired absorption of CSF may occur after a cerebral hemorrhage or infection in which the arachnoid villi become plugged.

When an obstruction occurs in the ventricular system or subarachnoid space, the cerebral ventricles dilate, stretching the ventricular surface and disrupting its ependymal lining. The underlying white matter atrophies and may be reduced to a thin ribbon. There is selective preservation of the gray matter, even when the ventricles have attained enormous size. The dilation process may be insidious or acute; acute dilation can cause a rapid rise in intracranial pressure.

CLINICAL MANIFESTATIONS

Acute hydrocephalus generally has the signs and symptoms of elevating intracranial pressure. Hydrocephalus that is more insidious may manifest itself with subtler symptoms, such as declining memory, inattentiveness, and apathy.

COMPLICATIONS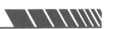

- Focal neurologic deficits
- Increased intracranial pressure
- Brain herniation
- Subdural hematoma (after shunt placement)
- Infection (after shunt placement)

DIAGNOSTIC STUDIES AND FINDINGS

Diagnostic test	Findings
Cerebral angiography	Vessel abnormalities caused by stretching; vascular lesions
Computed tomography (CT) scan/ magnetic resonance imaging (MRI) study	Variations in tissue density; presence of cysts or masses; visualization of ventricular system
Lumbar puncture (*Contraindication:* Elevated ICP)	For diagnosis of communicating hydrocephalus
Subdural or ventricular puncture (*Contraindication:* Elevated ICP)	For diagnosis of communicating hydrocephalus
Ventriculography	Visualization of ventricular system configuration; shows ventricular dilation with hydrocephalus

MEDICAL MANAGEMENT

GENERAL MANAGEMENT

ICP monitoring: May be indicated if patient's condition is rapidly deteriorating.

SURGERY

Correction of CSF obstruction such as resection of cyst, neoplasm, or hematoma.

Ventricular bypass into normal intracranial channel (i.e., Torkildsen procedure, in which CSF is shunted from lateral ventricle to cisterna magna) in noncommunicating hydrocephalus.

Ventricular bypass into extracranial compartment (i.e., ventriculoperitoneal or ventriculoatrial shunt): A catheter is placed in the lateral ventricle to transfer excess CSF into a body cavity (heart or peritoneum) (Figure 4-7).

Reduction of CSF production, as in third or fourth ventriculostomy, or endoscopic choroid plexus extirpation (plexectomy or electric coagulation).

DRUG THERAPY

Osmotic diuretic therapy: Mannitol, in initial management of severe increased ICP.

Corticosteroids: Dexamethasone (Decadron).

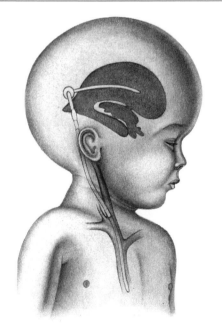

FIGURE 4-7
Placement of ventriculoatrial shunt. (From Neurosurgery wound closure, Ethicon, Inc.)

1 ASSESS

ASSESSMENT	OBSERVATIONS
Increased ICP	Restlessness, lethargy; change in level of consciousness (LOC); widened pulse pressure; bradycardia; change in respiratory patterns; pupillary changes; papilledema; worsening of focal neurologic signs; seizures; vomiting
Mental status	Apathy; inattentiveness; declining memory
Pediatrics	Severely enlarged head; irritability; vomiting; seizures; change in LOC; bulging fontanels; fixed downward gaze of eyes (sunset gaze); visible, distended scalp veins; radiation of light throughout accumulated CSF with transillumination; poor feeding behavior

2 DIAGNOSE

NURSING DIAGNOSIS	SUBJECTIVE FINDINGS	OBJECTIVE FINDINGS
Altered cerebral tissue perfusion related to enlarged/ dilated ventricular system	Complains of headache and anxiety	Restlessness, lethargy; change in LOC; focal neurologic deficits; pupillary changes; change in respiratory pattern; widening pulse pressure; bradycardia; seizures; vomiting

Other related nursing diagnosis: Potential for infection related to internalized shunting procedure.

3 PLAN

Patient goal

1. The patient will demonstrate optimum cerebral tissue perfusion.

4 IMPLEMENT

NURSING DIAGNOSIS	NURSING INTERVENTIONS	RATIONALE
Altered cerebral tissue perfusion related to enlarged/ dilated ventricular system	Assess neurologic status q 2-4 hprn; monitor for signs of increasing ICP.	Hydrocephalus can cause rapid rise in ICP.
	Maintain head position at appropriately pre-scribed head gauge.	During the initial postoperative period after placement of a shunt, the HOB may be kept flat to prevent decompression of the ventricular system. The HOB is gradually elevated.
	Avoid flexion of hip, isometric exercises, coughing, Valsalva maneuver, hypoxemia, and hypercapnia.	These activities elevate ICP.
	If patient has a shunt, pump shunt as pre-scribed	Shunting devices have a one-way valve to facilitate removal of CSF from the ventric-ular system.

NURSING DIAGNOSIS	NURSING INTERVENTIONS	RATIONALE
	Monitor sites of shunt placement for redness, tenderness, fluid collection, and bulging.	Infection and obstruction cause shunt malfunction.
	Position patient to avoid compressing shunt tubing.	To prevent obstruction of CSF flow through the shunting system.
Knowledge deficit	See Patient Teaching.	

5 EVALUATE

PATIENT OUTCOME	DATA INDICATING THAT OUTCOME IS REACHED
Patient maintains optimum cerebral tissue perfusion.	There are no signs of increased ICP and no focal neurologic deficits; internalized shunt procedure is effective.

PATIENT TEACHING

1. Be sure the patient and family know and understand the following:
   a. The nature of hydrocephalus, treatments, and procedures (explain as they occur)
   b. Care of shunt devices, if indicated
   c. The need to ambulate as tolerated
   d. The importance of having planned rest periods
   e. The names of medications, dosages, frequency of administration, purposes, and toxic or side effects
   f. The need to avoid taking over-the-counter medications without consulting the physician
   g. The possible residual effects such as headaches, sensory or motor deficits, and seizures
   h. The possibility that shunt revisions may be needed
2. Teach the patient and family members how to recognize seizure activity and the appropriate course of action:
   a. Help the patient sit or lie down.
   b. Do not try to stop the seizure or restrain the patient.
   c. Protect the patient from injury.
   d. Observe and record the body parts involved and the duration of seizure activity.
   e. Report seizures to the physician.
3. Teach the patient and family members the signs and symptoms of increasing intracranial pressure; emphasize the importance of seeking immediate medical attention.
4. Ensure that the patient and family understand the importance of ongoing outpatient care (i.e., physician's visits and physical therapy).
5. Teach the patient and family the importance of maintaining a well-balanced diet.

Seizure Disorder (Convulsions, Epilepsy)

Seizures, or convulsions, are paroxysmal episodes involving sudden, violent, involuntary contractions of a group of skeletal muscles and disturbances in consciousness, behavior, sensation, and autonomic functioning.

Seizures may be tonic or clonic, focal, and unilateral or bilateral. The term *epilepsy* denotes a group of neurologic disorders characterized by the repeated occurrence of any of the various forms of seizures. Approximately 2 million to 4 million Americans have epilepsy, and many of them are children. A seizure disorder can have significant social consequences, including possible loss of driving or educational privileges. Of those with epilepsy, 25% have recurrent seizures while receiving medication, 10% are institutionalized, and 5% are home bound.[137]

PATHOPHYSIOLOGY

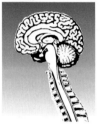

Seizure disorders can be classified as idiopathic or as resulting from pathologic processes, endogenous or exogenous poisons, metabolic disturbances, or fever. Pathologic processes include formation abnormalities (e.g., vascular anomalies), space-occupying lesions (e.g., brain abscess, tumors, hematomas), craniocerebral trauma, acute cerebral edema, infection (e.g., encephalitis), degenerative changes, vascular lesions (e.g., embolus, cerebrovascular accidents, and hemorrhages), and neuronal injury (e.g., anoxia from deficient oxygen).[29]

Toxic endogenous substances (e.g., uremia) or exogenous substances such as certain medications (e.g., phenothiazines), lead ingestion, and alcohol intoxication or sudden withdrawal may precipitate seizure activity.

Metabolic disturbances (e.g., electrolyte imbalances) that interfere with the delivery of crucial substances such as oxygen, glucose, or calcium to cerebral tissues can result in seizures.

Individuals with decreased neuronal thresholds may experience a seizure secondary to a febrile state.

Idiopathic seizures may occur without any identifiable cause. The basis of idiopathic seizure disorders may be a biochemical imbalance.

These causative agents are either genetic or acquired. Genetically, epilepsy is rarely a predictable inherited entity. The only well-defined inherited seizure pattern is that of the classic 2.5 to 3/s spike-and-wave pattern on the electroencephalogram (EEG).[76] Therefore, although inheritance may be a risk in developing

seizures, environmental risk factors (e.g., trauma) play a significant role. Acquired causes include pathologic processes (e.g., infection), trauma that produces epileptogenic lesions, toxic substances, metabolic disturbances, and febrile states.

Traditionally, seizures have been classified as grand mal, petit mal, psychomotor (temporal lobe), and focal motor (jacksonian). With advanced technology it became evident that many neurologic manifestations of seizures did not fit into these categories. In 1969 the International League Against Epilepsy formulated a revised classification that incorporated pathophysiologic principles of all types of seizure activity (box, p. 103).[29]

Partial seizures start with a localized activation of neurons and generally do not involve the whole brain or significantly impair consciousness or memory. Partial seizures with simple symptoms produce symptoms of which the individual is aware, including autonomic, sensory, or focal motor symptoms. Simple partial seizures start with focal motor symptoms (jacksonian seizures), generally in the contralateral precentral gyrus. Symptoms first occur in the part of the body controlled by that brain area and then can spread to involve the entire limb and frequently the entire half of the body. The seizure ends with a gradual reduction of clonic, jerking movements. Seizure activity that occurs usually in the hand or face and is continuous, clonic, and localized is called epilepsia partialis continua. Simple sensory seizures are uncommon, but when present, they originate from hyperexcitable neurons in the postcentral gyrus. Symptoms of a partial sensory seizure include various degrees of numbness and paresthesia. Autonomic seizures result from hyperexcitable neurons of the frontal, temporal, mesial, orbital, or insular cortices. These seizures may begin with disturbances in gastric motility, which may progress to nausea and vomiting, tenesmus, or sudden bowel evacuation.[48] Partial seizures with only autonomic symptoms are rare.

Partial seizures with complex symptoms generally produce some type of episodic loss of consciousness. This type of seizure may include cognitive, affective, psychosensory, or psychomotor symptoms. Events that trigger the seizure occur within the structures of the temporal lobe. Complex partial seizures begin with various types of auras such as sensory illusions, déjà vu, or

INTERNATIONAL CLASSIFICATION OF EPILEPTIC SEIZURES

Traditional terminology	New nomenclature
	I. Partial seizures (seizures beginning locally)

Focal motor; jacksonian seizures (occasionally become secondarily generalized)	A. Simple (without impairment of consciousness)
	  1. With motor symptoms
	  2. With special sensory or somatosensory symptoms
	  3. With autonomic symptoms
	  4. With psychic symptoms

Temporal lobe or psychomotor seizures	B. Complex (with impairment of consciousness)
	  1. Simple partial onset followed by impaired consciousness—with or without automatisms
	  2. Impaired consciousness at onset—with or without automatisms

	C. Secondarily generalized (partial onset evolving to generalized tonic-clonic seizures)
	II. Generalized seizures (bilaterally symmetrical and without local onset)
Petit mal	A. Absences
Minor motor	B. Myoclonic seizures
Limited grand mal	C. Clonic seizure
	D. Tonic seizure
Grand mal	E. Tonic-clonic seizure
Drop attacks	F. Atonic seizure
	G. Infantile spasms
	III. Unclassified seizures (because of incomplete data)
	IV. Status epilepticus (prolonged partial or generalized seizures without recovery between attacks)

From McCance.[98]

TERMINOLOGY FOR SEIZURE DISORDERS

Term	Definition
Aura	A peculiar sensation immediately preceding the onset of a seizure that may take the form of gustatory, visual, or auditory experience or a feeling of dizziness, numbness, or just "a funny feeling"
Prodrome	Early clinical manifestations such as malaise, headache, a sense of depression that may occur hours to a few days before the onset of a seizure
Tonic phase	A state of muscle contraction where there is excessive muscle tone
Clonic phase	A state of alternating contraction and relaxation of muscles
Postictal state	The time period immediately following the cessation of seizure activity

From McCance.[98]

unusual smells. The individual may recognize these auras, or memory of them may be lost in postictal amnesia. In complex partial seizures, EEG abnormalities are localized in temporal or frontotemporal areas, including rhinencephalic structures. Complex partial seizures are characterized by purposeful behavior that is inappropriate for the time and place.[13] Automatisms such as lip smacking, walking aimlessly, or picking at one's clothing are common. The individual with this type of seizure usually cannot remember the seizure, but consciousness is not lost totally.

Psychomotor seizures in children can be confused with absence attacks because of the relative paucity of memory patterns in the temporal lobe of the young child. Complex partial attacks in children can be distinguished from absence attacks by the fact that the psychomotor attacks occur much less frequently and are of longer duration.

Generalized seizures begin locally but almost immediately result in bilateral involvement of the corticoreticular and reticulocortical systems of the diencephalon. Generalized seizures are usually petit mal (absence seizures) or grand mal (tonic-clonic) in nature. Petit mal seizures usually affect children after the age of 4 years and before puberty,[65] and although rare, they can occur in adults up to 70 years of age. Petit mal seizures consist of a sudden cessation of conscious activity without convulsive motor activity or loss of postural control.[116] These absence attacks usually last for seconds or minutes. The brief lapses of consciousness may be accompanied by minor motor manifestations (e.g., eyelid flickering and isolated myoclonic jerks). After a petit mal seizure the individual quickly regains consciousness or awareness and usually experiences no postictal confusion.

Grand mal seizures are one of the most common epileptic paroxysms and may be generalized seizures or the result of secondary generalization of partial seizures. Grand mal seizures usually occur without warning and follow a common pattern: (1) tonic phase: forceful contraction of axial and appendicular muscles, loss of postural control, epileptic cry, cyanosis; usually lasts 2 or 3 minutes; (2) clonic phase: characterized by gradual transition from tonic contractions to intermittent bilateral brisk clonic movements; this phase represents recurring inhibition phases interrupting the initial tonic phase; (3) postictal phase: amnesia of seizure and possibly even retrograde amnesia.

Generalized seizures also can result from secondary generalization of focal cortical discharges and are identical to primary generalized seizures. These facts make it difficult to distinguish secondary generalized seizures from primarily generalized tonic-clonic seizures. With secondary generalized seizures, however, there are usually diffuse cerebral pathologic findings.[13]

Status epilepticus occurs when two or more seizures follow each other without time between the seizures for the person to fully regain consciousness. Status epilepticus usually is caused by an untreated or inadequately treated seizure disorder or the abrupt discontinuation of anticonvulsant medication. Status epilepticus is considered a medical emergency and is usually treated by intravenous anticonvulsants. If left untreated, it can cause cerebral anoxia and even death.

Generalized seizures such as myoclonic seizures, tonic seizures, infantile spasms, and atonic seizures usually occur during childhood and generally are associated with some type of genetic, perinatal, or metabolic brain disease. Myoclonic seizures may occur alone or coexist with other types of seizures. Individuals with severe and generalized myoclonus demonstrate evidence of disturbances in function of the reticular substance in relevant areas of the sensory cortex.

Tonic seizures are a less common type of primary generalized seizure marked by sudden rigid posturing of trunk and extremities, frequently with deviation to one side of the head and eyes. Tonic seizures are frequently of a shorter duration than tonic-clonic seizures and are not followed by a clonic phase. These seizures usually indicate a lesion in the area of the midbrain and are sometimes seen in individuals with severe cerebral palsy.

Infantile spasms are generalized seizures occurring between birth and approximately 12 months of age. They consist of brief synchronous contractions of the neck, torso, and arms.[116] Infantile spasms rarely occur in an apparently normal infant; rather, they usually occur in children with an underlying neurologic disorder (e.g., anoxic encephalopathy). Approximately 90% of children with infantile spasms develop mental retardation.

Atonic seizures consist of brief loss of consciousness and postural tone; these symptoms are not associated with tonic muscular contractions.[116] This type of seizure frequently is accompanied by other forms of seizure activity.

Unilateral seizure is a type of seizure in which clinical signs usually occur on one side of the body and the EEG discharges are recorded over the contralateral cerebral hemisphere.[13] Unilateral seizures may shift from one side to another but generally do not become symmetric.

Pseudoseizures appear much like regular seizures but do not show any observable changes in EEG waves. Pseudoseizures may be suspected if the presentation of the seizures varies from episode to episode; if the seizures are immediately preceded by an emotional event; if the seizures usually occur when someone is with the person; if the person can verbally respond during the seizure; and/or if the person can remember what happened during the seizure.

The microscopic changes leading to the pathologic processes that occur during the different types of seizure activities are essentially the same. The major alteration in the physiologic state is a hypersynchronous discharge in a localized area of the brain.[116] This localized area of hypersynchronized discharge is called the epileptogenic focus, producing a large, sharp EEG waveform known as the spike discharge.

Metabolic changes occurring within the cerebrum during the epileptic discharges include release of unusually large amounts of neuropeptides and neurotransmitters during the seizure, increased cerebral blood flow to primary involved areas, increased extracellular concentrations of potassium and decreased extracellular concentrations of calcium, changes in oxidative metabolism and local pH, and increased utilization of glucose.

Termination of seizure activity appears to be related

to the large and lasting hyperpolarization of the neuronal cell membrane. This hyperpolarization is possibly generated by an electrogenic sodium pump. As the hyperpolarization is sustained, the neuronal cells cease firing and the surface potentials of the brain are suppressed.[48]

COMPLICATIONS

Musculoskeletal trauma   Cerebral hypoxia
Aspiration   Death
Status epilepticus

DIAGNOSTIC STUDIES AND FINDINGS

Diagnostic test	Findings	Diagnostic test	Findings
Computed tomography (CT) scan	Structural changes	Electroencephalogram (EEG)	Grand mal: high, fast voltage spiked in all leads; petit mal: 3/s, rounded spike wave complexes in all leads; psychomotor (temporal lobe): square-topped 4-6/s spike wave complexes over involved lobe; delta waves: usually associated with destroyed brain tissue; theta waves: not always abnormal
Magnetic resonance imaging (MRI) study	Structural changes		
Skull x-ray	Evidence of fractures; shift of calcified pineal gland; bony erosion; separated sutures		
Echoencephalogram	Possible midline shifts of brain structures	Urine screening	Indicates presence and levels of certain medications
Cerebral angiography	Possible vascular abnormalities; evaluation of a subdural hematoma	Serum chemistry	Hypoglycemia; electrolyte imbalance; increased BUN; blood alcohol levels; elevated liver enzymes
		History and neurologic exam	Pattern of onset and characteristics of seizure activity; precipitating factors

MEDICAL MANAGEMENT

GENERAL MANAGEMENT

Suction and oxygen equipment set up at bedside; seizure precautions; serum drug levels of anticonvulsants; ketogenic diet; serum electrolytes, CBC, and liver function tests; heparin lock in place if significant risk of tonic-clonic seizure

SURGERY

Excision of epileptogenic focus

Stereotactic lesions (corpus callosotomy)

DRUG THERAPY

Anticonvulsants (dosage is regulated by therapeutic blood levels)

Grand mal, simple partial, and complex partial seizures: Phenytoin sodium (Dilantin); phenobarbital sodium; carbamazepine (Tegretol); valproic acid (Depakene); diazepam (Valium); primidone (Mysoline).

Petit mal seizures: Ethosuximide (Zarontin); clonazepam (Klonopin).

NURSING DIAGNOSIS	NURSING INTERVENTIONS	RATIONALE
	Keep side rails up at bedtime, after sedation, when patient is confused, and prn.	To decrease risk of patient falling out of bed.
	Keep brakes locked on bed, wheelchair, or stretcher when transferring patient.	To decrease risk of movement during transfers and to minimize risk of falls.
	Before seizure activity, maintain seizure precautions: oral airway at bedside; suction equipment at bedside; oxygen set up at bedside; bed rails padded.	To increase speed of response when seizure occurs.
	Maintain reliable method of communication with patient.	Patient may feel an aura but may be unable to call out verbally.
	During seizure activity: maintain patent airway; support and protect head; turn patient onto side; ease patient to floor if he is in chair; place pillows along rails if in bed; loosen constrictive clothing; provide privacy; stay with patient.	To prevent hypoxia, aspiration, and musculoskeletal trauma; to maintain patient's right to privacy; to assure patient's safety and necessary observations for documentation.
	Note frequency, time, involved body parts, and length of seizure.	To help identify type of seizure and changes in manifestations and to aid in accurate documentation.
	After seizure activity: maintain patent airway; suction as indicated; check vital signs and neurologic status; administer oxygen per protocol; reorient patient to environment; place patient in comfortable position; administer oral hygiene.	To prevent hypoxia and aspiration; to monitor patient's physiologic response after seizure; to reorient and reassure patient; to provide comfort; to remove oral secretions and check for blood from tongue lacerations.
Anxiety related to fear of seizures, embarrassment caused by seizures and/or incontinence, perceived threat to self-concept, perceived loss of significant others, change in environment, and/or perceived change in socioeconomic status	Increase time with patient; support present coping methods; speak slowly and calmly; do not make demands; minimize patient's decision making; assure patient that problems can be addressed.	To reassure and comfort patient.
	Simplify your speech; focus on the present; decrease noise and interruptions; minimize patient's contact with others who increase his anxiety; involve patient in simple tasks.	To decrease amount of sensory stimulation.
	Validate anxiety assessment; identify what precedes anxiety and usual coping methods; help patient evaluate perceived threats; identify possible alternative coping methods.	To help patient identify his own anxiety and begin problem solving.
	Specific interventions are determined by type of problem; nurse must recognize her own reactions and feelings about patient's coping methods.	To help patient reduce or eliminate problem coping methods and substitute adaptive coping methods.

NURSING DIAGNOSIS	NURSING INTERVENTIONS	RATIONALE
	Teach patient about seizures, their control, and how he might address identified problems.	Requires ongoing assessment of readiness to learn; use a variety of teaching methods, but take care not to bombard patient and increase his anxiety; provide printed material for patient to take home; include family or significant others in teaching.
	Consult other professionals as need is identified; refer patient for follow-up if necessary.	Temporary use of antianxiety medications may be prescribed by physician; consider consulting social worker, clinical nurse specialist, psychologist, psychiatrist, and pastor or priest.
Social isolation related to seizures and/or anxiety	Encourage patient to discuss feelings of loneliness, and help patient identify factors contributing to social isolation.	Good interaction skills and a therapeutic relationship are necessary.
	Help patient contact family, friends, and neighbors.	May be done by phone, cards, etc.; patient may lack initiative or need assistance.
	Help patient remove barriers to social interaction.	Specific interventions are determined by what barriers are identified.
	Help patient identify activities to do when feeling lonely or to prevent loneliness.	Diversional activities help fill time when social contacts are not likely.
	Identify potential contacts, groups, and outside activities for patient.	Patient may be unaware of potential social contacts.
	Refer patient to outside groups or for follow-up as necessary.	Patient may be unaware of how to initiate contact.
Knowledge deficit	See Patient Teaching.	

5 EVALUATE

PATIENT OUTCOME	DATA INDICATING THAT OUTCOME IS REACHED
Patient is free of injury related to seizures.	Patient has not fallen and has no evidence of musculoskeletal injury; there is no evidence of hypoxia or aspiration; patient can explain how to decrease risk of injury.
Patient can describe his anxiety patterns and potential coping methods and has begun to use effective coping strategies.	Patient describes causes of anxiety and usual coping methods; identifies and begins to use alternative adaptive coping methods; relates feelings of increased psychologic and physiologic comfort.

→ 〉 〉

PATIENT OUTCOME	DATA INDICATING THAT OUTCOME IS REACHED
Patient can identify why he feels isolated, has learned how to initiate and maintain relationships, and can identify activities of interest.	Patient identifies causes of feelings of isolation; initiates and begins to maintain relationships; identifies activities of interest and shows plans for follow-through.

PATIENT TEACHING

1. Instruct the patient in the nature of the seizure disorder and the need to adopt a positive attitude.
2. Stress the importance of expressing feelings of shame, humiliation, and anxiety and fears about seizure disorder. Clear up common fears and myths about epilepsy (e.g., it is not a form of insanity).
3. Emphasize the need to avoid overprotection.
4. Stress the need to continue with normal work and recreation routines. Assure the patient that activity may inhibit seizure activity.
5. Emphasize the need to avoid excessive stress or emotional excitement.
6. Teach the patient the importance of wearing a medical alert band or carrying a medical alert card at all times.
7. Stress the importance of a well-balanced diet and of avoiding excessive use of stimulants such as alcohol.
8. Emphasize the importance of identifying aura and the course of action to take.
9. Teach the patient about medications: name, action, side effects, dosage, and frequency of administration.
10. Stress the need to avoid taking over-the-counter medications without first consulting the physician.
11. Emphasize the importance of ongoing outpatient care.
12. Seek advice from a dietitian about devising a ketogenic diet (high intake of fats) for the patient if prescribed.
13. Teach the family first aid for seizures, and encourage the patient to share this information with friends, co-workers, teachers, and others.

Spinal Cord Trauma

Spinal cord trauma is an injury to the spinal cord caused by violent or disruptive action.

Approximately 15,000 to 20,000 people suffer spinal cord injuries each year in the United States, and vehicular accidents account for about 48% of these cases. Other major causes are falls (21%), violence (15%), and sports (14%). Diving accounts for 66% of sports-related spinal cord injuries, and football, snow skiing, surfing, and trampoline injuries as a group make up 16%. The highest incidence occurs between 16 and 30 years of age, and males are the victim in 82% of the cases. Approximately one third of those who suffer a spinal cord injury die before reaching an acute care facility. The National Spinal Cord Injury Association estimates that spinal cord injury costs the nation $6 billion annually. Lifetime costs can vary from $50,000 for a person with a low-level injury to nearly $2 million for a person with a severe injury.[150]

PATHOPHYSIOLOGY

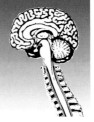

As with craniocerebral trauma, the spine (and spinal cord) can be injured by direct or indirect forces. Direct injuries such as falls on the head or buttocks can cause spinal cord lesions from fractured vertebrae or direct compression of the cord by depressed bone fragments. Indirect injuries (the major type of spinal cord injuries) can occur when excessive forces accelerate the cranium in relation to the trunk (i.e., whiplash injury) or when the trunk is suddenly decelerated in regard to the lumbar spine. Whether the forces are direct or indirect, the subsequent fractures of vertebrae seriously injure the neural elements of the spinal cord.

The most common sites of injury are the lower cervical region (C4-7 and T1) and the thoracolumbar junction (T12, L1, and L2). Trauma to the spinal cord causes concussion, contusion, laceration, hemorrhage, transection (partial or complete), or impairment in the spinal vascular supply.

Vertebral Injuries

The primary mechanisms of vertebral injury, occurring alone or in combination, include hyperextension, hyperflexion, vertical compression trauma, and rotation.[65]

Hyperextension injuries (commonly called **whiplash**) are common in the cervical region, and damage results from the forces of acceleration-deceleration and the sudden reduction in the anteroposterior diameter of the spinal canal. Since the spinal canal is full of neural tissue in the cervical area, injury can produce profound disability. With a hyperextension injury the cord can be compressed between the body of one vertebra and the leading edge of the laminal arch of adjacent vertebrae, causing complete or partial transection. In addition, the ligamentum flavum may be torn or may bulge inward, and intervertebral disks may tear. Severe hyperextension injuries can produce a complete transverse fracture of the vertebral body. With the compression and shearing forces of a hyperextension injury, gray matter of the cord is destroyed and microcirculation at and around the level of the injury is disrupted. (See Figure 4-8.)

Hyperflexion injury results in an overstretching, compression, and deformation of the spinal cord from sudden and excessive force that propels the neck forward or causes an exaggerated lateral movement of the neck to one side. Hyperflexion injuries can occur with wedge or compression fractures of the vertebral body with or without dislocation, fracture of the pedicle with or without dislocation of intraspinal ligaments, or fracture of the vertebral body and rupture of the intervertebral disks. (See Figure 4-9.)

Vertical compression trauma primarily occurs around the area of the thoracolumbar junction (T12 to L2) and results from a force applied along an axis from the top of the cranium through the vertebral bodies. With compression injuries the vertebral body bursts, compressing the spinal cord and damaging nerve roots with bony fragments. (See Figure 4-10.)

Rotation can involve all portions of the vertebral body, including pedicles, ligaments, and the articulation. Fracture of the pedicles or locked facets of the vertebrae can rupture ligaments and shear spinal cord tissue. (See Figure 4-11.)

Vertebral injuries can be classified as simple fractures, compressed or wedged fractures, comminuted fractures, or vertebral dislocation.[65] A **simple** fracture is a single break, usually affecting transverse or spinous processes. Vertebral alignment usually remains intact, and the spinal cord usually is not compressed.

Compressed, or **wedged,** vertebral fractures occur when the vertebral body is compressed anteriorly. The spinal cord may or may not be compressed with a wedged fracture.

Comminuted, or **burst,** fractures can seriously damage the spinal cord. The vertebral body shatters into several fragments, and these fragments may penetrate the spinal cord. Burst fractures occur in the cervical, thoracic, and lumbar regions.

Dislocation of a vertebra may rupture the ligamentum flavum, resulting in dislocation of the vertebral facets, which can be unilateral or bilateral. This dislocation disrupts alignment of the vertebral column, and the spinal cord may or may not be damaged. Partial dislocation of the vertebra is called **subluxation.**

Penetrating injuries are classified by the force of the impact of the penetrating object. A low-velocity impact injury, such as that caused by a knife, involves damage at the site of penetration and fairly localized damage to the spinal cord or spinal nerves, or both. A high-velocity impact injury, such as that caused by a bullet, involves damage at the site of penetration as well as disseminated damage to the spinal cord or spinal nerves, or both. A bullet also can shatter the vertebrae, causing secondary trauma to the spinal cord.

Spinal cord trauma also can be caused by spinal instability stemming from rheumatoid arthritis (usually involving the cervical spine), osteophytes in the spinal canal, or a congenital narrowing of the spinal canal.

Only a few cases of spinal fractures and dislocations result in spinal cord injury.[122] Only in rare cases does the spinal trauma lacerate or actually transect the spinal cord.

Spinal Cord Injuries

The neural elements of the spinal cord and spinal nerve roots are injured by compression from bone, disk herniation, hematoma, and ligaments; edema following compression or concussion; overstretching or disruption of neural tissue; and disturbances in spinal circulation.[48]

The sequence of pathologic processes following impact injury to the spinal cord is as follows: localized hemorrhaging, which advances from the gray to the white matter; reduced vascular perfusion and production of ischemic areas and decreased oxygen tension in tissue at the site of injury; edema; cellular and subcellular alterations; and tissue necrosis. Several minutes after the traumatic injury, microscopic hemorrhages appear in the central gray matter and in the pia-arachnoid. They increase in size until the entire gray

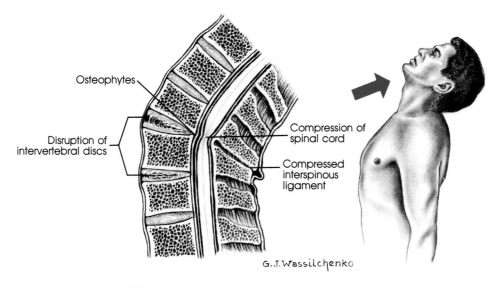

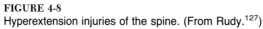

FIGURE 4-8
Hyperextension injuries of the spine. (From Rudy.[127])

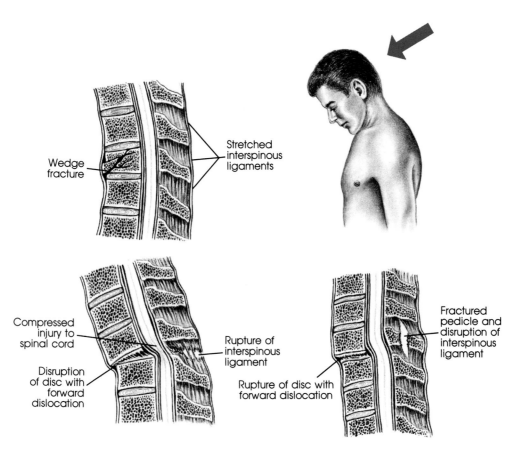

FIGURE 4-9
Hyperflexion injury of the spine. (From Rudy.[127])

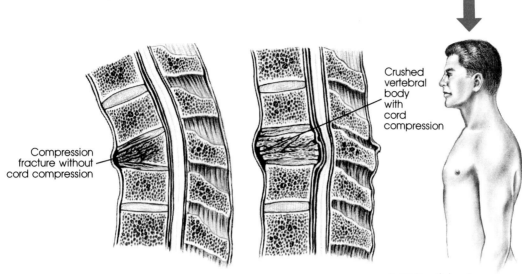

G. J. Wassilchenko

FIGURE 4-10
Vertical compression injuries of the spine. (From Rudy.[127])

matter is hemorrhagic and necrotic. Hemorrhaging and peritraumatic edema progress to the white matter, forming vacuolation and wedge-shaped foci that impair the microcirculation to the spinal cord. This impairment produces ischemia or vascular stasis.[29]

Circulation in the white matter returns to normal within approximately 24 hours, but circulation in the gray matter remains altered.[29]

Changes in the chemistry and metabolism of the traumatized regions include a transitory increase in tissue lactate, a rapid decrease in tissue oxygen tension within 30 minutes of the injury, and increased norepinephrine concentration. Increased concentrations of norepinephrine released to the cord tissue may produce ischemia, vascular rupture, or necrosis of neuronal tissue.[13]

Localized ischemia of neural tissue may result from compression on the vasculature of the cord or nerve roots by bony fragments or herniated disks. If the flow of blood from the vertebral artery to the anterior spinal artery or to the branches of the radicular arteries is impaired, severe cord ischemia results. Hemorrhage, other than with contusion and edema, usually does not produce significant neural impairment. Epidural and subdural hematomas rarely are large enough to cause serious compression. Although subarachnoid bleeding is usual, it is of little clinical significance. Larger intramedullary hematomas, on the other hand, may produce a tubular hematomyelia that can cause partial or complete interruption in spinal cord functioning.[29,48]

After the necrosis that occurs immediately after the injury, a phase of resorption and organization begins.

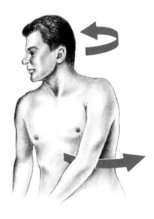

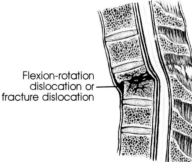

Flexion-rotation dislocation or fracture dislocation

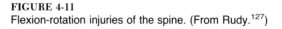

FIGURE 4-11
Flexion-rotation injuries of the spine. (From Rudy.[127])

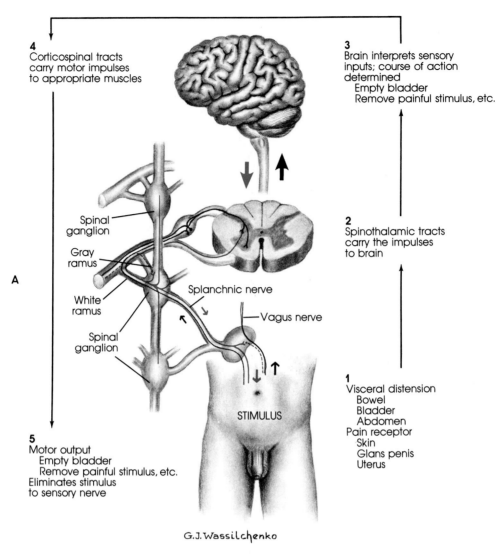

4
Corticospinal tracts
carry motor impulses
to appropriate muscles

3
Brain interprets sensory
inputs; course of action
determined
    Empty bladder
    Remove painful stimulus, etc.

A

Spinal
ganglion

Gray
ramus

White
ramus

Spinal
ganglion

Splanchnic nerve

Vagus nerve

2
Spinothalamic tracts
carry the impulses
to brain

1
Visceral distension
    Bowel
    Bladder
    Abdomen
Pain receptor
    Skin
    Glans penis
    Uterus

STIMULUS

5
Motor output
    Empty bladder
    Remove painful stimulus, etc.
Eliminates stimulus
to sensory nerve

G.J. Wassilchenko

FIGURE 4-12
A, Normal response pathway. **B,** Autonomic dysreflexia pathway. (From Rudy.[127])

This state is characterized by the appearance of phago-cytes within 36 to 48 hours after injury, proliferation of microglial and mesenchymal cells, and changes in astro-glias. Blood gradually is removed from the tissue by disintegration of red cells and resorption of hemor-rhages. Macrophages engulf degenerating axons in the first 10 days after injury.[13,29]

Gradually the traumatized section of the cord is re-moved, usually in the third to fourth week after the in-jury. It is replaced with acellular collagenous tissue, which connects the meninges to the cord and central canal. The scarring in the injured area consists mainly of thickened meninges and connective tissue.

Spinal Shock (Neurogenic Shock)

Spinal shock at the area of transection occurs after com-plete or incomplete severing of the spinal cord. It causes a complete loss of sensory, motor, autonomic, and reflex functioning below the level of the lesion. Spinal shock results from the loss of inhibition from de-scending tracts, continued inhibition of supraspinal im-pulses, and axonal degeneration of the interneurons. It is characterized by flaccid paralysis and loss of reflex ac-tivity below the level of the spinal cord injury, hypo-tension, bradycardia, and sometimes paralytic ileus. It can last several days to several months.[29]

Autonomic Hyperreflexia (Autonomic Dysreflexia)

Autonomic hyperreflexia usually occurs after spinal shock has resolved and reflex activity has returned (Fig-ure 4-12). Individuals most likely to experience auto-nomic hyperreflexia are those who have lesions at the level of T6 or above. The syndrome results from unin-hibited sympathetic discharge that usually is caused by

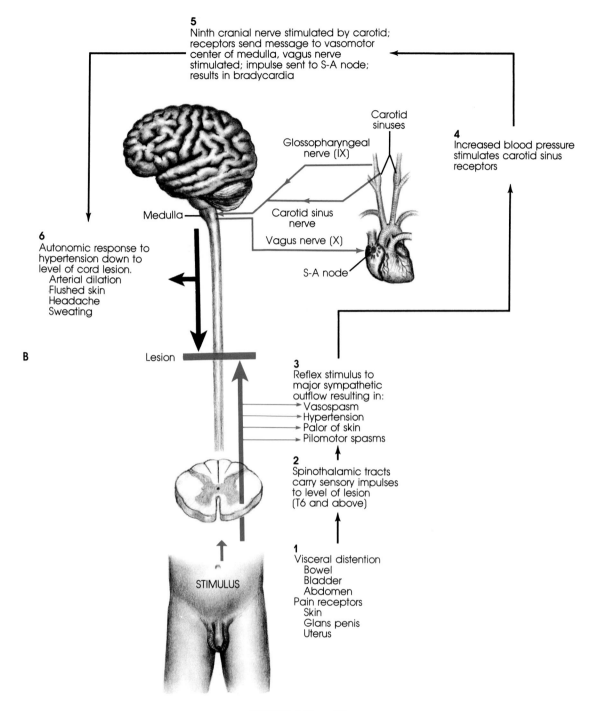

5
Ninth cranial nerve stimulated by carotid; receptors send message to vasomotor center of medulla, vagus nerve stimulated; impulse sent to S-A node; results in bradycardia

Carotid sinuses

Glossopharyngeal nerve (IX)

4
Increased blood pressure stimulates carotid sinus receptors

Medulla

Carotid sinus nerve

Vagus nerve (X)

S-A node

6
Autonomic response to hypertension down to level of cord lesion.
Arterial dilation
Flushed skin
Headache
Sweating

B

Lesion

3
Reflex stimulus to major sympathetic outflow resulting in:
→ Vasospasm
→ Hypertension
→ Palor of skin
→ Pilomotor spasms

2
Spinothalamic tracts carry sensory impulses to level of lesion (T6 and above)

STIMULUS

1
Visceral distention
Bowel
Bladder
Abdomen
Pain receptors
Skin
Glans penis
Uterus

FIGURE 4-12, cont'd.

bladder distention, fecal impaction, or other noxious stimulus below the level of the spinal cord lesion (such as tight clothing, an ingrown toenail, or a pressure ulcer). Symptoms include a pounding headache; elevated blood pressure; bradycardia (may lead to dysrhythmia); profuse sweating above the level of injury; cutaneous vasodilation, resulting in nasal congestion, flushed skin above the level of the lesion, and pallor below the level of the lesion; gooseflesh and piloerec-

tion; paresthesia; anxiety; and visual disturbances. The dangers of autonomic hyperreflexia are related to the consequent hypertension, which can cause changes in mental status, seizures, intracerebral hemorrhage, and even death.

Classification of Spinal Cord Injuries

Classification of spinal cord injuries not only aids professional communication, but also precisely determines

1. Complete (A)

The lesion is found to be complete, both motor and sensory, below the segmental level marked. If there is an alteration of level but the lesion remains complete below the new level, then the arrow would point up or down the complete column.

2. Sensory only (B)

There is some sensation present below the level of the lesion but the motor paralysis is complete below that level. This column does not apply when there is a slight discrepancy between the motor and sensory level but does apply to sacral sparing.

3. Motor useless (C)

There is some motor power present below the lesion but it is of no practical use to the patient.

4. Motor useful (D)

There is useful motor power below the level of the lesion. Patients in this group can move the lower limbs and many can walk with or without aids.

5. Recovery (E)

The patient is free of neurologic symptoms (e.g., no weakness, no sensory loss, no sphincter disturbance). Abnormal reflexes may be present.

From Frankel, H.L., Hancock, D.O., Hyslop, G., et al.[54]

any progression or improvement in the extent of injury. The classification system of the American Spinal Injury Association (ASIA) designates the spinal cord injury level as the lowest intact segment where the key muscle grade is fair (grade 3) or better. A more precise classification method is embodied in the Frankel Scale (see box). Care must be taken not to confuse the level of spinal injury with the level of the spinal cord injury. It is not uncommon for the spinal cord injury to extend above and below the level of spinal trauma as a result of edema and hemorrhage within the confines of the spinal canal.[42]

Terms commonly used to describe a spinal cord injury are **quadriplegia, paraplegia, complete injury,** and **incomplete injury.** Quadriplegia results from impairment or loss of motor or sensory function (or both) in the cervical segments of the spinal cord. This results in impaired functioning of the arms, trunk, legs, and pelvic organs. Paraplegia results from impairment or loss of motor or sensory function (or both) in the thoracic, lumbar, or sacral neurologic segments because of damage to the neural elements within the spinal canal, including the conus medullaris and the cauda equina. Paraplegia spares the arms but, depending on the level of injury, may involve the trunk, legs, and pelvic organs.[150]

A complete injury is one in which there is no motor or sensory function more than three segments below the level of neurologic injury. An incomplete injury is one in which there is some sensory or motor function (or both) more than three segments below the level of neurologic injury. Use of the terms quadriparesis and paraparesis is discouraged, because they are too imprecise.[150]

CORD SYNDROMES

Trauma to the spinal cord results in several syndromes that develop from the specific area of cord damaged and vary in severity, depending on the amount of cord compression or transection (Figure 4-13).

Anterior cord syndrome, the most common syndrome, occurs after an acute flexion injury to the cervical area. Damage to the anterior spinal artery or the ventral portion of the spinal cord, or both, accounts for the loss of motor function, pain, and temperature sensation below the lesion. Proprioception, touch, pressure, and vibration remain intact.

Posterior cord syndrome, which is rare, is associated with cervical hyperextension trauma. This type of lesion involves damage to the dorsal columns, resulting in loss of proprioception but preservation of pain, temperature sensation, and motor function below the level of the lesion.

Central cord syndrome may result from either hyperextension or flexion injuries, almost always in the cervical region. Central cord syndrome is characterized by central edema of the spinal cord and compression on the anterior horn cells. This produces greater weakness in the upper extremities than in the lower extremities. It also results in sacral sensory sparing but varying degrees of bladder dysfunction.

Brown-Séquard's syndrome results from rotation-flexion injuries in which subluxation or dislocation of the fracture occurs by unilateral pedicle-laminar injuries.[39] The lesion involves primarily one side of the cord. Neurologic deficits include ipsilateral paralysis and loss of touch, pressure, vibration, and proprioception, and contralateral loss of pain and temperature sensations below the level of the lesion.

Conus medullaris syndrome involves an injury of the conus medullaris of the sacral cord and the lumbar nerve roots within the neural canal. This usually results in an areflexic bladder and bowel and flaccid, areflexic lower extremities. Higher lesions within the conus medullaris may preserve the bulbocavernosus and micturition reflexes.[150]

Cauda equina syndrome occurs when the injury is below the conus medullaris, and the lumbosacral nerve roots within the neural canal are injured. This causes areflexia in the bladder, bowel, and lower extremities.

Herniated disk syndrome is a common spinal cord syndrome. Degenerative changes in the anulus fibrosus predispose the intervertebral disks to posterior displacement through a laceration of the anulus fibrosus and the posterior longitudinal ligament. The fibrocartilaginous material may extrude spontaneously or in response to activity or slight injury. The severity of symptoms depends on the quantity of herniated disk tissue, the number of involved disks, the amount of nerve root compression, and the amount of spinal canal narrowing.[65] (For further information, refer to page 224.)

Horner's syndrome occurs when there is an injury to the postganglionic sympathetic neurons of the superior cervical ganglion or the preganglionic sympathetic trunk. This results in the ipsilateral pupil being smaller than the contralateral pupil; a sunken ipsilateral eyeball; ptosis of the affected eyeball; and lack of perspiration on the ipsilateral side of the face.[98]

MOTOR NEURONS

Motor neurons are responsible for transmitting impulses from the brain or spinal cord to muscular or glandular tissue. Upper motor neurons originate in the cerebral cortex and brainstem, form tracts within the spinal cord, and terminate or synapse at all levels of the spinal cord in the anterior horn cells. Spinal cord trauma resulting in injury to upper motor neurons results in spastic paralysis and hyperreflexia, since the spinal reflex is still intact below the level of the injury. Lower motor neurons originate in the anterior horn cells of the spinal cord and terminate in skeletal muscles. Spinal cord trauma resulting in injury to lower motor neurons results in flaccid paralysis and hyporeflexia.[29]

RETURN OF FUNCTION

The degree of return of function after a spinal cord injury depends on the amount of direct destruction of the cord and the amount of secondary damage from hemorrhage and edema compressing the cord within the spinal canal. Any interventions to prevent secondary damage may reduce the extent of permanent damage to the spinal cord. A patient may regain one or even two levels of function over the first few months after injury. This has been attributed to the resolution of spinal cord edema. Patients often mistake the development of spasticity as the beginning of return of function.

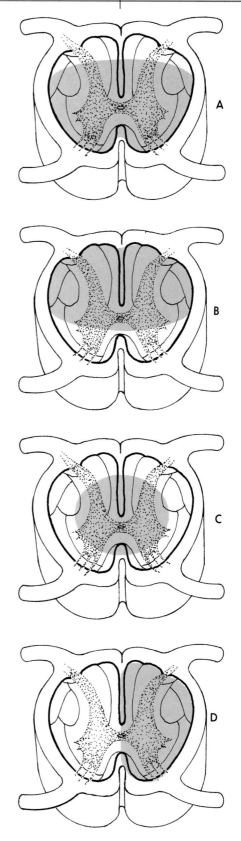

FIGURE 4-13
Anatomic classification of cord syndromes. **A,** Anterior cord syndrome. **B,** Posterior cord syndrome. **C,** Central cord syndrome. **D,** Brown-Séquard syndrome.

PATIENT OUTCOME AND REHABILITATION

The patient outcome after spinal cord trauma is determined by several factors. The most obvious is the level of the injury and the resulting neurologic deficits. Table 4-5 gives an excellent summary of the potential functional outcomes based on the identified level of injury. The rehabilitation process aims at training the person to strengthen and use what muscles are still under volitional control to learn adapted methods of doing various activities. If the person cannot do the activity independently, she learns how to direct others in providing the care or the activity for her. Although the involvement and education of family members are paramount, the person with a high-level injury may also need to learn the skills of hiring and training a personal care attendant.

Other physical factors that influence functional outcomes are the distribution of body weight, body proportions, spasticity, range of joint motion, strength, and flexibility. The development of various medical complications, such as pressure ulcers, also can impede the attainment of functional goals. Immobilization devices such as halo vests and chest shells temporarily limit some aspects of self-care while permitting earlier general mobilization. As with any type of disabling injury, the support of family, friends, and significant others is vital. This support sets the tone for the patient's attitude and motivation, not only during the acute and rehabilitation phases, but also after the patient leaves the hospital and returns home. A person's education, vocation, and life-style may also influence the outcome, with higher levels of education and some vocations allowing more flexibility for change. Financial resources often determine levels of independence, especially when electric wheelchairs, environmental controls, modified vans, and hired personal care attendants are needed.

KEY FUNCTIONAL MYOTOMES

Spinal cord level	Function
C1-6	Neck flexors
C1-T1	Neck extensors
C3-5	Diaphragm
C5	Elbow flexors
C6	Wrist extensors
C7	Elbow extension
C8	Wrist flexion
T1	Hand intrinsics
T1-6	Intercostals, chest musculature
T7-L1	Abdominal musculature
L1-4	Hip flexion
L2-4	Hip adduction
L4-S1	Hip abduction
L5-S2	Hip extension
L2-4	Knee extension
L4-S2	Knee flexion
L4-S1	Foot dorsiflexion, toe extension
L5-S2	Foot plantar flexion, toe flexion

Adapted from DeMeyer.[43]

KEY SENSORY DERMATOMES

Spinal cord level	Sensory area
C5	Deltoid
C6	Thumb
C7	Middle finger
C8	Little finger
T4	Nipple line
T10	Umbilicus
L5	Big toe
S1	Little toe
S2-5	Perineum

COMPLICATIONS

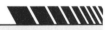

Neurogenic shock	Gastrointestinal bleeding	Osteoporosis
Severe bradyrhythmia	Aspiration	Fecal impaction or in continence
Hypoxia	Urinary tract infection	Contractures
Autonomic hyperreflexia	Urinary retention or incontinence	Sexual dysfunction
Deep vein thrombosis	Urinary tract calculi	Superior mesenteric artery syndrome
Pulmonary embolus	Pressure ulcer	Pain
Pneumonia	Spasticity	Syringomyelia
Atelectasis	Heterotopic ossification	
Spinal instability		
Orthostatic hypotension		
Paralytic ileus		

DIAGNOSTIC STUDIES AND FINDINGS

Diagnostic test	Findings	Diagnostic test	Findings
X-rays (anterior-posterior and lateral)	Vertebral fractures	**Magnetic resonance imaging (MRI) study**	Spinal cord edema and compression
Serum chemistry	Hypoglycemia or hyperglycemia; electrolyte imbalance; possibly decreased hemoglobin and hematocrit	**Spinal puncture**	Establishes presence or absence of spinal block; blood in spinal fluid
		Myelography	Establishes presence of spinal block
Computed tomography (CT) scan	Spinal cord edema	**Urodynamic studies**	Coordination of bladder filling and emptying

Table 4-5

FUNCTIONAL OUTCOMES FOR PATIENTS WITH COMPLETE SPINAL CORD INJURIES

Level of injury	Pulmonary hygiene	AM care	Feeding	Grooming	Dressing	Bathing	Bowel & bladder routine
C3-C4	Totally assisted cough	Total dependence	May be unable to feed self. Use of BFOs with universal cuff and adapted utensils indicated; drinks with long straw after set up	Total dependence	Total dependence	Total dependence	Total dependence
C5	Assisted cough	Independent with specially adapted devices with set up	Independent with specially adapted equipment for feeding after set up	Independent with specially adapted equipment for grooming after set up	Assist with upper extremity dressing; dependent for lower extremity dressing	Total dependence	Total dependence
C6	Some assistance required in supine position; independent in sitting position	Independent with equipment	Independent with equipment; drinks from glass	Independent with equipment	Independent with upper extremity dressing; assistance needed for lower extremity dressing	Independent in upper and lower extremity bathing with equipment	Independent for bowel routine; assistance needed with bladder routine
C7	As above	Independent	Independent	Independent with equipment	Potential for independence in upper and lower extremity dressing with equipment	Independent with equipment	Independent
C8-T1	As above	Independent	Independent	Independent	Independent	Independent	Independent
T2-T10	T2-6 as above T6-10 independent	Independent	Independent	Independent	Independent	Independent	Independent
T11-L2	Not applicable	Independent	Independent	Independent	Independent	Independent	Independent
L3-S3	Not applicable	Independent	Independent	Independent	Independent	Independent	Independent

From DeLisa.[42]   *Continued.*

Table 4-5—cont'd

Level of injury	Bed mobility	Pressure relief	Wheelchair transfers	Wheelchair propulsion	Ambulation	Orthotic devices	Transportation	Communications
C3-C4	Total dependence	Independent in powered recliner wheelchair; dependent in bed or manual wheelchair	Total dependence	Independent in pneumatic or chin control-driven power wheelchair with powered reclining feature	Not applicable	Upper extremity: external powered orthosis, dorsal cockup splint, BFOs	Dependent on others in accessible van with lift; unable to drive	Read with specially adapted equipment; specially adapted phone; unable to write, types with special adaptions
C5	Assisted by other and by equipment	Most require assistance	Assistance of one person with or without transfer board	Independent in powered chair indoors and outdoors; short distances in manual wheelchair with lugs indoors	Not applicable	As above	As above	As above
C6	Independent with equipment	Independent	Potentially independent with transfer board	Independent in manual wheelchair with plastic rims or lugs indoors; assistance needed outdoors and with elevators	Not applicable	Wrist-driven orthosis	Independent driving specially adapted van	Independent with phone; writes with equipment; types with equipment; independent in turning pages
C7	Independent	Independent	Independent with or without transfer board including car except to/from floor with assistance	Independent in manual wheelchair indoors and outdoors, except curbs, stairs	Not applicable	None	Independent driving car with hand controls or specially adapted van; independent wheelchair into car placement	Independent with equipment for phone, typing, and writing; independent in turning pages
C8-T1	Independent	Independent	Independent including to/from floor and car	Independent in manual wheelchair indoors and outdoors; curbs, escalators	Not applicable	None	As above	Independent
T2-T10	Independent	Independent	Independent	Independent	Exercise only (not functional with orthoses); requires physical assist or guarding	Knee/ankle/foot orthoses with forearm crutches or walker	As above	Independent

Table 4-5—cont'd

Level of injury	Bed mobility	Pressure relief	Wheelchair transfers	Wheelchair propulsion	Ambulation	Orthotic devices	Transportation	Communications
T11-L2	Independent	Independent	Independent	Independent	Potential for independent functional ambulation indoors with orthoses; some have potential for stairs using railing	Knee/ankle/ foot orthoses or ankle/foot orthoses with forearm crutches	As above	Independent
L3-S3	Independent	Independent	Independent	Independent	Community ambulation; independent indoors and outdoors with orthoses	Ankle/foot or- thoses with forearm crutches or canes	As above	Independent

MEDICAL MANAGEMENT

GENERAL MANAGEMENT

Acute phase: Mechanical ventilation; Stryker or Foster frame bed; skeletal traction; vital capacity and tidal volume measurements; splints and braces; phrenic nerve stimulator; bed board and firm mattress; cardiac monitoring; intermittent urinary catheterization; intake and output recording; dietary consultation; sexual counseling; psychosocial counseling for individual and family; cervical collar (soft or hard); immobilization with sandbags; serial measurement of arterial blood gases; urine sugar and acetone; guaiac; antiembolus stockings or sequential compression devices; nasogastric tube.

Rehabilitation phase: Specific to level of spinal cord injury; prevent long-term complications; increase mobil- ity: wheelchair and/or ambulation; increase self-care skills; establish bladder management program; establish bowel management program; determine or establish effective respiratory function program; maintain skin in- tegrity; sexual counseling; psychologic counseling and peer support; patient and family education; home ac- cessibility; driving evaluation and training; evaluate and retrain in vocational and avocational skills.

SURGERY

Laminectomy; tracheostomy; spinal fusion for stabilization; wound debridement; suturing of lacerations; cer- vical tongs (i.e., Cone, Vinke, Crutchfield, Gardner-Wells); halo traction; halo with femoral traction; body casts; spinal cord cooling; myotomies, tenotomies, neurectomies, rhizotomies, and muscle transplants (treatment for spasticity); Harrington rod insertion for stabilization of thoracic deformities; sphincterotomy.

DRUG THERAPY

Corticosteroids (to control cord edema): Methylprednisolone sodium succinate (Solu-Medrol); dexamethasone (Decadron).

Antihypertensives (to control BP in acute autonomic hyperreflexia): Diazoxide (Hyperstat); hydralazine hydro- chloride (Apresoline).

Antihypertensives (autonomic hyperreflexia prophylaxis): Phenoxybenzamine hydrochloride (Dibenzyline); prazosin hydrochloride (Minipress); clonidine hydrochloride (Catapres); mecamylamine hydrochloride (In- versine); guanethidine monosulfate (Ismelin).

Continued.

MEDICAL MANAGEMENT—cont'd.

Antianginals (to control BP in acute autonomic hyperreflexia): Nitroglycerin: 2% ointment; nifedipine (Procardia).

Vasodilators (to control BP in acute autonomic hyperreflexia): Amyl nitrite, prn.

Anticoagulants (deep vein thrombosis prophylaxis): Heparin sodium, SQ.

Skeletal muscle relaxants: Baclofen (Lioresal); dantrolene sodium (Dantrium); diazepam (Valium).

Cholinergics (to increase detrusor tone): Bethanechol chloride (Urecholine).

Spasmolytics (useful in detrusor hyperreflexia): Oxybutynin chloride (Ditropan); flavoxate hydrochloride (Urispas).

Anticholinergics (to decrease bladder activity): Propantheline bromide (Pro-Banthine).

Antidepressants (to increase tone in bladder neck, decrease tone in bladder dome): Imipramine hydrochloride (Tofranil).

Antihistamines (to stimulate beta-receptors of urethra and bladder): Phenylpropanolamine hydrochloride/chlorpheniramine maleate (Ornade Spansules).

Antiulcer agents: Ranitidine hydrochloride (Zantac).

Stool softeners: Docusate sodium (Colace).

Laxatives: Bisacodyl (Dulcolax).

Parathyroid-like agents (heterotopic ossification prophylaxis): Editronate disodium (Didronal).

1   ASSESS

ASSESSMENT	OBSERVATIONS
Respiratory system	Respiratory compromise (mild to life-threatening, depending on level of injury); decreased vital capacity and minute volume
Cardiovascular system	Bradycardia; hypotension; cardiac dysrhythmias; hemorrhage or bleeding around fracture site (leading to tachycardia and weak, thready pulse); dependent edema; orthostatic hypotension

ASSESSMENT	OBSERVATIONS
Neurologic status	Score on Glasgow Coma Scale (up to 20% of spinal cord injuries have head injury)
Motor function	Partial or complete loss of motor control below level of lesion; quadriplegia; paraplegia; determine level of motor function (see box on page 118)
Deep tendon reflexes	Spinal shock: loss of all reflexes below level of lesion; postspinal shock: hyperreflexic if upper motor neuron (UMN) lesion, flaccid if lower motor neuron (LMN) lesion
Sensory function	Partial or complete loss of sensation below level of lesion (see dermatome chart on page 16 and box on page 118); partial or complete loss of visceral and somatic sensations below level of lesion; patient may report hyperesthesia immediately above level of lesion; pain; tingling or burning below level of lesion if paraplegic
Autonomic function	Impaired vasomotor tone below level of injury; loss of ability to perspire below level of injury; impaired thermoregulation
Autonomic hyperreflexia (level T6 or above)	Pounding headache; elevated blood pressure; bradycardia; profuse sweating above level of injury; nasal congestion; flushed skin above level of lesion; pallor below level of lesion; gooseflesh and piloerection on arms; paresthesia; anxiety; visual disturbances
Gastrointestinal system	Delayed gastric emptying; neurogenic bowel; paralytic ileus: absence of bowel sounds, gastric distention; stress ulcer: guaiac-positive stool; bowel incontinence or bowel impaction
Urinary system	Neurogenic bladder: urinary retention; reflex incontinence; overflow incontinence
Musculoskeletal system	Muscle atrophy; decreased range of motion
Skin	Reddened areas over bony prominences (caused by pressure)
Sexual function	Varies from normal function to complete impotence; reflex erections; menstrual irregularities or amenorrhea
Psychosocial factors	Crisis reaction by patient, family, and significant others; identify resources, both psychosocial and financial

2 DIAGNOSE

NURSING DIAGNOSIS	SUBJECTIVE FINDINGS	OBJECTIVE FINDINGS
Ineffective airway clearance and **Potential for aspiration** related to ineffective cough, positioning for spinal stabilization	States she cannot cough or expresses fear of choking	Ineffective cough; inability to remove airway secretions; abnormal breath sounds; abnormal respiratory rate, rhythm, or depth; inability to reposition patient because of spinal stabilization

→ 〉 〉

NURSING DIAGNOSIS	SUBJECTIVE FINDINGS	OBJECTIVE FINDINGS
Ineffective breathing pattern related to impaired innervation to intercostals, respiratory accessory muscles, and/or diaphragm	States she cannot catch her breath; may report feeling faint	Tachypnea; tachycardia; bounding pulse; elevating blood pressure (BP); anxious facial expression
Decreased cardiac output related to vasodilation and bradycardia secondary to sympathetic blockade of spinal shock following spinal cord injury at T6 or above	May state that she feels faint	Postural hypotension; systolic blood pressure (SBP) < 90 mm Hg or below patient's norm; decreased pulmonary artery pressure (PAP), PAD, and pulmonary capillary wedge pressure (PCWP); decreased cardiac index; decreased systemic vascular resistance (SVR), bradycardia; cardiac dysrhythmias; decreased urine output; impaired thermoregulation
Altered spinal cord tissue perfusion related to compression, contusion, and/or edema	Reports loss or increasing loss of sensation and motor function; may report bowel/bladder incontinence	Neurologic examination reveals loss or increasing loss of sensation, motor function; bowel/bladder incontinence may be noted
Impaired physical mobility related to quadriplegia/paraplegia	Reports inability to move body parts normally; cannot walk	Neurologic examination reveals loss of motor function; quadriplegia or paraplegia
Total/partial self-care deficit related to quadriplegia/paraplegia	Reports impaired ability to bathe, groom, feed, dress, and/or use toilet	Patient cannot independently do own activities of daily living (ADL)
Altered urinary elimination related to neurogenic bladder	May report wetting self; inability to urinate and/or lack of feeling need to urinate	Patient has urinary retention and/or incontinence; may be unaware of urinary incontinence
Altered bowel elimination related to neurogenic bowel and immobility	May report inability to control bowel movements and/or not having a bowel movement recently; may also report lack of feeling need to have a bowel movement	Patient has bowel incontinence; may also have impacted stool in rectum; may be unaware of bowel incontinence
Potential impaired skin integrity related to impaired sensation, immobility, bowel and/or bladder incontinence	Reports decreased or loss of sensation over heels/ankles, sacrum, trochanters, and/or other bony prominences; reports impaired ability to move; loss of bowel/bladder control	Patient has increased risk of developing pressure ulcers or other skin breakdown because of impaired sensation, impaired mobility, and/or bowel/bladder incontinence

NURSING DIAGNOSIS	SUBJECTIVE FINDINGS	OBJECTIVE FINDINGS
Altered sexuality patterns and **Sexual dysfunction** related to impaired innervation of reproductive organs, impaired sensation, impaired mobility, and/or decreased self-esteem	Patient reports actual or anticipated sexual function problems such as impotence, impaired sensation of genitalia and/or other sensual areas, impaired physical mobility, decreased ability to see self as a sexual being	Neurologic examination reveals impaired sensation of genitalia; impaired sensation of other areas of body; impaired physical mobility; impotence; impaired ability to attain/maintain erection and/or ejaculate; may not interact with spouse or friends, especially those of opposite sex
Potential impaired adjustment related to change in body image, role performance, and/or depression	States she cannot or will not accept body and/or life-style changes related to effects of spinal cord trauma	Lengthened period of shock, disbelief, or anger; shows no interest or involvement in working toward independence and/or future goals
Potential for autonomic hyperreflexia related to uninhibited autonomic response to noxious stimuli after spinal cord injury at or above T6	Reports a history of hyperreflexia or reports its signs and/or symptoms	Spinal cord injury at or above T6 level

Other related nursing diagnoses: Impaired thermoregulation related to impaired vasomotor control and impaired ability to sweat secondary to spinal cord injury; **Impaired gas exchange** related to alveolar hypoventilation secondary to loss of accessory muscle function; and/or related to ventilation-perfusion inequality secondary to stasis of secretions; **Ineffective breathing pattern** related to deconditioning of respiratory muscles secondary to mechanical ventilation; **Ineffective airway clearance** related to impaired cough secondary to loss of glottic closure with tracheostomy or endotracheal tube; **Activity intolerance** related to prolonged immobility and loss of vasomotor tone; **Body image disturbance** related to actual changes in body structure, function, and/or appearance; **Altered role performance** related to inability to resume previous roles; **Self-esteem disturbance** related to feelings of guilt regarding traumatic injury or present physical condition; **Powerlessness** related to loss of control of body functions, inability to do own ADL independently, regimen of hospital/caregiver environment; **Ineffective individual/family coping** related to crisis situation, changes in body integrity, unsatisfactory support systems; **Hopelessness** related to perceptions of personal failure or deteriorating health; **Altered health maintenance** related to lack of perceived threat to personal health; **Knowledge deficit (patient/family) regarding self-care after a spinal cord injury** related to lack of prior need or exposure to the information; **Impaired physical mobility** related to inaccessibility of home, work, school, or community environment; **Potential for injury** related to motor and/or sensory deficits.

3 PLAN

Patient goals

1. The patient will have a patent airway.
2. The patient will demonstrate an effective breathing pattern.
3. The patient will have adequate cardiac output.
4. The patient will have adequate perfusion of spinal cord tissue.
5. The patient will have the optimum level of mobility.
6. The patient will be able to direct her own activities of daily living.
7. The patient will have an effective bladder management program.

→ > >

NURSING DIAGNOSIS	NURSING INTERVENTIONS	RATIONALE
	Administer crystalloid IV fluids using fluid challenge technique as prescribed.	Involves infusing precise amounts of fluid (usually 5-20 ml/min) over a 10-min period; monitor cardiac loading pressures to determine success of fluid challenge.
	Anticipate administration of colloids and vasopressors.	May be necessary if fluid challenge is ineffective.
	Monitor cardiac rhythm, especially during suctioning.	Vagal stimulation during suctioning can cause severe bradycardia.
	Anticipate administration of atropine per protocol.	For symptomatic bradycardia.
	Maintain normothermia with blankets and by adjusting room temperature. Avoid electric warming blankets and lamps if patient has impaired sensation and peripheral blood flow.	To compensate for impaired autonomic thermoregulation; impaired sensation and peripheral blood flow increase risk of burns.
Altered spinal cord tissue perfusion related to compression, contusion, and/or edema	Do neurologic assessment q 15-30 min and prn.	To monitor for any change in neurologic status, and to detect progression of spinal cord tissue trauma.
	Maintain skeletal traction as prescribed.	To relieve pressure on spinal cord and prevent further bony impingement on cord (see page 278).
	Maintain strict body alignment. Keep body straight with head flat; do not move head or spinal column; use sandbags if needed to maintain alignment; after placement of halo traction device or internal stabilization surgery, log roll patient to prevent torsion on spinal column.	To prevent further trauma to the spinal cord.
	Use special beds when prescribed.	To facilitate turning patient without interfering with traction and body alignment (see page 277).
	Use special orthoses when prescribed.	Braces provide support and maintain vertebral alignment until bony healing occurs (see page 278 for description of common braces and related nursing care).
	Administer medications as prescribed.	Steroids are administered to control cord edema; guaiac stool, to detect occult blood and monitor blood glucose levels; phytonadione (vitamin K) may be ordered to control bleeding tendency; antacids and/or antiulcer medications may be prescribed.

NURSING DIAGNOSIS	NURSING INTERVENTIONS	RATIONALE
	Administer parenteral fluids per protocol.	To maintain hydration and prevent shock.
	Measure fluid intake and output every hour. Immediately report urine output < 30 ml/h.	To monitor kidney function and fluid volume status.
Impaired physical mobility related to quadriplegia/ paraplegia	Perform active/passive ROM exercises q 2-12 h, depending on need.	To promote circulation and prevent contracture formation.
	Turn patient q 2 h maintaining alignment and promoting comfort.	Adjust turning schedule and positioning according to the patient's skin tolerance to pressure and spasticity.
	Consult and collaborate with physical therapist and occupational therapist.	To gradually increase patient's activity tolerance, balance and mobility skills, and independence in ADL; maintain communication with therapist to ensure follow-through of learned skills in daily activities and proper use of ambulatory aids and adapted equipment.
	Gradually increase the patient's time up out of bed.	To increase activity tolerance and encourage patient to get out of room to socialize.
	Monitor patient's complaints of pain and/or fatigue.	May indicate overexertion; scheduling rest periods may help.
	Teach or reinforce safe bed mobility and transfer skills.	Ensure that bed brakes are locked at all times; side rails up on bed aid in turning; if patient can do her own bed and wheelchair transfers, keep wheelchair next to bed at all times; properly position sliding board and use transfer belt to improve safety; transfer patient with halo cautiously, since halo vest makes patient top heavy; patient wearing a chest shell or brace may have difficulty with balance because of limited trunk flexibility.
	Ensure that patient and family use wheelchair and mobility aids safely.	Brakes on wheelchair should be locked during all transfers; a seat belt or chest belt should be used if balance is a problem (especially over rough terrain); antitip bars may be needed on back of wheelchair; proper use of recliner mechanisms is necessary; teach battery precautions on electric wheelchairs; teach getting on and off elevators "straight on," so that front wheels are not caught in gap; place canes and crutches away from elevator gap; teach proper follow-through on ambulation techniques.

NURSING DIAGNOSIS	NURSING INTERVENTIONS	RATIONALE
	Monitor spasticity and its effects on physical function.	Mild to moderate spasticity can be useful in doing ADL and transfers if patient learns how to control and trigger it; uncontrolled or severe spasticity can cause falls and decreased function; monitor for effectiveness of antispasticity medications.
	Measure and record calf and thigh circumferences daily while patient is supine and before daily activities; observe for lower extremity edema in morning and afternoon or after being up; check for reddened streaks or differences in skin temperature or pulses of lower extremities; note any changes in spasticity.	To monitor for signs and symptoms of deep vein thrombosis.
	Do not give injections or administer IV fluids in legs unless other alternatives are unavailable; protect legs from injury during transfers, turning, or other activities; ensure proper fit of support stockings.	To protect legs from trauma.
Total/partial self-care deficit related to quadriplegia/ paraplegia	Set aside sufficient time for patient to do as much of her own care as possible.	Patient is unhurried and more likely to spend effort to try new techniques; caregivers are less likely to do for patient.
	Consult and collaborate with physical therapist and occupational therapist concerning appropriate ADL techniques and adaptive equipment.	Special ADL techniques and adaptive equipment allow patient more independence; good communication facilitates follow-through on learned techniques.
	Help patient with activities not yet learned or with those components patient cannot do.	Providing appropriate level of assistance decreases patient's frustration and maintains self-esteem; stand-by assistance may be needed for safety while patient learns new skills.
	Secure call light to bed, bedside commode, or bathroom safety bars.	To keep call light within reach.
	Consider use of overbed trapeze; side rails up or down.	May aid mobility at first; continued use is determined by patient's need and availability in home setting.
	Acknowledge progress, and encourage continued effort.	Progress may be slow; continued strengthening of muscles and improving balance aid ADL performance.
	Involve patient in setting short-term ADL goals.	To encourage more commitment to self-determined goals.
	Encourage patient to direct others in aspects of care with which she needs assistance.	Patient's ability to direct others in her care permits care to be done as she prefers without losing self-esteem.

NURSING DIAGNOSIS	NURSING INTERVENTIONS	RATIONALE
Altered urinary elimination related to neurogenic bladder	Assess and address any current urinary tract infection (UTI).	UTI affects effectiveness of bladder management program and poses health risk.
	Discuss urinary elimination options with physician and patient.	Options include indwelling urethral catheter, intermittent catheterization (IMC), reflex voiding, bladder expression, suprapubic catheter, or a combination of techniques; sterile IMC is usual choice for inpatients, clean IMC for home is usually acceptable; patient's and caregiver's abilities also must be considered.
	Evaluate current fluid intake patterns and modify to about 150 ml/h from waking until about 7 PM.	To assure adequate hydration and consistent bladder filling; dependent edema is mobilized when patient reclines, so stopping fluids around 7 PM prevents bladder overdistention at night; patient catheterizes at bedtime and may not need to catheterize again until morning.
	Evaluate current urinary output patterns; if indwelling urethral catheter is in place, remove per hospital protocol.	Clamping of catheter before removal is not necessary and may be contraindicated.
	Provide privacy while discussing or doing bladder management procedures.	To honor patient's right to privacy.
	Institute intermittent catheterization program as prescribed or per protocol.	Usually done q 3-4 h; residual urine of 50 ml or less is usual goal for reflex voiding; residual urine no greater than 350 ml if patient is continent between catheterizations; sterile technique followed in hospital, clean technique acceptable at home.
	Apply condom catheter and leg bag for men; use incontinence pad, sanitary napkin, or adult diaper only if necessary for women. Closely monitor skin under collection device; allow skin under device to be open to air for 30 min bid.	If goal is continence between catheterizations, external collection device may be unnecessary.
	Monitor and record patient's pattern of incontinence and catheterization results.	To provide basis for decisions on frequency of catheterization.
	Administer bladder program medications as prescribed; observe for effects and side effects.	To judge effectiveness of medications.
	Perform bladder stimulation techniques if patient has UMN lesion and has recovered from spinal shock.	Includes tapping on abdomen above bladder, stroking inner thighs, tugging pubic hairs, anal stretch.
	Have patient perform Valsalva's or Credé's maneuver if patient has LMN lesion, unless contraindicated.	Increased intraabdominal pressure overcomes sphincter pressure; contraindicated if there is risk of ureteral reflux.

→ › ›

NURSING DIAGNOSIS	NURSING INTERVENTIONS	RATIONALE
	Check patient for bladder distention q 2 h when beginning bladder program.	To detect overfilling if patient has no sensation.
	Encourage patient to do her own bladder management program as soon as possible (if able).	To return control of basic body function to patient, increasing independence and self-esteem.
	Monitor for autonomic hyperreflexia in patient with spinal cord injury at T6 or above.	Distended bladder can cause autonomic hyperreflexia.
	Observe and report any signs or symptoms of UTI.	Instruct patient also to observe and report signs and symptoms of UTI.
Altered bowel elimination related to neurogenic bowel and immobility	Ensure patient's privacy	To honor patient's right to privacy.
	Assess patient's preinjury bowel elimination habits, and establish routine time for bowel evacuation.	Initially try timing similar to patient's preinjury habits; best time is ½ h after a meal; daily routine and time must be adhered to closely; frequency can be modified on the basis of program results.
	Evaluate patient's diet, and be sure that she receives adequate dietary fiber; identify foods causing gas, constipation, and diarrhea.	Fiber modifies stool consistency.
	Evaluate daily fluid intake, and ensure daily intake of 1,800-2,000 ml unless contraindicated.	To prevent constipation.
	Evaluate current bowel elimination patterns, and address any problems.	Check for impaction; address cause of any diarrhea.
	Auscultate bowel sounds bid.	To check bowel motility.
	Evaluate patient's balance, mobility, and hand dexterity skills.	Patient should be as independent as possible; check ability to maintain balance on commode, transfer on and off commode, get clothes up and down; consider need to do bowel program in bed while positioned on left side; check ability to do own rectal stimulation and/or suppository insertion.
	Institute daily bowel program.	Usually consists of rectal stimulation with or without suppository administered 15-30 min before; best position is upright on commode or on left side in bed.
	Use adaptive equipment as appropriate.	An adapted suppository inserter, rectal stimulation device, and toilet paper holder are available; open-elevated commode seat, roll-over commode shower chair, and bathroom grab bars may be needed.

NURSING DIAGNOSIS	NURSING INTERVENTIONS	RATIONALE
	Avoid use of oral laxatives, enemas, and diapers.	Laxatives and enemas cause unpredictable results, and chronic use results in chronic irritation and loss of bowel tone; diapers are not necessary with an effective bowel program, lead to decreased self-esteem, and may cause skin breakdown.
	Observe and record the appearance, consistency, and amount of stool with bowel program and any episodes of stool incontinence.	To determine if modifications in diet, fluid intake, or bowel program are needed.
	Encourage patient to be as active as possible.	Increased movement facilitates peristalsis.
	Encourage patient to do her own bowel program as soon as possible (if able).	To return control of basic body function to patient, increasing independence and self-esteem.
	Monitor for autonomic hyperreflexia in patient with spinal cord injury at T6 or above.	Rectal stimulation, suppository use, and/or distended bowel can cause autonomic hyperreflexia.
	Evaluate and report any rectal bleeding and/or discomfort during bowel program.	May be caused by too vigorous stimulation or suppository irritation.
Potential impaired skin integrity related to impaired sensation, immobility, bowel and/or bladder incontinence	Determine patient's risk factors that may lead to skin breakdown; modify risk factors as possible.	Risk factors include immobility, loss of sensation, bowel and bladder incontinence, possible dry or macerated skin; use standardized risk assessment tool, such as Braden or Norton scales; modify risk by establishing bowel and bladder management programs, etc.
	Apply appropriate special mattress or mattress topper to bed.	To allow more body surface contact with special surface, distributing body weight over larger surface area and lowering interface pressure over bony prominences.
	Obtain seat pad for use in chair or wheelchair.	To distribute body weight over larger body surface area; decreases pressure on ischial tuberosities.
	Turn patient q 2 h, and modify schedule according to absence or presence of reddened areas; use all positions, building up tolerance for prone position during day and evening while someone is with patient; record specifics of turning schedule on care plan.	To develop turning and positioning schedule according to patient's special needs and skin tolerance to pressure.
	Encourage patient who can to do weight shifts and/or lift ups while in wheelchair.	To provide needed periodic pressure relief.

→ 〉 〉

NURSING DIAGNOSIS	NURSING INTERVENTIONS	RATIONALE
	Development of therapeutic relationship necessary.	Patient must develop trust before feeling safe and sharing personal feelings and concerns.
	Monitor family's and significant others' response to patient's situation.	Rate and method of adjustment to a disability differ among family members and friends.
	Encourage patient, family, and friends to visit and ask questions.	Fear and anxiety increase with lack of knowledge.
	Identify factors influencing (positive/negative) adjustment.	To decrease controllable patient stressors and reinforce and encourage positive coping.
	Establish routine for daily care and therapy; assign routine caregivers.	So patient will know what to expect and will develop therapeutic relationships with caregivers.
	Encourage patient and family to participate in organized educational and support groups.	Group participation offers mutual support, sharing, and learning, also follow-up on identified issues.
	Identify and address dysfunctional coping mechanisms.	Drug and alcohol use, denial, and prolonged anger or depression need skilled professional interventions; helps identify resources available within facility as well as for follow-up after discharge.
	Teach patient skills to promote optimum independence; identify more effective coping strategies.	Self-care or ability to direct others in providing care gives person more control over herself and environment.
	Carry out care in unhurried manner, allowing time to listen to patient's concerns; if busy, acknowledge patient's concern and make arrangements to return to discuss issue.	Allow patient to express her feelings.
	Encourage patient to take evening, overnight, and weekend passes when ready.	To allow patient to try new skills and interact with family and friends with reassurance of returning to supportive, accessible, professional environment.
	Refer patient for counseling and follow-up during hospitalization and after discharge if needed.	Coping with a permanent disability is an ongoing process, often taking years for full adjustment.

NURSING DIAGNOSIS	NURSING INTERVENTIONS	RATIONALE
Potential for autonomic hyperreflexia related to uninhibited autonomic response to noxious stimuli after a spinal cord injury at/above T6	Discuss autonomic hyperreflexia causes, signs, and symptoms with patient and family; impress on them the need to notify the nurse if signs or symptoms appear.	Usual causes are distended bladder, distended bowel, or infection, or are treatment related (kinked catheter, rectal stimulation during bowel program or impaction removal); signs and symptoms: headache; sweating, flushed skin and piloerection above level of lesion; pallor below level of lesion; bradycardia and sudden elevation of BP above patient's postinjury norm.
	Initiate bowel and bladder management programs; establish skin care regimen.	To prevent precipitating factors.
	Observe for signs of autonomic hyperreflexia.	Ensure that others working with patient also know signs and symptoms of hyperreflexia and importance of quick intervention.
	If signs of hyperreflexia occur: return patient to bed, elevate head of bed; loosen or remove restrictive clothing (such as antiembolism stockings, leg bandage wraps, abdominal binders, and tight-waisted pants).	To induce some orthostatic hypotensive effects, slightly lowering BP until cause can be determined and addressed.
	Monitor blood pressure, pulse, and respiration q 3-5 min.	To monitor effectiveness of interventions.
	Notify physician of episode of hyperreflexia.	Each case may be handled individually, or unit or facility protocol may be followed.
	Bladder: check for distention; check for kinks in indwelling catheter (if clogged, slowly irrigate with 30 ml sterile normal saline and/or replace catheter); gently catheterize patient, pinching off catheter after each 500 ml to monitor patient's response if distended; bowel: gently check rectum for stool, give suppository or gently remove stool; topical anesthetic (such as Nupercaine) can be used as lubricant on catheter or for bowel program to decrease worsening of hyperreflexia.	To identify cause, and try to resolve the problem.
	Administer pharmacologic treatment as prescribed if signs and symptoms do not resolve or if noxious stimuli cannot be identified and eliminated.	Monitor patient for response to medication and potential hypotension.
	If signs and symptoms of hyperreflexia do not resolve or continue to worsen, notify physician again, monitor neurologic status, and continue to monitor vital signs.	Uncontrolled hyperreflexia can lead to seizures, stroke, or even death.

→ 〉 〉

NURSING DIAGNOSIS	NURSING INTERVENTIONS	RATIONALE
	Reassure patient during process; inform patient of actions being taken and their effectiveness.	Entire episode can be frightening, especially if patient cannot do her own intervention or if it is her first episode.
Knowledge deficit	See Patient Teaching.	

5 EVALUATE

PATIENT OUTCOME	DATA INDICATING THAT OUTCOME IS REACHED
Patient has a patent airway.	There is no evidence of aspiration; patient has effective coughing and improved air exchange in lungs; breath sounds are normal; there are no subjective or objective findings of shortness of breath, air hunger, or dyspnea on exertion.
Patient demonstrates an effective breathing pattern.	An effective respiratory rate has been established; gas exchange has improved; there are no signs of respiratory distress or skin cyanosis. Arterial blood gases are within normal limits.
Patient has adequate cardiac output.	SBP is >90 mm Hg or within patient's norm; patient has no fainting or dizziness with position change; <10 mm Hg DBP drop after changing positions; heart rate is 60-100 beats per minute; <20 beats per minute change in heart rate after position change; PAP of 4-6 mm Hg; PCWP of 4-12 mm Hg; PAD of 8-14 mm Hg; SVR of 950-1,300 dynes/sec/cm; cardiac index is 2.5-4; urinary output >30 ml/h; normothermia.
Patient has adequate perfusion of spinal cord tissue.	Neurologic function does not worsen, but stabilizes or improves; spinal column is immobilized, body alignment is maintained.
Patient achieves the optimal level of mobility.	Patient is free of contractures and is as mobile as possible considering residual loss of motor function; mobility includes bed mobility, transfers into and out of bed, ambulation and/or wheelchair mobility.
Patient can do or direct her own ADL.	Patient can either independently do or correctly direct others in doing her own bathing, grooming, dressing, feeding, and/or toileting (including bowel and bladder management programs).
Patient has an effective bladder management program.	Patient has medically acceptable urinary bladder residual (usually <50 ml) or catheterization results (≤450 ml); patient has no symptomatic infection.
Patient has an effective bowel management program.	Patient has regular evacuation of soft-formed stool; there is no bowel incontinence between bowel programs.
Patient has normal skin integrity and does her own skin care or can direct others in doing it.	Patient's skin is intact with no burns, bruises, abrasions, redness, or pressure ulcers; patient inspects her own skin, does her own turns and pressure reliefs and other aspects of skin program or can direct others to do so.
Patient reports satisfying sexual activity.	Patient discusses ways to conduct future sexual encounters and reports satisfying sexual activity.

PATIENT OUTCOME	DATA INDICATING THAT OUTCOME IS REACHED
Patient demonstrates adjustment to altered life-style.	Patient identifies and discusses short-term and long-term problems and goals.
Patient is free of episodes of autonomic hyperreflexia.	Patient does not experience episodes of autonomic hyperreflexia; she knows its causes, signs, and symptoms and can direct others in doing necessary interventions.

PATIENT TEACHING

1. Keep the patient and family informed about diagnostic tests, results, and interventions carried out.
2. Teach the patient and family about the spine and spinal cord, and how trauma has affected their function and therefore other bodily functions.
3. Teach the patient and family about each aspect of self-care: a. Turning and positioning; b. Bed mobility; c. Transfers into and out of bed, on and off the commode, into and out of a car, and from a wheelchair to a standing position and back; d. Good body mechanics; e. Range-of-motion exercises; f. Bowel management program and related skills of suppository insertion, rectal stimulation, and self-cleansing; g. Bladder management program and related skills of catheterization, irrigation, condom catheter application, donning leg bag and making connection, and emptying leg bag; h. How to recognize and resolve bowel and bladder complications: incontinence episodes, diarrhea, constipation, impaction, and urinary tract infections; i. Use and care of special mattresses, mattress toppers, and wheelchair seat pads; j. Skin checks; k. Pressure relief lifts and tilts; l. Recognition of skin breakdown (including ingrown toenails) and appropriate interventions; m. Preventive skin care, precautionary measures (such as turning down temperature on water heater, insulating exposed pipes under sinks, proper trimming of toenails); n. Monitoring spasticity and interventions to control spasticity; o. Discuss sexuality and sexual functioning concerns; p. Discuss parenting, fertility, and birth control concerns; q. Teach the signs and symptoms of respiratory infection (especially important for quadriplegics); r. Teach percussion and postural drainage, assisted quad cough, and the Heimlich maneuver; s. Encourage quadriplegics to obtain influenza and pneumococcal vaccinations at recommended intervals; t. Teach muscle strengthening exercises, including respiratory muscle exercises; u. Teach the patient and family about autonomic hyperreflexia (if applicable) and how to prevent and treat it; v. Teach the patient about her medications: their purpose, dose, frequency, administration, and potential side effects to report; w. Teach the care and maintenance of any orthotics, adaptive aids, ambulation aids, and/or wheelchairs; x. Teach the patient how to obtain and care for any supplies and equipment she will be using; y. Teach the patient and family how to hire and train an attendant (if applicable); z. Discuss nutrition and any special diet guidelines, such as an acid-ash diet to acidify urine or a high-protein diet to heal a wound.
4. Discuss the importance of keeping follow-up appointments.
5. Encourage the patient to contact a national spinal cord injury organization and to participate in a local group.
6. Tell the patient about available driver training and vocational rehabilitation resources.

Spinal Cord Tumors

Spinal cord tumors, although less common than intracranial tumors, are similar in pathologic types. They can arise from spinal nerve roots, the meninges, parenchyma of the cord, vertebral column, or the spinal vascular network.

Spinal cord tumors frequently affect young and middle-aged adults, and most often involve the thoracic (50%), cervical (30%), and lumbosacral (20%) areas. The tumors are rare in children and elderly people. Spinal cord tumors are classified according to their location; those occurring within the spinal cord tissue are called intramedullary tumors, and those outside the spinal cord are called extramedullary tumors. Extramedullary tumors are further categorized as intradural, extradural, or extravertebral. Spinal lesions constitute approximately 1% of all tumors in the general population. Men and women are affected about equally, except that meningiomas affect women more frequently. Approximately 85% of intraspinal tumors are benign. Secondary spinal tumors arise from the lungs, breasts, prostate, kidneys, and gastrointestinal tract.

Intramedullary tumors arise primarily from astrocyte or ependymal cells. Expanding intramedullary lesions may compress the spinal cord and nerve roots and destroy the parenchyma. Extramedullary tumors can occur inside or outside the dural sac and can cause spinal cord and spinal nerve root compression. Lesions outside the dural sac are called extradural tumors and include herniated intervertebral disks, acute and chronic infections, metastatic lesions, meningiomas, schwannomas, and epidural hemorrhages. Tumors within the dural sac but outside the spinal cord and nerve roots are extramedullary intradural tumors and include several types of glial tumors, most meningiomas and schwannomas, hemorrhages, and embryonic or congenital lesions. Extramedullary extravertebral tumors commonly are associated with destruction of vertebral bodies (Figure 4-14) (see boxes on page 141).[65]

Meningiomas constitute approximately 22% of all primary spinal cord tumors. Most meningiomas are extramedullary. Eighty percent of meningiomas affect women, usually in the fourth, fifth, or sixth decade of life. These tumors can appear anywhere in the spinal canal but are most common in the region of the nerve roots, particularly in the thoracic region (two thirds of meningiomas occur in this area). Symptoms initially are caused by traction or irritation of the nerve roots (i.e., radicular pain) and progress to long motor tract signs (i.e., spasticity) as a result of compression. Meningiomas can undergo malignant changes.[13]

Schwannomas are the spinal cord tumors that most commonly arise from the nerve sheath, and they can be found in all portions of the spinal cord. A schwannoma appears as a firm, encapsulated, rounded mass that contains many small cysts. Schwannomas can compress cervical, mediastinal, or abdominal tissue.[13]

Ependymomas make up approximately 13% of all spinal cord tumors. They arise from the lining of the internal spaces of the central nervous system and usually are intramedullary. Ependymomas are found throughout the spinal cord but commonly are located caudally in the conus medullaris and the filum terminale (cauda equina ependymoma). They are more common in men, generally appearing in the fourth or fifth decade of life. These tumors occur as loculated masses in the spinal canal, frequently with fusiform swelling. Microscopically, an ependymoma appears as a crowded mass of polygonal-type cells. In the filum it appears as a central core of connective tissue and blood vessels surrounded by a single layer of ependymal cells. Ependymomas may extend to 10 vertebral spaces in length and produce symptoms resulting from cord compression.[13]

Astrocytomas and oligodendrogliomas are similar clinically. Oligodendrogliomas are a rare type of spinal cord tumor. Astrocytomas are less common than ependymomas, generally intramedullary, and more common in men. Astrocytomas appear as elongated, fusiform swellings of the spinal cord. Symptoms result from compression of the long tracts of the spinal cord.

PATHOPHYSIOLOGY

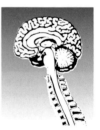

The pathologic processes occurring with any spinal cord tumor can result from destruction and infiltration of the spinal cord, displacement and compression of the cord, irritation and compression of the spinal nerve roots, disruption of the spinal blood supply, or disruption of cerebrospinal fluid (CSF) circulation.[65,121]

CLINICAL MANIFESTATIONS

The clinical symptoms of spinal cord tumors are related to the tumor's cell type and location. Symptoms of intramedullary tumors are related to direct invasion and compression of the spinal cord. Extramedullary tumors produce symptoms by compressing the spinal cord and nerve roots or occluding the spinal blood vessels.[121,126]

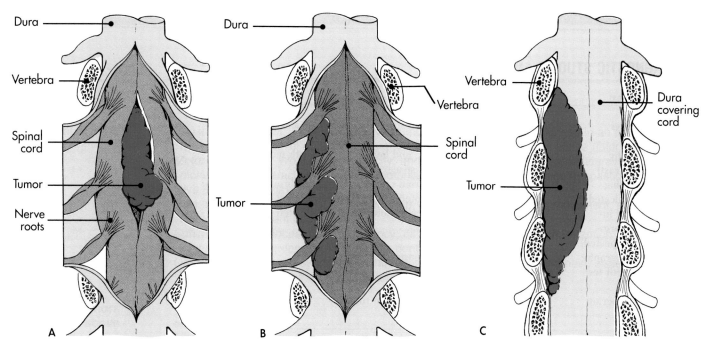

FIGURE 4-14
Spinal cord tumors. **A,** Intramedullary tumor. **B,** Intradural-extramedullary tumor. **C,** Extradural-extramedullary tumor.

CLASSIFICATION OF SPINAL CORD TUMORS

Intramedullary tumors

Ependymoma
Astrocytoma
Oligodendroglioma
Hemangioblastoma

Extramedullary tumors

Intradural
  Meningioma
  Neurofibroma
  Congenital (dermoid, epidermoid)
Extradural
  Metastatic carcinoma
  Lymphoma
  Multiple myeloma

The severity of neurologic symptoms depends on the tumor's rate of growth and the degree of compression. With slower-growing tumors, the spinal cord can accommodate the mass by compressing itself into a slender, ribbonlike tissue. Such a slow-growing tumor may produce minimum deficits. Fast-growing tumors can produce sudden cord compression, edema, and severe neurologic deficits.[61]

COMPLICATIONS

Spinal cord compression
Paralysis and motor loss
Sensory loss
Respiratory failure

CHARACTERISTICS OF SPINAL CORD TUMORS

Intramedullary tumors

Ependymomas and astrocytomas are most common types
Usually extend over many spinal cord regions
Most have slow, progressive onset
Cord compression occurs on central fiber tracts rather than on nerve roots
Sensory loss of pain and temperature
Tumors in caudal region may cause bowel, bladder, and sexual dysfunction

Extramedullary tumors

Intradural
  Most common spinal cord tumor
  Meningiomas and neurofibromas are most common types
  Thoracic spine is frequent site
  Slow, gradual onset
  Local and radicular pain may be present, but isn't always
  Symptoms of cord compression may be gradual
Extradural
  Mostly malignant
  Rapid onset of symptoms
  Local pain at area of tumor and along spinal nerve dermatomes
  Increased pain with bed rest, movement, and straining
  Pain appears before symptoms of spinal cord dysfunction

Adapted from Rudy.[127]

Parkinson's Disease (Paralysis Agitans)

Parkinson's disease is a chronic, slowly progressive degeneration of the brain's dopamine neuronal systems; it is characterized by the clinical systems of masklike facies, trunk-forward flexion, muscle weakness and rigidity, shuffling gait, resting tremors, finger pill-rolling, and bradykinesia.

The progressive, degenerative course of Parkinson's disease varies from individual to individual. Approximately 10% to 15% of those with Parkinson's disease develop dementia.

Parkinson's disease occurs throughout the world in all racial and ethnic groups. Population surveys indicate an incidence of about 130 per 100,000 standard population. The disorder is uncommon in individuals under 40 years of age, and the mean age of onset is 60 years. The prevalence of Parkinson's disease increases with age, and statistics indicate that it is the leading cause of neurologic diseases in individuals over 60 years of age.[126] Family studies show that approximately 2% of the adult siblings of individuals with Parkinson's disease also have the disorder.

PATHOPHYSIOLOGY

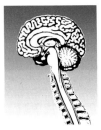

The exact cause of Parkinson's disease (parkinsonism) is unknown. In most cases, the cause is idiopathic. However, symptomatic or secondary parkinsonism is associated with a variety of nervous system disorders such as toxic agent poisoning, brain tumors in the region of the basal ganglia, cerebral trauma, infection, cerebral arteriosclerosis, and drug induction. The recent discovery that the chemical MPTP (n-methyl 4-phenyl-1236 tetrahydropyridine) produced clinical and neuropathologic findings similar to those in Parkinson's disease has focused a considerable amount of research on the possibility of an environmental cause. Environmental toxins such as fertilizers, pesticides, and herbicides have been proposed as causes.[58,126]

Parkinson's disease results from the deterioration of dopaminergic neurons in the substantia nigra (Figure 4-15), the part of the basal ganglia that produces and stores the neurotransmitter dopamine. The substantia nigra plays a critical role in the extrapyramidal motor system, which is responsible for controlling posture and the coordination and refinement of voluntary motor movements.

The basal ganglia comprises the caudate nucleus,

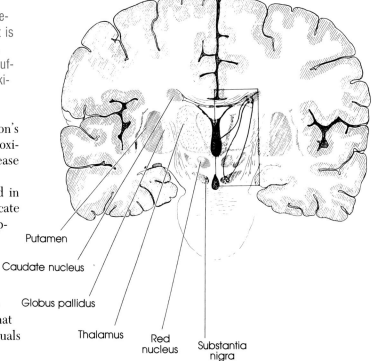

Putamen

Caudate nucleus

Globus pallidus

Thalamus   Red nucleus   Substantia nigra

FIGURE 4-15
Coronal section of the brain shows the basal ganglia. Pathways controlling normal and abnormal motor function are depicted in portion of basal ganglia named in the drawing. (From Cutler.[40])

putamen, and globus pallidus. Below these structures are smaller nuclei, including the subthalamic nuclei, red nucleus, and the substantia nigra. Normally stimulation of the basal ganglia results in the refinement of voluntary motor activity via the relative balance of the neurotransmitters acetylcholine and dopamine.

Dopamine, which is produced in the substantia nigra, is transmitted to the putamen and caudate nucleus and has an inhibitory effect on movement. Acetylcholine, which is produced throughout the basal ganglia, has an excitatory effect on movement. The deterioration of the substantia nigra results in an imbalance of excitatory acetylcholine and inhibitory dopamine. The relative depletion of dopamine results in the predominance of cholinergic activity, producing the characteristic symptoms of rigidity, tremors, and bradykinesia.[23]

CLINICAL MANIFESTATIONS

Tremor, rigidity, and bradykinesia are the classic triad of symptoms of Parkinson's disease. However, disturbances in posture, equilibrium, and autonomic function occur with equal frequency. Symptoms often are subtle and occur in varying combinations. Often early symptoms, such as generalized slowness and fatigue, are attributed to advancing age.

Tremor, the most recognizable symptom, occurs in approximately 75% of patients with parkinsonism. However, it is the least disabling symptom.[142] The tremor often includes the distinctive "pill-rolling" action of the thumb and forefinger. Tremor occurs at rest and dissipates with movement. It usually begins unilaterally but can spread to involve other body segments.

Rigidity is almost always present in parkinsonism and is attributed to an increase in muscle tone at rest. Stiffness of the trunk, head, and shoulders is evident. A lack of arm swing when walking may be evident. Cogwheel rigidity, described as a ratchetlike movement caused by a tremor breaking through rigidity, can be observed.[58] Initially rigidity may be mild and limited to a few muscle groups. However, it usually progresses to involve other areas.

Bradykinesia and poverty of movement result in large delays in the execution of movement. The patient may describe a feeling of being "frozen in place." This motor impairment may affect a wide variety of movements, such as eye blinking, facial movements (producing the masklike facies), and walking gait, and cause voice disturbances. The patient's frustration often is compounded by the intermittent and paradoxic nature of this symptom, referred to as "paradoxic akinetic reaction," because a patient may very suddenly move normally.

Postural disturbances in Parkinson's disease are readily recognizable. The head is bowed, and the trunk is bent forward. The shoulders appear drooped, and the arms are flexed. The parkinsonian gait is one of shuffling with small steps (festination) (Figure 4-16). Changes in balance give rise to a tendency to fall forward (propulsion) and backward (retropulsion).

Autonomic dysfunction can cause urinary incontinence, constipation, orthostatic hypotension, overactivity of sweat glands, and eczematous eruption.

Behavior and mentation also change. Dementia is estimated to occur in 10% to 15% of patients with parkinsonism. In a few cases mild impairment of memory and dementia have been reported to precede most symptoms. Depression, social withdrawal, and generalized apathy often accompany Parkinson's disease.[126]

COMPLICATIONS
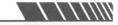

Motor disturbances	Dysarthria
Impaired gait, balance, and posture	Dysphagia
	Dementia
Autonomic dysfunction	Depression

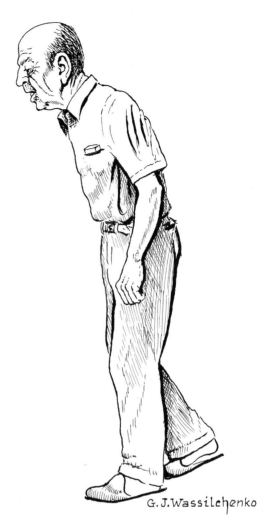
G.J.Wassilchenko

FIGURE 4-16
Posture and shuffling gait associated with Parkinson's disease. (From Rudy.[127])

DIAGNOSTIC STUDIES AND FINDINGS

There is no definite test to diagnose Parkinson's disease; diagnosis is based on the history and physical examination.

Diagnostic test	Findings
Chest x-rays	Slight scoliosis
Skull x-rays	Normal
Computed tomography (CT) scan	Normal (with history of chronic dementia, may show cerebral atrophy)
Electroencephalography	Normal or shows minimum slowing and/or disorganization (with marked dementia and bradykinesia, may show moderate to marked slowing and diffuse disorganization)
Cineradiographic study of swallowing	Abnormal pattern: delayed relaxation of cricopharyngeal muscles

2 DIAGNOSE

NURSING DIAGNOSIS	SUBJECTIVE FINDINGS	OBJECTIVE FINDINGS
Impaired physical mobility related to muscle tremors and rigidity, gait disturbance, and bradykinesia	Reports inability to complete or participate in ADL, as well as muscle spasms and freezing	Tremors; poverty of movement; bradykinesia; shuffling gait; rigidity; freezing
Altered nutrition: less than body requirements related to tremors and rigidity of muscles of mastication, dysphagia, and side effects of medications	Reports difficulty swallowing and chewing, and nausea	Choking; drooling; rigidity of facial muscles; weight loss; dehydration; lack of appetite; vomiting
Potential for injury related to gait disturbance, rigidity and tremors of muscles, cognitive impairments, and orthostatic hypotension	Reports falling frequently and difficulty maintaining balance	Gait disturbances; tremors; rigidity; impaired judgment and confusion; orthostatic hypotension
Ineffective individual coping related to lack of control over disease process and changes in body image/function	Reports having difficulty coping with disease	Lack of appetite; irritability; insomnia; apathy; lack of interest in social activity

Other related nursing diagnoses: Impaired communication related to dysarthria; **Self-care deficit** related to muscle rigidity, tremors, and bradykinesia.

3 PLAN

Patient goals

1. The patient will demonstrate maximum mobility within limitations of disease.
2. The patient will demonstrate adequate or improved nutrition for his age and size.
3. The patient will remain free of any injuries associated with disability.
4. The patient will demonstrate effective coping.

4 IMPLEMENT

NURSING DIAGNOSIS	NURSING INTERVENTIONS	RATIONALE
Impaired physical mobility related to muscle tremors and rigidity, gait disturbance, and bradykinesia	Assess muscle rigidity/tremors, gait disturbance, bradykinesia q 4-8 h prn.	Deficiency of dopamine causes these symptoms in Parkinson's disease.
	Administer prescribed medications in a timely manner; observe and document patient's response.	Medications must be given on time to avoid aggravation of symptoms; dosages are individualized to patient's response.

NURSING DIAGNOSIS	NURSING INTERVENTIONS	RATIONALE
	Perform active and passive ROM exercises.	To prevent joint contractures and stiffness.
Altered nutrition: less than body requirements related to tremors and rigidity of muscles of mastication, dysphagia, and side effects of medications	Assess patient's usual dietary preferences, the extent of rigidity and tremors involving the muscles of chewing, and dysphagia.	Muscles necessary for chewing and swallowing can be affected in parkinsonism.
	Administer medications such that they peak around mealtime.	To decrease rigidity and tremors of muscles needed to chew and swallow.
	Take precautions to prevent aspiration and/or choking: raise head of bed, keep head slightly flexed; have suction equipment at bedside.	Risk of choking and aspiration increases considerably as the disease progresses.
	Give patient semisoft foods if he has difficulty swallowing.	These are easier to swallow than liquids.
	Give foods high in calories.	To maintain adequate nutritional intake.
	Provide small, frequent meals; encourage patient to take small bites.	Small meals may be easier than larger ones, and this helps decrease frustration.
	Consult occupational therapist if hand tremors interfere with patient's ability to feed himself.	Assistive devices are available (i.e., wrist braces) that allow patient to maintain his independence.
Potential for injury related to gait disturbance, rigidity and tremors of muscles, cognitive impairments, and orthostatic hypotension	Assess the extent of the patient's disability; assess for orthostatic hypotension and for any cognitive impairments.	The extent of disability varies considerably; orthostatic hypotension is a side effect of the medications given to treat parkinsonism.
	Teach patient to change position slowly.	To prevent dizziness.
	Use chairs that have armrests and backs; use sidebars in bathroom and handrails in hall.	To help reduce the risk of falling.
	Teach patient to walk erect, using a wide-based stance.	To try to minimize abnormal gait.
	Maintain clutter-free environment; remove objects that could cause falls.	To reduce risk of falling.
	Place side rails up when patient is in bed, and put call bell within reach.	To assure patient's safety and security.
Ineffective individual coping related to lack of control over disease process and changes in body image/function	Assess patient's coping mechanisms and behavior.	Parkinson's disease is a chronic, progressive disease that requires life-style adjustments; depression and dementia are symptoms of advanced parkinsonism.
	Give patient the opportunity to express his fears and concerns.	To help reduce tension.

Multiple Sclerosis

Multiple sclerosis (MS), or disseminated sclerosis, is a chronic, progressive neurologic disease characterized by disseminating demyelination of nerve fibers of the brain and spinal cord.

Multiple sclerosis is the most prevalent of the human demyelinating diseases, with an incidence of 40 to 60 per 10,000 people in the United States and Canada. Women are affected with the disorder slightly more often than men. The onset of symptoms occurs between 20 and 40 years of age in 75% of the cases. The disease is rare in childhood and fairly uncommon in old age. The severity, duration, and prognosis of multiple sclerosis vary. The survival rate of individuals with multiple sclerosis is approximately 85% of that for the general population. The diagnosis of this disorder is made on the presence of multiple lesions in the central nervous system and dissemination over time.

Studies show an association between the prevalence of multiple sclerosis and distance from the equator. Multiple sclerosis is most prevalent in western Europe, southern Canada, southern Australia, and New Zealand.[126] Within the United States, the prevalence of multiple sclerosis is higher in the Great Lakes region, the northern Atlantic states, and the Pacific Northwest.

Studies have shown that people who move from areas of higher prevalence to areas of lower prevalence after 15 years of age retain the risk of multiple sclerosis at the level of their previous environment. Individuals under 15 years of age acquire the risk prevalence of the new environment.[126]

PATHOPHYSIOLOGY

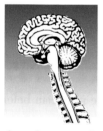

The cause of multiple sclerosis is unknown. Etiologic hypotheses include genetic, virologic, epidemiologic, and immunologic features. Studies indicate that first-degree relatives of a family member with multiple sclerosis have a 15 times greater incidence of the disease than the general population. A person with an identical twin with multiple sclerosis has a 20% risk of the disease, 300 times greater than in the general population.

Individuals with multiple sclerosis have elevated (i.e., up to twofold) serum and cerebrospinal fluid (CSF) titers of antibodies to many viruses, including the herpes simplex type I, parainfluenza, rubella, mumps, measles, and Epstein-Barr viruses.

Approximately 90% of individuals affected with multiple sclerosis have abnormalities of the cerebrospinal fluid, particularly increased IgG and oligoclonal bands. Suppressor lymphocyte function is altered, and acute deteriorations are accompanied or perhaps preceded by defective immunoregulation, allowing unimpeded damage to the myelin membrane and oligodendrocytes. Remission is accompanied by a rebound elevation in suppressor function.[76]

The neuropathologic changes in multiple sclerosis include multifocal plaques of demyelination distributed randomly within the brainstem, cerebellum, spinal cord, optic nerve, and cerebrum.

During the demyelination process (called primary demyelination), the myelin sheath and the myelin sheath cells are destroyed. The demyelination process leads to four significant central disturbances: a decrease in nerve conduction velocity, nerve conduction block (frequency related), differential rate of transmission of impulses, and complete failure of impulse transmission. These disturbances account for the variety of clinical signs and symptoms. Symptom remission occurs when demyelinated areas are healed by sclerotic tissue. However, when the nerve fiber degenerates, symptoms become permanent.[65]

CLINICAL MANIFESTATIONS

The clinical signs and symptoms of multiple sclerosis vary considerably and are marked by the chronic yet unpredictable nature of the disease. Exacerbations and remissions are seen in 75% of patients. Symptoms during an exacerbation may last several weeks or just brief moments. Subjective physical symptoms often are described as bizarre and may be unsubstantiated by physical examination, making diagnosis even more difficult. The course of multiple sclerosis has been categorized into four distinct patterns (see box on page 159).

The symptoms of multiple sclerosis are diverse and depend on the area of the central nervous system that is affected. Some neurologists classify the symptoms simply as spinal, brainstem, cerebellar, and cerebral (see box on page 159).

Spinal syndrome describes symptoms that involve damage to the corticospinal tracts and dorsal column. Motor symptoms often begin with weakness of the lower extremities and may progress to the upper extremities. Spastic paraparesis can occur. Fatigability of

COURSE OF MULTIPLE SCLEROSIS

Benign: (20% of cases) mild exacerbations with complete or near complete remissions, minimum or no disability

Exacerbation-remitting: (25% of cases) more frequent attacks early in the illness with less complete remissions; there are long periods of stability and some disability

Chronic-relapsing: (40% of cases) fewer remissions as the disease progresses and disability becomes cumulative

Chronic-progressive: (15% of cases) insidious onset with steady progression of symptoms and no remissions

From Rowland.[126]

INITIAL SYNDROMES OF MULTIPLE SCLEROSIS

Cerebral syndrome

Optic neuritis
Intellectual and emotional changes
Seizures
Hemiparesis, hemisensory loss, dysphasia

Cerebellar syndrome

Motor ataxia
Hypotonia
Asthenia

Brainstem syndrome

Intranuclear ophthalmoplegia (INO)
Nystagmus
Dysarthria

Spinal syndrome

Spastic paresis
Bowel and bladder dysfunction
Paresthesia

From McCance.[98]

the muscle is a common complaint. Bowel and bladder disturbances can occur with major spinal cord involvement. Paresthesia and disturbances in vibration, position and two-part discrimination reflect involvement of the dorsal column.[98]

Brainstem syndrome describes symptoms that reflect damage to cranial nerves III through XII. Ocular disturbances are relatively common and may include diplopia, blurred vision, loss of visual acuity, eye pain, and nystagmus. Other symptoms of brainstem origin include dysarthria, vertigo, tinnitus, and facial weakness. Scanning speech, defined as slow speech with pauses between syllables, occurs in late stages of the disease.[98]

Cerebellar syndrome reflects involvement of the cerebellum and involves ataxia, hypotonia, and asthenia (weakness). Charcot triad (dysarthria, intention tremor, and nystagmus) may be observed.[98]

Cerebral syndrome is characterized by optic neuritis. Optic neuritis often is an early sign of multiple sclerosis and involves visual clouding, loss of part of the visual field, and pain. Emotional and intellectual disturbances can occur. Depression, euphoria, and emotional lability are most common. Dementia can occur later in the disease.[98]

Paroxysmal attacks, described as sensory or motor symptoms that are abrupt and brief (lasting seconds to minutes), occur daily with some patients (e.g., Lhermitte's sign, an electric-like shock sensation that extends down the trunk and limbs when the neck is flexed).[98]

Exacerbation of symptoms in multiple sclerosis has been correlated with several factors: infection, emotional stress, pregnancy, physical injury, cold temperatures, hot baths, and fatigue.

COMPLICATIONS

Varying degrees of sensory and motor loss
Bowel and bladder dysfunction
Speech deficits
Visual disturbances, blindness
Infection
Decubitus ulcers
Pneumonia
Thrombus formation

NURSING DIAGNOSIS	NURSING INTERVENTIONS	RATIONALE
	Encourage family to participate in patient's care.	To help reduce anxiety that may be associated with patient's nursing care needs.
	Help family identify resources to facilitate their short- and long-term needs.	MS has a tremendous impact on the family system; the emotional and financial effects require most families to consider seeking community help.
Knowledge deficit	See Patient Teaching.	

5 EVALUATE

PATIENT OUTCOME	DATA INDICATING THAT OUTCOME IS REACHED
Patient demonstrates increased participation in activities.	The patient shows improved interest in participating in activities and performs activities within her physical limitations.
Patient demonstrates maximum mobility within limitations of disease.	The patient understands her exercise and physical therapy regimens; she has no contractures, skin breakdown, or thrombus formation; her mobility is appropriate to her physiologic status.
Patient demonstrates optimum vision and use of eyes.	The patient has no diplopia, visual field cut, nystagmus, or eye pain.
Patient demonstrates effective communication.	The patient can express her needs clearly; she develops alternative communication methods if necessary.
Patient demonstrates adequate urinary elimination.	The patient has urinary continence; she has no frequency, urgency, pain on urination, incontinence, or nocturia; her bladder is not distended, and her intake and output are balanced.
Patient is free of injuries.	The patient has no injuries and is aware of the risk factors associated with falls.
Patient is free of pain/discomfort.	The patient says that she is more comfortable; she shows no facial grimacing or irritability, and her vital signs are stable.
Patient demonstrates effective methods of coping.	The patient openly expresses her concerns and feelings of grief and loss; she participates in decision making about her care; she expresses positive feelings about herself and acknowledges the changes in her self-image.

PATIENT OUTCOME	DATA INDICATING THAT OUTCOME IS REACHED
Patient and family demonstrate adjustment to changes in patient's family role.	The family understands the disease process; the patient and family have identified alternative family roles as needed; family members interact appropriately with the patient and each other and encourage the patient to participate in family decision making.

PATIENT TEACHING

1. Teach the patient and family about multiple sclerosis and the treatment modalities (explain procedures as they occur).
2. Stress the importance of routines for activities of daily living.
3. Emphasize the importance of avoiding fatigue, overwork, and emotional stress.
4. Stress the importance of regular exercise and planned rest periods.
5. Emphasize the importance of diversional activities.
6. Stress the importance of speech therapy, physical therapy, and occupational therapy.
7. Encourage the patient to talk about her feelings.
8. Emphasize the need for socialization with significant others.
9. Stress the need for independence and self-care to level of tolerance: a. Support the patient when ambulating; b. Help the patient to walk with a wide base.
10. Teach the patient and family the symptoms of disease progression to report to the physician.
11. Emphasize the need to avoid persons with upper respiratory infections.
12. Stress the need to avoid extremes of hot and cold.
13. Teach the patient and family the names of medications, the dosage, frequency of administration, purpose, and toxic or side effects.
14. Emphasize the importance of avoiding over-the-counter medications.
15. Stress the importance of ongoing outpatient care: visits to the physician, physical therapy, speech therapy, occupational therapy, and home nursing services.
16. Ensure that the patient and family demonstrate the following: active and/or passive range-of-motion exercises; proper techniques of ambulation; proper techniques for turning, positioning, and transfer; proper bowel and bladder management; application of hand splints and braces; methods for maintaining patient safety.
17. Teach the patient about factors that exacerbate symptoms of multiple sclerosis (i.e., overexertion, hot baths, fever, emotional stress, cold, high humidity, and pregnancy); consult physician before receiving any immunizations.
18. Refer the patient and family to the MS Society.

Alzheimer's Disease

Alzheimer's disease is a chronic neurologic disorder characterized by progressive and selective degeneration of neurons in the cerebral cortex and certain subcortical structures.

Alzheimer's disease was named for German neuropsychiatrist Alois Alzheimer, who first described the disorder in 1907. It is the fourth leading cause of death in the United States. The disease can affect anyone over 40 years of age, but it is most common in those over the age of 65. It is estimated that more than 3 million Americans over age 65 have Alzheimer's disease. The annual cost of care is estimated at $40 billion.[29]

Both men and women may be affected, but the incidence is higher in women. Current research indicates that Alzheimer's disease is age related; it is uncommon in young people and rare in middle age. However, as age increases, so does the incidence of the disorder, such that its prevalence in individuals over 80 years of age is estimated at more than 20%.[29]

To date, only genetics and female gender have been identified as risk factors for Alzheimer's disease. The genetic factor is believed to be inherited in the form of an autosomal dominant trait. The risk associated with female gender has been attributed to two factors. First, Alzheimer's disease is age related, and women live longer than men. Second, it is believed that development of Alzheimer's disease is sometimes related to a gene on the X chromosome.[21,149]

The onset of Alzheimer's disease usually is subtle and insidious. The duration and rate of progression vary, but for patients who are well cared for, the average survival rate from onset is approximately 8 to 9 years.

PATHOPHYSIOLOGY

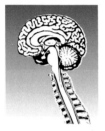 Grossly, the primary pathologic feature of Alzheimer's disease is the degeneration and loss of selective neuronal cells in the cerebral cortex, which ultimately results in symmetric and extensive convolutional atrophy, particularly in the frontal and medial temporal regions. This cerebral atrophy is accompanied by an enlargement of the cerebral ventricles, which is not severe unless concomitant hydrocephalus exists.

Characteristic microscopic lesions in the brain tissue of individuals with Alzheimer's disease include neuritic plaques, neurofibrillary tangles, granulovacuolar degeneration, and Hirano bodies. Neuritic plaques consist of degenerated intracortical foci of clustered and thickened neurites (axons and dendrites) that surround a spherical deposit of amyloid (starchlike protein) fibrils.[21] These plaques usually are found most prominently in the frontal cortex and hippocampus. Neurofibrillary tangles (neurofibrils) consist of masses of twisted and tangled intracellular protein that are deposited primarily in the cytoplasm of neuronal cell bodies. These neurofibrils are found primarily in the hippocampus and adjacent areas of the temporal lobe and are most abundant in areas of severe neuronal loss. Granulovacuolar degeneration consists of membrane-bound vacuoles containing fine granular material that is found most prominently in the pyramidal neurons of the hippocampus. Hirano bodies are found in the neurophil and consist of intracytoplasmic eosinophilic rods. Cell loss in the hippocampus is believed to correlate with the memory loss of Alzheimer's disease.[21,29]

Characteristic cell loss found in the brain of an individual with Alzheimer's disease includes both cortical and subcortical structures. Cell loss in the cortex includes the larger cells of the association cortex and cholinergic cells at the rostal portion of the reticular activating system (RAS). The loss of cholinergic cells results in re-duced levels of the neurotransmitter acetylcholine. Recent studies have suggested that deficiencies in cholinergic transmission may lead to a breakdown of neuronal structures and may play a role in the clinical expression of Alzheimer's disease. Cell loss in subcortical structures includes noradrenalin cells in the locus ceruleus and dopamine-secreting cells of the pars compacta of the substantia nigra.[21,149]

The basic pathophysiologic processes of brain damage that occur with Alzheimer's disease are not known. One proposed cause is related to chronic aluminum toxicity. However, recent studies indicate that although aluminum apparently does accumulate in tangle-bearing neurons, it does not appear that such an accumulation is a necessary condition for Alzheimer changes in the cell. Further, epidemiologic data do not indicate a higher incidence of Alzheimer's disease in individuals who chronically ingest aluminum (e.g., antacids).[21,29]

One possible reason that brain cells degenerate and die may be the reduced rate in overall cerebral metabolism in Alzheimer's disease. This cerebral metabolic reduction is approximately 25% compared to age- and sex-matched cognitively intact controls. Another possibility is that the disease may be linked to some type of generalized membrane abnormalities or abnormal cellular calcium metabolism.[21]

Researchers also are investigating the seemingly higher incidence and earlier onset of Alzheimer's disease in individuals who have had a head injury.[27]

DIAGNOSTIC STUDIES AND FINDINGS

Diagnostic test	Findings
Computed tomography (CT) scan (serial)	Cerebral ventricular and subarachnoid space enlargement because of diffuse brain atrophy (later stages)
MRI study	Same as CT scan
Electroencephalography	Diffuse slowing of brain waves and diminished voltage (advanced stages)
Comprehensive history	Symptoms listed in assessment section for this disorder; family history of similar disorders; careful attention to medication history
Psychometric and behavioral rating scales*	Scores indicate increasingly impaired cognitive functioning, fluctuating signs of depression
PET scan	Significant decrease in metabolic activity of brain
Brain biopsy	Confirms presence of neurofibrillary tangles and neuritic plaques (usually done at postmortem only to confirm diagnosis)

*Mini Mental State (MMS); Mental Status Questionnaire (MSQ); Haycos behavior scale; Hamilton depression scale; Wechsler's Adult Intelligence Scale (WAIS).

NOTE: A variety of other tests may be done to rule out treatable causes of dementia (e.g., cardiac workup; CBC; serum electrolyte, folate, and vitamin B_{12} levels; liver and thyroid function tests; drug toxicity screen; and serologic test for syphilis).

COMPLICATIONS

Any of the complications of immobility, most notably:

Pneumonia	Bladder incontinence
Bowel incontinence	Contractures
	Pressure ulcers

STAGES OF ALZHEIMER'S DISEASE

Initial stage (lasts 2 to 4 yr)

Absentmindedness
Lack of spontaneity
Time and spatial disorientation
Loss of memory and emotional control
Changes in affect
Depression
Diminished ability to concentrate
Perceptual alterations
Neglectfulness in appearance
Careless actions
Poor judgment
Delusions (transitory) of persecution
Muscle twitching
Epileptiform seizures

Middle stage (lasts 2 to 12 yr)

Nocturnal restlessness

From Thompson.[139]

Apraxia (impaired ability to perform purposeful activity)
Alexia (inability to comprehend written words)
Astereognosis (inability to identify objects by touch)
Auditory agnosia (total or partial inability to recognize familiar objects by the sense of sound)
Agraphia (inability to write)
Hypertonia
Increased aphasia
Hyperorality
Complete disorientation
Unsteady gait
Progressive memory loss
Increase in socially unacceptable behavior

Decreased ability to comprehend
Perseveration (repetitive actions such as chewing, tapping)

Terminal stage (lasts up to 1 yr)

Seizures (rare)
Marked weight loss; emaciation
Decreased appetite
Bulimia
Apraxia
Visual agnosia
Incontinence (bowels and/or bladder)
Hyperorality
Paraphasia
Hypermetamorphosis
Increased irritability
Feelings of helplessness
Bedridden
Unresponsive or comatose

MEDICAL MANAGEMENT

GENERAL MANAGEMENT

Electroconvulsive therapy; cardiac monitoring; support of vital functions (with ventilator) if indicated; nutritional support: soft or liquid diet; social services consultation; physical therapy; psychologic counseling and support; community referrals; occupational therapy; home nursing services; extended care facility referrals.

SURGERY

None

DRUG THERAPY

Antipsychotics: Haloperidol (Haldol).

Sedative-hypnotics: Chloral hydrate.

Antianxiety agents: Lorazepam (Ativan); diazepam (Valium); alprazolam (Xanax).

Antidepressants (anticholinergic side effects may impair cognition): Amitriptyline hydrochloride (Elavil); nortriptyline hydrochloride (Aventyl or Pamelor).

Laxatives/stool softeners: Docusate sodium (Colace).

though the precise mechanism of tumor development is not well understood. CNS neoplasms attributed to AIDS include primary CNS lymphoma, systemic non-Hodgkin's lymphoma, and metastatic Kaposi's sarcoma.

Before the AIDS epidemic came to light about 10 years ago, primary CNS lymphoma was extremely rare, accounting for fewer than 1.5% of all brain tumors. Primary CNS lymphoma is a large cell lymphoma that may have some link to the Epstein-Barr virus. The clinical manifestations of primary CNS lymphoma can be attributed to the intracranial mass lesions that develop and expand rapidly. The lesions appear as multicentric in the brain parenchyma and do not metastasize to extracranial sites.[124]

CNS involvement can be attributed to invasion of the meninges caused by systemic non-Hodgkin's lymphoma. Metastasis to the cranial nerves and spinal cord can occur. Although Kaposi's sarcoma is the most common neoplasm seen in AIDS patients, metastasis to the central nervous system is rare.[124]

Cerebrovascular complications of AIDS include multifocal ischemic infarction, hemorrhagic infarction, hemorrhage into tumors, transient ischemic attacks, subdural hematomas, and epidural hematomas. Although the precise mechanisms are unknown, hematologic factors that cause a hypercoagulable state may account for these complications.[85]

The complexity of the CNS syndromes seen in AIDS is compounded by reported neurologic symptoms caused by AIDS therapy, including extrapyramidal movements, myoclonus, dysphasia, delirium, and acute myelopathy. Furthermore, multiple CNS pathologic conditions have been reported to be as high as 30%.[85]

Although less common, AIDS-related diseases of the peripheral nervous system (PNS) do occur. Four clinical syndromes have been identified: distal symmetric peripheral neuropathy, chronic inflammatory demyelinating polyradiculoneuropathy, mononeuropathy multiplex, and progressive polyradiculopathy. The cause of peripheral nerve disease remains unclear; however, HIV has been cultured from nerves.[85]

CLINICAL MANIFESTATIONS

The neurologic manifestations of AIDS are extensive and reflect the increasingly vast number of clinical symptoms. Table 4-6 lists the clinical manifestations of the AIDS-related neurologic diseases.

COMPLICATIONS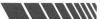

Pneumocystis carinii pneumonia (PCP)
Kaposi's sarcoma (KS)
Oral candidiasis
Diarrhea
Hepatitis
Biliary dysfunction
Anorectal disease
Cytomegalovirus retinitis

DIAGNOSTIC STUDIES AND FINDINGS

Diagnostic test	Findings
Enzyme-linked immunosorbent assay (ELISA)	Identifies HIV antibodies (can yield false positive)
Western Blot	Identifies HIV antibodies (confirms positive results from ELISA)
Complete blood count (CBC)	Leukocytopenia; neutropenia; anemia
Total T cell count	Reduced T4 count (< 400/mm)
T4/T8 ratio (T helper cells to T suppressor cells)	Low (< 1:2)
Immunoglobulin level	May have elevated IgG and IgA
Chest x-ray	May reveal pneumonia, infiltrates
Cerebrospinal fluid (CSF) sampling	Culture and sensitivity may reflect infecting organism; elevated protein; elevated WBC
CT and MRI studies	Distinguishes focal from diffuse lesions and enhancing from nonenhancing lesions; may show white matter abnormalities
Electroencephalography	May show focal or diffuse slowing
Brain biopsy	Offers definitive diagnosis of cerebral lesions
Electromyography	Disturbances in nerve conduction

```
┌─────────────────────────────────────┐
│  NERVOUS  SYSTEM  DISORDERS          │
│  RELATED  TO  HIV  INFECTION         │
└─────────────────────────────────────┘
```

Primary Viral (HIV) Syndromes

Central nervous system
  AIDS-related dementia
  Atypical aseptic meningitis
  Spinal vacuolar myelopathy
Peripheral nervous system
  Mononeuritis multiplex
  Distal symmetric peripheral neuropathy
  Inflammatory demyelinating polyradiculoneuropathy
  Progressive polyradiculopathy

Opportunistic Viral Infections

Progressive multifocal leukoencephalopathy (JC papovavirus)
Meningitis/encephalitis (cytomegalovirus, herpes simplex virus types 1 and 2, herpes varicella-zoster virus)

Opportunistic Nonviral Infections

Toxoplasmic meningoencephalitis *(Toxoplasma gondii)*
Meningitis/encephalitis/brain abscess *(Cryptococcus neoformans, Candida albicans, Aspergillus fumigatus, Coccidioides immitis, Mycobacterium tuberculosis hominis, Mycobacterium avium-intracellulare, Listeria monocytogenes, Nocardia asteroides)*

Adapted from Rosenbaum et al.[124]

Neoplasms

Primary CNS lymphoma
Metastatic Kaposi's sarcoma
Systemic lymphoma with CNS metastasis

Cerebrovascular Complications

Cerebral infarction
Cerebral hemorrhage
Cerebral vasculitis

CNS Complications Related to AIDS Therapy

Extrapyramidal movements
Myoclonus
Dysphasia
Delirium
Acute myelopathy

Table 4-6

CLINICAL MANIFESTATIONS OF AIDS-RELATED CNS SYNDROMES

Syndrome	Symptoms	Cause
AIDS dementia complex (ADC)	Inattention; loss of concentration; general mental slowness to global dementia; apathy; social withdrawal; mutism; disturbances in balance and eye-hand coordination; tremors; motor weakness; dysarthia	Primary HIV infection
Atypical aseptic meningitis	Headache; fever; meningeal irritation; cranial neuropathies; elevated intracranial pressure	Primary HIV infection
Spinal vacuolar myelopathy	Leg weakness; incontinence; paraparesis; spasticity; ataxia	Primary HIV infection
Progressive multifocal leukoencephalopathy	Headaches; alteration in level of consciousness or cognition; blindness; aphasia; hemiparesis; ataxia	JC papovavirus
Herpes group infections	Headaches; fever; seizures; focal neurologic deficits; altered mental status	Herpes simplex Herpes zoster Cytomegalovirus
Cerebral toxoplasmosis	Headache; fever; altered mentation or cognition; lethargy; focal neurologic signs; seizures	Protozoa; *T. gondii*
Cryptococcal meningitis	Headache; lethargy; altered mentation; meningeal signs	Soil fungus, *Cryptococcus neoformans*
Primary CNS lymphoma	Altered mental status or cognition; headache; seizures; focal weakness; aphasia; incontinence	Primary CNS lymphoma

3 PLAN

Patient goals

1. The patient will not develop additional opportunistic infections.
2. The patient will demonstrate improved or stable mental status within physiologic limitations.
3. The patient will demonstrate improved or stable self-care abilities within physical limitations.
4. The patient will demonstrate improved nutritional status.

4 IMPLEMENT

NURSING DIAGNOSIS	NURSING INTERVENTIONS	RATIONALE
Potential for infection related to immunosuppression	Monitor vital signs, CBC with differential, T4/T8 count.	To determine physiologic response to infection.
	Monitor skin integrity and invasive lines for signs of infection.	Immunosuppressed patients may not mount the usual physiologic response to infection; meticulous care must be provided to all open areas.
	Institute isolation precautions as recommended by the Centers for Disease Control (CDC); wash hands meticulously before and after providing care; provide a low-microbial diet, and do not allow patient to have plants or flowers if absolute granulocyte count is <500 cells/cm^3.	Meticulous hand washing is essential to minimize cross-contamination; plants, flowers, and ingestion of raw produce can introduce bacteria, virus, and fungus into the body.
	Wear gloves, mask, gown, and goggles when direct contact with body fluids is anticipated; dispose of needles and sharps in rigid puncture-resistant containers; handle linen, body fluid containers, soiled dressings, and specimens per hospital policy.	The CDC and hospitals have outlined specific guidelines to protect health care providers from contracting AIDS; HIV is not transmitted via casual contact.
	Assess patient frequently for signs and symptoms of new infection.	AIDS patients are susceptible to a wide variety of opportunistic infections.
	Obtain cultures as ordered.	To identify the causative agent of infection.
	Administer antibiotics and antiinfectives as prescribed.	To treat appropriate organisms.
	In the event of fever, monitor patient closely for signs of dehydration, and administer antipyretic as prescribed; provide adequate hydration, and place patient on hypothermic blanket.	Hyperthermia, night sweats, and chills may accompany infections.

NURSING DIAGNOSIS	NURSING INTERVENTIONS	RATIONALE
Altered thought processes related to HIV infection of CNS, opportunistic CNS infections, CNS neoplasms, and side effects of medications	Assess patient's general behavior and appearance: face, posture, eye contact, speech.	Many of the CNS manifestations of AIDS are subtle.
	Assess patient's reality orientation and problem-solving ability.	Impaired problem-solving ability and other neuropsychiatric complications are often seen with ADC.
	Monitor patient for any patterns of confused behavior and/or anxiety.	Dementia may vary from periods of confusions to complete dementia.
	Assess patient's medication regimen.	Many of the medications given to treat AIDS and the opportunistic infections can cause alterations in mental status.
	Monitor patient's neurologic status q 2-4 h prn; observe for meningeal irritation, increasing headache, motor weakness, sensory loss, and any signs of increasing ICP.	Neurologic diseases associated with AIDS often begin with subtle symptoms (e.g., headache, neck pain).
	Speak to patient slowly and clearly.	To facilitate patient's ability to comprehend.
	Reduce extraneous stimuli; place familiar objects in patient's room.	To reduce excess noise and distraction and facilitate reality orientation.
	Reorient patient as needed.	To reassure patient and decrease anxiety.
	Assess patient's potential for self-injury; maintain a safe environment.	Confusion, disorientation, and poor judgment require that the patient's environment be supervised.
	Provide support to patient and significant others.	Family and friends may have difficulty coping with changes in patient's personality and mental status.
Self-care deficit related to impaired mental status, motor and sensory loss, and generalized fatigue	Assess the extent of cognitive, physical, and/or emotional limitations and ability to provide self-care safely.	To determine cause of self-care deficit (infection, depression, and side effects of medications can all contribute to deficit).
	Identify with patient his physical and nursing care needs; negotiate with patient how care will be provided.	Feelings of powerlessness may accompany a self-care deficit; allowing the patient to identify care needs enhances self-esteem.
	Consult with physical therapist and occupational therapist about adaptive devices to enhance self-care.	Adaptive devices may facilitate patient's independence.
	Teach family and friends how to help with patient's physical care needs.	Involving family and friends in care can minimize social isolation.

tive and usually follows a viral illness, most commonly the mumps. Lymphocytic infiltration of the pia-arachnoid layers occurs, but the clinical severity varies. Progression to encephalitis can occur, but the disease usually is self-limiting.[118]

CLINICAL MANIFESTATIONS

A headache, often described as severe, usually is the initial symptom of meningitis. An elevated temperature (38.3°-40° C [101°-104° F]) is evident with bacterial meningitis. The patient usually complains of generalized malaise, and the level of consciousness may begin with drowsiness and decreased attention span, which can progress to stupor and coma. Confusion, agitation, and irritability may be evident.

Signs of meningeal irritation are present. Severe neck pain on flexion (nuchal rigidity) and a stiff neck are evident. The patient may lie in the opisthotonos position. Kernig's sign is elicited by flexing the hip at a 90-degree angle (Figure 4-17, A). A positive sign is noted when pain is observed on extension of the knee. Brudzinski's sign is considered positive when flexion of the neck elicits flexion of the thigh and knee (Figure 4-17, B). Photophobia or extreme light sensitivity may be evident. A skin rash with petechial hemorrhage is evident with meningococcal meningitis.

Cranial nerve deficits may be caused by inflammation. Most often involved are cranial nerves III, IV, VI, VII, and VIII, resulting in ocular palsies, pupillary abnormalities, ptosis, diplopia, facial paresis, deafness, and vertigo. Progression of the infection can result in signs of increased intracranial pressure, attributed to purulent exudate, cerebral edema, and hydrocephalus. Seizures may develop as a result of irritation of the cerebral cortex.[65]

The clinical symptoms of viral meningitis are similar to those of bacterial meningitis: headache, mild photophobia, neck pain, and generalized malaise. However, the symptoms are considerably less severe with the viral form.[98]

COMPLICATIONS

Increased intracranial pressure (ICP)
Hydrocephalus
Cerebral infarction
Cranial nerve deficits
Encephalitis
Syndrome of inappropriate secretion of antidiuretic hormone (SIADH)
Brain abscess
Visual impairment
Deafness
Intellectual deficits
Seizures
Endocarditis
Pneumonia

Table 4-7

OVERVIEW OF MENINGITIS

	Meningococcal meningitis	Pneumococcal meningitis	Haemophilus meningitis	Viral meningitis
Microorganism	*Neisseria meningitidis*	*Streptococcus pneumoniae*	*Haemophilus influenzae*	Most viruses (mumps, polio, herpes)
Reservoir	Humans	Humans	Humans	Humans
Transmission	Direct contact with droplets from respiratory passages of infected persons and carriers	Direct and indirect contact with respiratory secretions	Direct contact with respiratory secretions	Not transmitted
Incubation period	2-10 days	1-3 days	2-4 days	Depends on virus
Period of communicability	Until organism is not present in secretions; within 24 h of antiinfective therapy	Until organism is not present in secretions; 24-48 h after antiinfective therapy	Prolonged; until organism is not present in secretions	Depends on virus

From Grimes.[60]

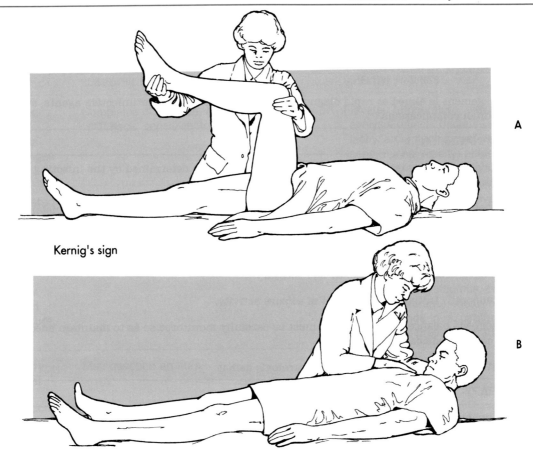

Kernig's sign

Brudzinski's sign

FIGURE 4-17
Kernig's and Brudzinski's signs are tests of meningeal irritation. **A,** Kernig's sign. Flex one of the patient's legs at the hip and knee, then straighten the knee. Note resistance or pain. **B,** Brudzinski's sign. With the patient recumbent, place your hands behind the patient's head and flex the neck forward. Note resistance or pain. Watch also for flexion of the patient's hips and knees in reaction to your maneuver.

DIAGNOSTIC STUDIES AND FINDINGS

Diagnostic Test	Findings	
	Bacterial	Viral
Lumbar Puncture		
Cerebrospinal fluid (CSF) appearance	Turbid	Clear
Leukocytes	500-20,000/mm^3	10-500/mm^3
Cell type	Neutrophils	Lymphocytes
Protein	Increased	Increased
Glucose	Decreased	Normal
Gram's stain	Positive for bacteria	Absence of bacteria
Blood cultures	Positive for *H. influenzae*	
	Positive for *N. meningitidis*	
Respiratory cultures	Positive for *H. influenzae*	
	Positive for *N. meningitidis*	
	Positive for *S. pneumoniae*	
Skull/sinus x-rays	May indicate original site of infection	
Computed tomography (CT)/magnetic resonance imaging (MRI) studies	May indicate hydrocephalus	

Brain Abscess

A **brain abscess** is a suppurative infection consisting of a collection of pus within the parenchyma of the brain.

The incidence of brain abscesses is site specific, depending on such factors as the size of the area and the amount of cerebral blood flow. As a result, 80% of abscesses are found in the cerebrum, and 20% are found in the cerebellum. Statistics indicate that 5% to 20% of brain abscesses occur in more than one site. The individual with a brain abscess presents a difficult clinical situation, since a 30% to 60% mortality is associated with the disorder. Surgical intervention may reduce the mortality, but this depends on the accessibility of the abscess and the patient's general condition. Morbidity after a brain abscess presents continued difficulties. Individuals surviving brain abscesses may experience different types of neurologic deficits, including paralysis and seizures.[29]

PATHOPHYSIOLOGY

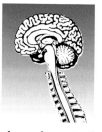

Most brain abscesses are caused by extension of chronic middle ear, sinus, or mastoid infections. The bacteria of these infections can invade the cranial vault directly through the bone, through the spinal dura mater, across the subdural and subarachnoid spaces, or along venous channels, as in the extension of a septic thrombophlebitis. Suppuration from the ear accounts for one third to one half of all brain abscesses and produces disease either in the ipsilateral cerebellar hemisphere or in the temporal lobe. Extended infections from the frontal sinuses primarily affect the anteroinferior parts of the frontal lobes. Sphenoidal sinusitis may extend to the frontal or temporal lobes, and ethmoid sinusitis may extend to the frontal lobes.[29]

Penetrating head injuries, compound skull fractures, and osteomyelitis of the skull also may lead to the formation of a brain abscess. Patients with right-to-left cardiac shunts are susceptible to the formation of brain abscesses because of polycythemia, which causes cerebral ischemia and necrosis. Patients with suppressed immune systems, particularly those with acquired immunodeficiency syndrome (AIDS), are particularly susceptible to brain abscesses.[29]

Organisms commonly isolated as the cause of brain abscesses include streptococci, aerobic Enterobacteriaceae, and the staphylococci. Anaerobic bacteria (e.g., *Bacteroides fragilis*) and aerobic Enterobacteriaceae (e.g., *Escherichia coli*, *Klebsiella* organisms) are found in suppurative ear infections. Anaerobic and microaerophilic streptococci, *Bacteroides*, *Fusobacterium*, and *Veillonella* species are found in suppurative lung infections. Staphylococci frequently are associated with penetrating head injuries and endocarditis. In the AIDS patient, *Toxoplasma gondii*, a protozoal organism, may cause brain abscesses.[29]

After the initial implantation of bacteria, a localized inflammatory reaction develops (e.g., cerebritis or encephalitis), which is characterized by local edema, hyperemia, leukocyte infiltration, and parenchymal softening. Several days to weeks after bacterial invasion of the brain tissue, central liquefaction and necrosis of brain tissue occur, producing a cystic mass of pus. The cystic mass is encapsulated by a wall of granulated tissue from migration of fibroblasts. Continued fibroblastic activity and gliosis result in replacement of granulation tissue of the abscess wall by collagenous connective tissues. The encapsulation process usually is completed within about 3 weeks (Figure 4-18).

CLINICAL MANIFESTATIONS

A severe headache is the most common early symptom of a brain abscess. This usually is accompanied by a low-grade temperature and nuchal rigidity. Confusion and lethargy may be evident.

Other symptoms are dictated by the size and location of the abscess and may be insidious in nature. Later clinical symptoms may include focal motor deficits and seizures. Edema of the surrounding tissue often is significant, resulting in rapidly elevating intracranial pressure (ICP) and brain herniation.

COMPLICATIONS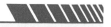

Altered mentation	Focal neurologic deficits
Paralysis	Hydrocephalus
Seizures	Brain herniation

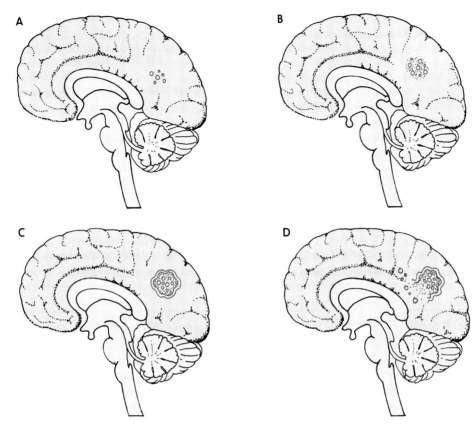

FIGURE 4-18
Brain abscess. **A,** Initial implantation of bacteria. **B,** Central liquefaction and necrosis, which form a cystic mass of pus. **C,** Cystic mass becomes encapsulated by collagenous connective tissue. **D,** Without treatment the encapsulated mass can break, spreading the infection.

DIAGNOSTIC STUDIES AND FINDINGS

Diagnostic Test	Findings	Diagnostic Test	Findings
X-rays: skull, sinuses, mastoid processes, chest	Helpful in locating associated suppurative processes	Brain scan	Locates abscesses over 1 cm in size; sensitive in early cerebritis when local alteration in permeability of blood-brain barrier can be visualized
Computed tomography (CT) scan	Locates well-formed and encapsulated abscesses and visualizes ventricle size and midline displacement	MRI study	Same as CT scan without radiation
		EEG	Marked slowing at sites of abscess
Lumbar puncture (Contraindication: May precipitate brain herniation if ICP is severely elevated.)	CSF results may show slight increase in pressure; increase in WBC; normal glucose; increased protein; CSF cultures may be nonspecific	Brain biopsy	Isolates pathogen

such as response to trauma or as a result of medical disorders such as cervical arthritis. Traction-inflammatory headaches may result from infection, intracranial or extracranial lesions, occlusive vascular disorders, diseases of facial structures, and medical disorders such as arteritis.[39]

PATHOPHYSIOLOGY

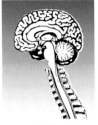 Headache pain can originate from an intracranial or extracranial source. Structures within the cranium that are sensitive to pain include the three divisions of the trigeminal nerve (cranial nerve V), the facial nerve (cranial nerve VII), the glossopharyngeal nerve (cranial nerve IX), the vagus nerve (cranial nerve X), and the first three cervical nerves, cranial blood vessels, venous sinuses, and the dura at the base of the brain. The skull, the brain tissue, most of the dura and pia-arachnoid, and the ventricular system are insensitive to pain.

Intracranial causes of headaches, such as mass lesions, cause pain through compression, inflammation, distortion, or traction of the venous sinuses, the large arteries at the base of the brain, the intracranial arteries, the pain-sensitive structures within the cranium, and the pain-sensitive cranial and cervical nerves.

Extracranial causes of headaches may be attributed to dilation and distortion of extracranial vessels. Other extracranial causes include muscle tension, sinusitis, dental abscess, mastoiditis, and eye and ear diseases.

VASCULAR HEADACHES
Migraine Headaches

There are several subdivisions of migraine headaches, including the classic migraine, the common migraine, and cluster headaches. Migraine headache generally begins in childhood, adolescence, or early adult life and is found in approximately 5% of the general population. It frequently is familial. Young women appear most susceptible, particularly just before or during the menstrual period. Migraine is characterized by a paroxysmal, throbbing, unilateral head pain that frequently is accompanied by autonomic symptoms such as nausea and vomiting. Attacks generally decrease in frequency and intensity with advancing age.

The exact pathogenesis of migraine is unknown. The initial physiologic change is that of vasospasm in the intracranial and extracranial arteries and their branches on one side of the head. Ten to 30 minutes later, the same vessels dilate. The constriction of the arteries is responsible for the symptoms of the aura, whereas vessel dilation produces the headache part of the syndrome. In headache-free intervals, the cranial vessels of the migraine patient are hypersensitive to inhalation of carbon dioxide and intravenously administered histamine.[116, 146]

Recent studies indicate that serotonin levels rise during the prodromal phase and drop during the headache phase. Also, the urinary excretion of 5-hydroxyindoleacetic acid (5-HIAA), a metabolite of serotonin, is increased during the migraine episodes. Platelet aggregability, which increases just before a migraine attack, is thought to be responsible for the release of serotonin.[76]

Agents and circumstances thought to precipitate migraine attacks include emotional stress and tension, menstruation, too much or too little sleep, and dietary agents such as tyramine, nitrate, and glutamate. However, none of these affect all individuals or consistently produce attacks in the same individual.[38] There is no evidence to support allergy or autonomic disorders as the cause of migraine attacks.

Cluster Headaches

Cluster headaches (Horton's syndrome, histamine headache, migrainous neuralgia, or paroxysmal nocturnal cephalalgia) are intense, repetitive vascular events. Cluster headaches are five times more common in men and generally occur in the third and fourth decades of life.[146] They are characterized by a distinct episode of excruciating pain, usually unilateral, which lasts from 30 minutes to 1 hour and is accompanied by ipsilateral lacrimation, nasal stuffiness, and drainage. Usually the same side of the head is involved in the cluster of attacks. There is no prodrome and usually only slight nausea. The attack may occur at any time (generally they are nocturnal), and multiple attacks are common.[146]

Headaches may occur in an episodic or chronic pattern. The episodic pattern of cluster headaches is characterized by recurring headaches for several weeks to months, followed by months to years during which no headaches occur.

Chronic cluster headaches are either primary or secondary in type. The primary chronic pattern is characterized by persistent, repetitive attacks for years at a time. The secondary chronic type occurs when the episodic attacks evolve into chronic, unremitting attacks.[38]

The exact mechanism of cluster headaches is unknown. Increased histamine with resultant vasodilation has been implicated.

TENSION HEADACHES
Muscle Contraction Headaches

Muscle contraction headaches are the most common type of head pain. Research studies indicate a preponderance of muscle contraction headaches in women and a higher incidence in adults from 20 to 40 years of age.

This type of headache usually is bilateral and may be diffuse or confined to the frontal, temporal, parietal, or occipital area. The onset of an attack is more gradual than with a migraine, and the duration varies considerably but may extend for several days up to several months or years.

Muscle contraction headaches frequently are accompanied by contraction of skeletal muscles of the face, jaw, and neck. Concurrent arterial vasodilation may contribute further to the discomfort. There are no structural changes in the involved muscle groups.

Traumatic Headaches

A posttraumatic, or postconcussion, headache, which consists of dull, generalized pain, may develop after a head injury and may be coupled with other symptoms such as lack of concentration, giddiness, or dizziness. The symptoms are much the same whether the head injury is mild or severe. Traumatic headaches usually are nonfocal, appear for at least part of every day, and persist over days, weeks, or months. The headache is aggravated by coughing or straining, which raises the pressure in both intracranial and extracranial venous systems. Posttraumatic headaches are thought to be caused by vascular dilation, muscle contraction, or direct injury to the scalp.

TRACTION-INFLAMMATORY HEADACHES
Traction Headaches

Traction headaches may result from increased intracranial pressure, cerebral hemorrhage, decreased intracranial pressure (e.g., lumbar puncture), and inflammatory processes (e.g., encephalitis, meningitis). The discomfort caused by traction headaches stems from referred pain, when the pain-sensitive structures (e.g., cranial nerves, arteries) are stretched or displaced by a mass lesion.

Temporal Arteritis

Temporal arteritis, also called cranial arteritis or giant cell arteritis, generally affects individuals over 60 years of age. This headache most often is located in the temporal area and may be accompanied by visual loss, which results from involvement of the ophthalmic artery. Temporal arteritis is thought to result from an autoimmune mechanism and is included in the group of collagen-vascular diseases. The temporal arteries may be palpated as firm, tender cords or may be seen as tortuous, enlarged vessels.[76]

CLINICAL MANIFESTATIONS

The symptoms of headaches vary according to the cause and type of headache (see Table 4-9).

Table 4-9

CLINICAL MANIFESTATIONS OF HEADACHES

Type	Pain	Location	Onset	Duration	Other
Classic migraine	Throbbing, high-intensity	Usually unilateral in temporal area, but may occur in any area of the head	Hours	Hours to days	Prodrome/aura: visual disturbances, sensory symptoms, mild paresis, nausea, vomiting
Common migraine	Throbbing, intense pain; progresses to generalized nonthrobbing pain	Usually frontal or temporal region	Gradual	Hours to days	No aura; nausea; vomiting
Cluster	Sudden, usually awaking patient at night	Orbitotemporal area Usually unilateral	Sudden	½ to 1 hour; occurs in clusters	No prodrome; lacrimation; rhinorrhea; nasal congestion; flushing of face; Horner's sign
Muscle contraction	Aching, tightness, or pressure	Suboccipital, occipital, frontal, temporal, parietal	Gradual	Hours to days (variable)	Muscle tension
Traumatic headaches	Dull, generalized pain	Varies	Gradual	Varies	Intensified by physical exertion; lack of concentration; dizziness
Traction headaches	Deep, dull, steady ache	Varies	Varies	Varies	Varies
Temporal arteritis	Variable intensity; unilateral or bilateral tenderness of painful area	Temporal, occipital, frontooccipital areas	Gradual	Hours to days	Visual loss

COMPLICATIONS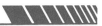

Chronic pain
Depression

DIAGNOSTIC STUDIES AND FINDINGS

Diagnostic Test	Findings	Diagnostic Test	Findings
Neurologic history and examination	Identifies precipitating influences; effects of activities of daily living (ADL); neurologic deficits	Provocative histamine test	Positive test indicates a vascular component to headache
Cervical and skull x-rays	Detects abnormalities at base of brain	CT scan	Possible intracranial lesions
Funduscopic eye examination	Possible irritation of iris and ciliary body	MRI study	Same as CT scan
Serum	Increased sedimentation rate; anemia (lithium serum level *not* to exceed 1 mEq/L)	Cerebral angiography	Detects vascular abnormalities

MEDICAL MANAGEMENT

GENERAL MANAGEMENT

Nutrition: Diet counseling to eliminate foods that may provoke headaches (e.g., vinegar, chocolate, pork, onions, sour cream, alcohol, excessive caffeine, citrus fruits, bananas, yogurt, figs, cheese, cured sandwich meats, chicken livers, broad bean pods, fermented or marinated foods, avocados, and MSG).[146]

Application of heat or cold to affected area.

Psychologic counseling: Behavioral modification, stress management, and biofeedback.

DRUG THERAPY

Drug therapy for migraine headaches is used for prophylactic treatment (Table 4-10), symptomatic treatment (Table 4-11), or both.

Analgesic/antiinflammatory agents: Ergot preparations (see Table 4-11).

Adrenergic agents: Isometheptene mucate (Midrin, Octinum).

Psychotherapeutic agents: Chlorpromazine (Thorazine); promethazine (Phenergan); hydroxyzine (Vistaril); lithium carbonate (Lithane).

Analgesic/antipyretics: Acetaminophen (Tylenol).

Narcotic analgesics: Meperidine (Demerol).

Glucocorticosteroids: Dexamethasone (Decadron).

Beta-adrenergic blocking agents: Propranolol (Inderal); methysergide maleate (Sansert).

Antihypertensive agents: Clonidine hydrochloride (Catapres).

Antianginal agents: Dipyridamole (Persantine).

Nonsteroidal antiinflammatory agents: Sulfinpyrazone (Anturane).

Antidepressants: Amitriptyline (Elavil); imipramine (Tofranil); desipramine (Norpramin).

Table 4-10

PROPHYLATIC MEDICATIONS FOR MIGRAINE HEADACHES[146]

Medication	Dosage	Medication	Dosage
Beta blockers		**Nonsteroidal antiinflammatory agents**	
Propranol (Inderal)	40 mg tid-qid	Naproxen (Anaprox)	550 mg bid with meals
Methysergide maleate (Sansert)	2 mg tid with meals		
Tricyclic antidepressants		**Calcium channel blockers**	
Amitriptyline (Elavil)	10-100 mg qhs	Verapamil (Calan, Isoptin)	80 mg tid-qid
Imipramine (Tofranil)	10-75 mg in divided doses	**Monoamine oxidase inhibitors**	
Desipramine (Norpramin)	25-75 mg in divided doses	Phenelzine sulfate (Nardil)	15 mg tid-qid

Table 4-11

SYMPTOMATIC MEDICATIONS FOR MIGRAINE HEADACHES[146]

Medication	Dosage
Ergotamine tartrate (Ergostat, Ergomar)	1 tablet sublingual at onset of migraine; may repeat in 20-30 min Maximum dosage: 3 tablets/24 h 6 tablets/wk
Ergotamine tartrate with caffeine (Cafergot)	Tablets: 1-2 PO at onset of headache, may repeat 1 tablet in 30 min Maximum dosage: 6 tablets/24 h 12 tablets/wk Suppository: 1 at onset of migraine; may repeat in 1 h Maximum dosage: 2 suppositories/24 h 5 suppositories/wk
Isometheptene/dichloralphenazone/ acetaminophen (Midrin)	2 capsules at onset of migraine; may repeat 1 capsule in 1 h Maximum dosage: 5 capsules/12 h
Naproxen sodium (Anaprox)	275 mg tablets: 3 tablets at onset, may repeat 2 tablets in 1 h Maximum dosage: 5 tablets/24 h

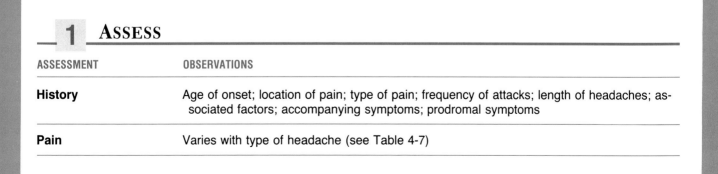

1 ASSESS

ASSESSMENT	OBSERVATIONS
History	Age of onset; location of pain; type of pain; frequency of attacks; length of headaches; associated factors; accompanying symptoms; prodromal symptoms
Pain	Varies with type of headache (see Table 4-7)

ASSESSMENT	OBSERVATIONS
Neurologic	Focal neurologic signs; visual field deficits; ophthalmoplegia; carotid/orbital bruits; Horner's syndrome
Other	Sinusitis; dental abscess; ear infection; nausea; vomiting
Psychosocial	Irritability; apathy; depression

2 DIAGNOSE

NURSING DIAGNOSIS	SUBJECTIVE FINDINGS	OBJECTIVE FINDINGS
Pain related to severe headache	Complains of severe, intense pain	Grimacing; crying; photophobia (variable); elevated BP and heart rate; nuchal rigidity; muscle tension; restlessness
Ineffective individual coping related to severe pain and altered life-style	Reports feelings of helplessness, anxiety	Anxiety; irritability

Other related nursing diagnosis: Sleep-pattern disturbance related to insomnia and/or awakening from pain.

3 PLAN

Patient goals

1. The patient will demonstrate an improved comfort level.

2. The patient will demonstrate effective coping.

4 IMPLEMENT

NURSING DIAGNOSIS	NURSING INTERVENTIONS	RATIONALE
Pain related to severe headache	Assess and document prodromal symptoms, degree of pain, location, duration, and associated symptoms.	Prodromal symptoms often precede migraine headaches; drug therapy trial may be prescribed on basis of patient's pain history.
	Instruct patient to report pain immediately.	Medication administered immediately upon onset of pain may reduce severity of attack.
	Promote rest and relaxation in quiet environment; decrease noxious stimuli.	To promote comfort.
	Massage head and neck if patient can tolerate it.	To promote relaxation and reduce muscle tension.

NURSING DIAGNOSIS	NURSING INTERVENTIONS	RATIONALE
	Apply cold compresses or dry heat to head and neck.	Applying cold compresses can cause vaso-dilation, which can reduce pain in vascular headache; heat can increase circulation and reduce muscle tension.
	Encourage patient to investigate alternative pain therapies: biofeedback, therapeutic touch.	Many headache patients have found these methods helpful.
	Administer drug therapy as prescribed, and document response.	Drug therapy must be given as prescribed to maintain effectiveness (often prescribed based on the patient's response).
Ineffective individual coping related to severe pain and altered life-style	Assess patient's behavior and response to condition.	Patients with severe headache often have to make life-style changes that may elicit feelings of grief, anger, and depression.
	Assess patient's coping mechanisms; discuss how patient copes with condition.	To determine effectiveness of coping behaviors.
	Encourage patient to express fears and concerns.	To promote a therapeutic relationship; talking about feelings can decrease anxiety.
	Offer patient support, and provide her with accurate, realistic information.	To facilitate patient's knowledge of treatment and reduce feelings of powerlessness.
Knowledge deficit	See Patient Teaching.	

5 EVALUATE

PATIENT OUTCOME	DATA INDICATING THAT OUTCOME IS REACHED
Patient's pain has been relieved.	The patient openly talks about feelings of discomfort when they occur and can use measures to decrease discomfort; the patient confirms a decrease in subjective feelings of discomfort, and objective findings of pain are decreased.
Patient demonstrates effective coping mechanisms.	The patient openly expresses concerns and feelings of grief and discomfort and identifies effective coping behaviors to deal with pain and anxiety.

PATIENT TEACHING

1. Review the patient's pain history, encouraging the patient to identify any triggering factors that can be avoided.
2. Teach the patient the names of medication, dosage, time of administration, and side effects; reinforce the necessity of taking drugs exactly as prescribed.
3. Stress need to avoid over-the-counter medications.
4. Review the patient's dietary limitations.
5. Encourage patient to keep a "headache diary" to document relationships between activities, emotions, drugs, and life-style and patient's headaches.

Peripheral Nervous System Disorders

Myasthenia Gravis

Myasthenia gravis is a neuromuscular disease characterized by abnormal weakness of voluntary muscles that improves with rest and the administration of anticholinesterase drugs.[34]

The voluntary muscles most commonly affected in myasthenia gravis are the oculomotor, facial, laryngeal, pharyngeal, and respiratory muscles. The severity of the disease varies; at its most extreme, it may result in severe muscular weakness and respiratory failure, a phenomenon known as crisis.[34]

The cause of myasthenia gravis is unknown, although considerable data suggest that it is a systemic autoimmune disease. Myasthenia gravis is not a hereditary condition, but 12% of infants born to myasthenic mothers manifest transitory symptoms lasting from 7 to 14 days after birth.[126] The incidence of myasthenia gravis is 3 to 6 per 100,000 individuals. The two characteristic ages of onset are between 20 and 30 years of age, and late middle age. When the disorder begins in the second or third decade, women are more commonly affected than men. When the disorder begins in late middle age, both sexes are equally affected.[126] Epidemiologic studies have not produced any specific socioeconomic or racial factors.

PATHOPHYSIOLOGY

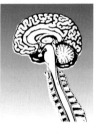

The basic physiologic defect in myasthenia gravis is the inability of nerve impulses to pass onto the skeletal muscle at the neuromuscular junction. The problem occurs at the neuromuscular junction, specifically the postsynaptic membrane. Studies of myasthenic muscles demonstrate a 70% to 89% reduction in the number of acetylcholine receptors per neuromuscular junction.[109] Research findings suggest that an anti-receptor antibody is responsible for this phenomenon, and 85% to 90% of myasthenic patients have serum anti-receptor antibody titers.[126] Thus it is believed that the reduced numbers of receptor sites result in diminished muscle depolarization, with the clinical symptoms of muscle weakness.

The specific role of the immune system in the development of myasthenia gravis is still the subject of much debate. Studies of the thymus gland of myasthenic patients have found pathologic changes in 75% of these individuals. Within this group, 85% show thymic hyperplasia and 15% have thymomas.[34]

CLINICAL MANIFESTATIONS

The clinical symptoms of myasthenia gravis may vary from patient to patient. Often the initial signs are intermittent double vision (diplopia) and droopy eyelids (ptosis). If symptoms do not progress beyond this state, the diagnosis of "ocular myasthenia gravis" is given.[34]

Many patients begin to develop facial weakness, as well as difficulty chewing, swallowing, and speaking. Weakness of the neck and limbs frequently develops later. Patients often complain of not being able to climb stairs or perform activities of daily living. Generally, symptoms are evident upon awakening in the morning and grow more prominent throughout the day. Myasthenia gravis often is distinguished by its high degree of variability, with notable fluctuation in strength from day to day. Remissions and exacerbations may occur frequently.[34]

In severe cases palatal and pharyngeal muscle weakness compromises the patient's ability to handle oral secretions, placing the patient at high risk for aspiration pneumonia. Weakness of the neck muscles interferes with the patient's ability to elevate and support the head. Compromise of the diaphragm and intercostal muscles may result in diminished ventilatory capacity.[34]

In myasthenia gravis, *crisis* is a term used to describe a rapid decline in neuromuscular function with marked weakness of the respiratory muscles. Crisis can be dramatic and can have life-threatening consequences. In the myasthenic patient, crisis may be of two types, *"myasthenic"* or *"cholinergic."* *"Myasthenic crisis"* is caused by an insufficiency of acetylcholine and often is induced by a change in or withdrawal of medication, emotional and physical stress, infection, or surgery. *"Cholinergic crisis"* is caused by an excess of acetylcholine, usually as a result of drug overdosage.

Paradoxically, the symptoms of myasthenic and cholinergic crises are very similar (see box). In both cases acute weakness of respiratory muscles, generalized muscle weakness, apprehension, and restlessness occur. It is difficult to distinguish between the two conditions by physical examination alone; the diagnosis often is confirmed by the patient's recent history of anticholinesterase use and the Tensilon test. In the case of myasthenic crisis, the edrophonium chloride (Tensilon) test response is positive; in cholinergic crisis, the response is negative. [34,78]

COMPLICATIONS

Myasthenic crisis
Cholinergic crisis
Pneumonia
Sepsis
Complications related to immobility

SIGNS AND SYMPTOMS OF MYASTHENIC AND CHOLINERGIC CRISES

Myasthenic crisis	Cholinergic crisis
Increased blood pressure	Decreased blood pressure
Tachycardia	Bradycardia
Restlessness	Restlessness
Apprehension	Apprehension
Increased bronchial secretions, lacrimation, and sweating	Increased bronchial secretions, lacrimation, and sweating
Generalized muscle weakness	Generalized muscle weakness
Absent cough reflex	Fasciculations
Dyspnea	Dyspnea
Difficulty swallowing	Difficulty swallowing
Difficulty speaking	Difficulty speaking
	Blurred vision
	Nausea and vomiting
	Abdominal cramps and diarrhea

From Chipps.[34]

DIAGNOSTIC STUDIES AND FINDINGS

Diagnostic Test	Findings
Chest x-ray, computed tomography (CT) scan of chest	May indicate presence of thymoma
Edrophonium chloride (Tensilon) test	2 mg of edrophonium chloride (Tensilon) is injected intravenously; if no symptoms develop, an additional 8 mg is injected, and the patient is observed for improvement in muscle tone; in 30 seconds to 1 minute, patients with myasthenia gravis demonstrate marked improvement in muscle tone that lasts 4 to 5 minutes
Electromyogram	Muscle fiber contraction with progressive decremental response
Serum anti-ACHR antibody titer	May be elevated

MEDICAL MANAGEMENT

Modern treatment has significantly improved the prognosis of patients with myasthenia gravis. However, medical management of the disorder is still difficult.

GENERAL MANAGEMENT

Plasmapheresis (The process of separating blood into component parts so that circulating anti-acetylcholine receptor antibodies can be removed): Blood is withdrawn by a venous catheter and anticoagulated. The blood is then circulated through a cell separator, and the plasma, which contains anti-acetylcholine receptor antibodies, is removed. The blood is replaced with donor plasma or another colloidal substance, which is returned via venous access to the patient (see Plasmapheresis, page 268).

Physical activity: Continuous monitoring of muscle strength with planned periods of rest and activity.

Mechanical ventilation: May be indicated in the event of respiratory failure secondary to either myasthenic or cholinergic crisis.

Nutrition: If dysphagia is severe, tube feeding may be indicated.

DRUG THERAPY

Anticholinesterase drugs: (These drugs are the mainstay of medical treatment. The optimum dose often is achieved through trial and error, since a single, fixed-dose schedule may not benefit all patients. The drugs must be given promptly, because delay may leave the patient too weak to swallow.) Neostigmine (Prostigmin), pyridostigmine (Mestinon), ambenonium chloride (Mytelase).

Corticosteroids: Prednisone.

Immunosuppressive agents: Azathioprine (Imuran), cyclophosphamide (Cytoxan).

SURGERY

Thymectomy (surgical removal of the thymus gland):   The mechanism by which the thymectomy reduces clinical symptoms is unclear. Controversy exists regarding the indication for a thymectomy.

1 ASSESS

ASSESSMENT	OBSERVATIONS
Eye muscles	Diplopia; ptosis; ocular palsy
Facial muscles	Masklike expression or facial weakness; weak, nasal voice that may fade; dysphagia and choking; drooling
Neck muscles	Difficulty maintaining head position
Respiratory muscles	Breathlessness; shortness of breath; respiratory failure with reduced tidal volume and vital capacity; weak, ineffective cough
Other muscles	Skeletal muscle weakness of trunk and extremities
Nutrition	Difficulty swallowing selected foods; weight loss
Psychosocial effects	Anxiety; fear of breathlessness

→ > >

6. Emphasize the need to wear a medical alert tag.
7. Stress the importance of avoiding individuals with an upper respiratory infection.
8. Teach the patient the symptoms of upper respiratory infection to report to the physician (i.e., chills, cough, low-grade fever).
9. Stress the need to avoid alcohol, tobacco, and prolonged exposure to heat or cold.
10. Emphasize the need for adequate nutrition:
    a. Give diet as tolerated.
    b. Arrange food and utensils so they can be managed more easily.
    c. Cut food into small pieces, chew thoroughly, and eat slowly.
11. Stress the need for activity and exercise as the patient is able:
    a. Plan activities of daily living.

b. Maintain rest periods as planned.
c. Do active and passive range-of-motion exercises.
d. Get at least 8 hours of sleep at night.
12. Encourage use of an eye patch if double vision is a problem.
13. Stress the need for diversional activities.
14. Emphasize the importance of avoiding physical and emotional stress.
15. Emphasize the need for speech therapy.
16. Stress the importance of avoiding constipation.
17. Emphasize the importance of ongoing outpatient care.
18. Provide information on available agencies (e.g., Myasthenia Gravis Foundation).
19. Give outpatient or home nursing care referrals.

Guillain-Barré Syndrome

Guillain-Barré syndrome is an acute syndrome characterized by widespread inflammation or demyelination of ascending or descending nerves in the peripheral nervous system.

Guillain-Barré syndrome has an incidence of 0.62 to 1.9 per 100,000 persons.[126] Of those affected by Guillain-Barré syndrome, 85% have complete functional recovery. The recovery period usually lasts several weeks, but it may last months or even years. The remaining 15% of affected individuals have some degree of permanent neurologic deficit.

Guillain-Barré syndrome is also known as acute idiopathic polyneuritis, acute polyradiculoneuropathy, postinfectious polyneuritis, Landry-Guillain-Barré-Strohl syndrome, infectious neuronitis, infectious polyneuritis, acute polyradiculitis, acute idiopathic polyradiculoneuritis, and acute inflammatory polyradiculoneuropathy.

The exact cause of Guillain-Barré syndrome is not known. However, more than half of those affected have had a nonspecific infection 10 to 14 days before the onset of Guillain-Barré symptoms, suggesting that sensitized lymphocytes may produce demyelination. A significant number of people have developed symptoms characteristic of Guillain-Barré syndrome after being inoculated for the swine flu. The syndrome occurs in both sexes and can affect people of any age.

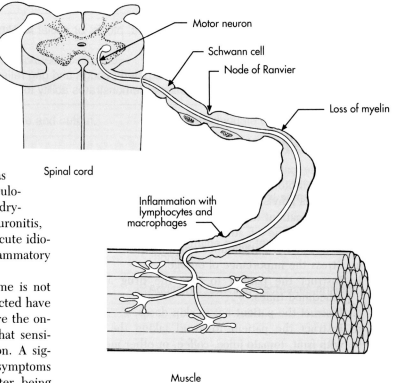

FIGURE 5-1
Demyelination of nerve segments in Guillain-Barré syndrome.

PATHOPHYSIOLOGY

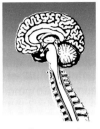

The pathogenesis of Guillain-Barré syndrome is thought to be caused by a cell-mediated immunologic reaction occurring on the peripheral nerves. The disease affects the peripheral nervous system and can involve both spinal and cranial nerves.[98]

The myelin sheaths surrounding the peripheral nerves are responsible for insulating these nerves. The spaces between the myelin sheaths, called the nodes of Ranvier, facilitate rapid conduction of nerve impulses.

It is hypothesized that lymphocytes migrate into areas adjacent to the nerve and attach to the myelin sheath. A local inflammatory response ensues, which alters the myelin sheath protein. This causes demyelination of nerve segments, resulting in delay in nerve conduction[98,117,127] (Figure 5-1).

Most patients recover completely over several weeks to months. Interestingly, recovery of function often mimics the steplike fashion of function loss. Recovery is attributed to regeneration of peripheral nerves.

CLINICAL MANIFESTATIONS

A thorough history usually reveals a recent nonspecific infection. The severity of symptoms may vary from patient to patient. However, most patients report a lower extremity weakness that can progress in an ascending pattern to the upper extremities and face. Complete flaccid paralysis with respiratory failure can occur within 48 hours. The paralysis usually is symmetric in nature and can progress for 2 to 3 weeks. Paresthesia may accompany the paralysis. Sensory loss may occur, but it generally is less common than motor loss. Involvement of cranial nerves VII (facial), IX (glossopharyngeal), X (vagus), XI (spinal accessory), and XII (hypoglossal) may cause facial weakness, dysphagia, and laryngeal paralysis.[127]

Autonomic dysfunction stemming from involvement of the sympathetic and parasympathetic nervous systems may cause hypertension, hypotension, dysrhythmias, and circulatory collapse. Respiratory failure can occur secondary to paralysis of respiratory muscles.[127]

COMPLICATIONS

Cardiac failure
Respiratory failure
Infection and sepsis
Venous thrombosis
Pulmonary embolus
Syndrome of inappropriate secretion of antidiuretic hormone (SIADH)

DIAGNOSTIC STUDIES AND FINDINGS

Diagnostic Test	Findings
Cerebrospinal fluid sampling	Albuminocytologic dissociation: decreased protein initially (15-45 mg), then increases as high as 600 mg, followed by return to normal Lymphocyte count normal
Electromyography	Reduced nerve conduction velocity when tested near peak of illness (usually 4-8 wk after onset); low voltage potentials; fibrillations and positive sharp waves (more common in late stages)
Pulmonary function tests	Below patient's anticipated baseline for height and weight

MEDICAL MANAGEMENT

There is no definitive cure. Medical management focuses on preventing the complications of immobility, infection, and respiratory failure.

GENERAL MANAGEMENT

Respiratory care: Directed at anticipation and recognition of respiratory failure. Mechanical ventilation may be necessary. Vital capacity should be measured at the bedside q 2 h during the acute period. A vital capacity < 15 ml/kg may indicate the need for assisted ventilation. Arterial blood gases should be drawn with any clinical change in respiratory status.

Herniated Intervertebral Disk

A herniated intervertebral disk is one in which the gelatinous substance (nucleus pulposus) has protruded through the fibrocartilaginous substance (anulus fibrosus).[127]

The herniation of the intervertebral disk is a major cause of chronic back pain. Intervertebral disk disease is most common in the lumbar region, followed by the cervical region. These two regions are the most flexible areas of the spine and the most susceptible to injury. Most lumbar disk disorders develop at the L4 to L5 to S1 levels. The C6 to C7 and C5 to C6 levels are the most commonly affected cervical regions. Thoracic herniations are relatively rare. Disk disease is more common in men than in women, and most patients with disk disease are 30 to 50 years of age.[65]

PATHOPHYSIOLOGY

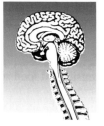

A herniated intervertebral disk often results from trauma, degenerative disk disease, or a combination of both. The intervertebral disk consists of three parts: the nucleus pulposus, the anulus fibrosus, and the cartilaginous endplates. The nucleus pulposus is a gelatinous mass that is surrounded by an outer laminated fibrocartilaginous structure, the anulus fibrosus. The anulus fibrosus holds the vertebral bodies together and is attached to the vertebral body, the cartilage endplates, and the vertebral ligaments.

The intervertebral disk begins to lose its hydraulic and elastic properties with age as a result of decreases in collagen fibers and the water content of the nucleus. In the normal disk, the nucleus can accommodate a wide variety of movements and high-compression loads. With age and degeneration of the disk, the nucleus cannot tolerate and absorb stress. As the nucleus begins to weaken with sufficient stress, the nucleus ruptures through the anulus fibrosus (Figure 5-2). Often herniation of the disk is precipitated by minor traumatic movements such as twisting, bending, sneezing, or coughing.

CLINICAL MANIFESTATIONS

Neurologic symptoms result from compression of the spinal cord or spinal nerve roots or both. Symptoms reflect the nerve or nerves affected.

Most herniated disks occur in the lumbar region. Pain is the most characteristic symptom, generally in the lower back with radiation to the buttocks, thigh, and leg. The pain often is aggravated by lifting and twisting and may vary in intensity, causing mild to se-

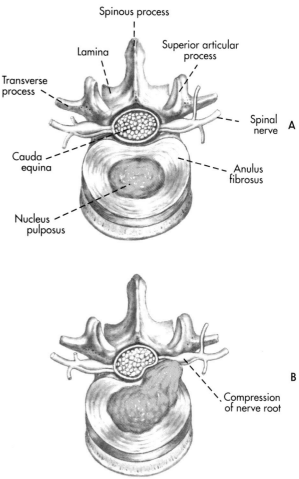

FIGURE 5-2
A, Normal intervertebral disk of lumbar vertebra. B, Herniation of nucleus pulposus.

vere discomfort. Normal lumbar lordosis may be absent, and one iliac crest may be elevated. Abnormal posture may be evident as a mechanism to compensate for discomfort. The gait often is stiff. Mild motor weakness of the foot, hamstring, and quadriceps muscles may be evident. Urinary and bowel elimination and sexual functioning also may be altered. Sensory impairments may include paresthesia and numbness of the leg and foot, and ankle and knee reflexes may be diminished.[65]

A herniated intervertebral disk in the cervical region results in pain in the neck, shoulders, and upper arm. Weakness and paresthesia may be evident.[86]

COMPLICATIONS

Motor weakness
Sensory loss
Loss of sexual function
Bowel and bladder incontinence

DIAGNOSTIC STUDIES AND FINDINGS

Diagnostic test	Findings
Spinal x-rays	May reveal narrowing of disk space (evident only in 50% of patients) and degenerative changes
Myelography	Reveals presence of herniated disk and level of herniation
Cerebrospinal fluid analysis	Protein levels may be elevated
Queckenstedt's test	May reveal partial or complete blockage of CSF in spinal subarachnoid space
Electromyography	May reveal neural or muscle damage; may indicate specific nerve root affected
Discography	May reveal herniation of specific disk (use is controversial)
Computed tomography (CT)	Reveals herniated disk
Magnetic resonance imaging (MRI)	Reveals herniated disk

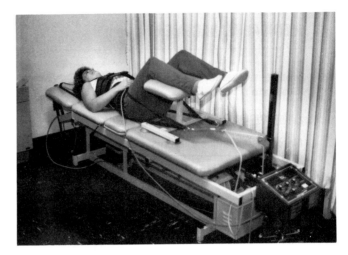

FIGURE 5-3
Patient positioned in pelvic traction.

MEDICAL MANAGEMENT

GENERAL MANAGEMENT

Treatment follows two approaches: initial treatment is conservative, aimed at rest and reducing stress; if conservative treatment is unsuccessful, surgery may be indicated.

Bed rest: Periods of bed rest on a firm mattress or back board in semi-Fowler's position with knees slightly flexed. This relieves compression of nerve roots and minimizes spinal flexion.

Physical therapy: An extensive exercise program is prescribed to strengthen back and abdominal muscles. This is begun after acute symptoms have subsided.

Traction: Used to increase the intervertebral space, which relieves spasm. Pelvic traction: A canvas girdle is applied to pelvis and hips. Straps are attached to girdle, and weights are attached (Figure 5-3). Cervical halter traction: A canvas sling is placed under the chin and occiput. Straps attached to the sling are attached to a pulley and weight system. Gravity lumbar traction: Patient is placed in a chest harness, which is attached to a CircOlectric bed. The bed is elevated gradually, and traction is applied by means of the patient's own weight. Cervical collar: Supports the neck in a neutral or slightly flexed position.

Nutrition: Weight loss or weight control is recommended.

SURGERY (SEE ALSO SPINAL SURGERY, page 245)

Laminectomy: Removal of vertebral lamina and degenerated disk, thus removing pressure on nerve root.

Lumbar/cervical microdiscectomies: Removal of degenerated disk using microsurgical techniques.

Spinal fusion: Performed to stabilize a vertebral column. Disk material is removed between two vertebral bodies, and a bone graft taken from the iliac crest is inserted between the vertebrae.

DRUG THERAPY

Analgesics: Aspirin, acetaminophen.

2 DIAGNOSE

NURSING DIAGNOSIS	SUBJECTIVE FINDINGS	OBJECTIVE FINDINGS
Pain related to damage to cranial nerve VII	Complains of severe pain in facial area	Increased heart rate and blood pressure; facial grimacing (may not be evident because of paralysis); guarding of facial muscles; restlessness
Potential for injury related to inability to close eyes	Complains of dry, sore eyes	Inability to close eyes completely; red eyes; corneal ulceration
Potential altered nutrition: less than body requirements related to inability to chew, sip, and loss of taste	Complains of inability to chew, sip, and taste	Weight loss; loss of interest in food

Other related nursing diagnosis: Body image disturbance related to onset of facial paralysis

3 PLAN

Patient goals

1. The patient will have no pain or discomfort.
2. The patient will have no eye injury.

3. The patient will maintain adequate nutrition.

4 IMPLEMENT

NURSING DIAGNOSIS	NURSING INTERVENTIONS	RATIONALE
Pain related to damage to cranial nerve VII	Establish baseline of patient's perception of discomfort.	To determine the patient's perception of the pain.
	Provide gentle massage as needed.	To relieve pain and promote relaxation.
	Provide electrical stimulation per protocol.	To relieve severe pain.
	Apply facial sling as needed.	To prevent muscle stretching and facilitate eating.
	Teach the patient to perform facial exercises three to four times daily for 5 minutes: wrinkling brow, grimacing, whistling, puffing out cheeks, forcing eyes closed.	To promote muscle tone.
	Administer pain medication as prescribed.	To relieve pain.
Potential for injury related to inability to close eyes	Assess eyes for muscle paralysis, dryness, excessive tearing, and ulcerations.	To establish the extent of eye involvement.
	Provide eye care with artificial tears or lubricants q 1-2 h or prn.	To prevent cornea from drying and injury.

NURSING DIAGNOSIS	NURSING INTERVENTIONS	RATIONALE
	Apply eye pads as needed.	To prevent injury and minimize eye strain.
	Provide patient with sunglasses.	To prevent eye strain.
Potential altered nutrition: less than body requirements related to inability to chew, sip, and taste	Assess patient's ability to chew and swallow.	To determine extent of facial paralysis.
	Offer patient frequent small meals.	To assure adequate caloric intake.
	Provide soft diet as needed.	To minimize choking.
	Avoid hot foods and fluids.	To prevent burns to insensitive areas.
	Provide patient adequate privacy and time for meals.	To minimize anxiety and embarrassment.
	Apply facial sling.	To improve lip alignment.
	Teach the patient to take foods on unaffected side.	Saliva and food can collect on paralyzed side.
Knowledge deficit	See Patient Teaching.	

5 EVALUATE

PATIENT OUTCOME	DATA INDICATING THAT OUTCOME IS REACHED
The patient has minimum discomfort.	The patient can use measures such as a facial sling and warm massage as needed; the patient openly expresses feelings of discomfort when they occur; the patient can perform facial exercises as indicated.
The patient has no eye injury.	The patient's eyes remain clear and white, and she can open and close her eyes adequately.
The patient demonstrates adequate nutritional status.	The patient's weight pattern is stable: normal for height, age, sex, and previous baseline; intake and output are balanced and stable; diet is appropriate to age; skin turgor is good; fluid and electrolyte balance is maintained, and dietary supplements are used as appropriate.

PATIENT TEACHING

1. Instruct the patient in the possible causes, involvement, symptoms, treatments, and usual course of Bell's palsy (explain procedures as they occur).
2. Teach the patient the signs of complications and progression of the disorder.
3. Teach the patient special techniques such as using facial slings, massage, dietary adjustments, and exercises to minimize discomfort.
4. Stress the importance of continued eye care.
5. Teach the patient safety measures for minimizing trauma to insensitive areas.
6. Teach the patient the names of medications, dosage, frequency of administration, purpose, and side effects.
7. Stress the importance of ongoing outpatient care: physician's visits, physical therapy and exercise programs, and support groups.

CHAPTER 6

Surgical and Therapeutic Interventions

Cranial Surgery

CRANIOTOMY

A **craniotomy** is a neurosurgical procedure in which an opening is made into the cranium. The skull is opened, and a flap is made by leaving the bone attached to the muscle (Figure 6-1). The dura mater is excised, exposing the brain tissue. After the intended treatment has been completed, closing is done in layers (i.e., dura, muscles, fascia, galea, and scalp). A turban dressing is wrapped tightly around the head, and a Hemovac-type drain may be inserted to prevent or remove fluid accumulation under the skin (Figure 6-2).[89] Craniotomies can be classified into two major categories, supratentorial and infratentorial. A **supratentorial craniotomy** involves brain structures above the tentorium, including the frontal, temporal, parietal, and occipital lobes. The incision is made behind the hairline. An **infratentorial craniotomy** involves structures below the tentorium, including the cerebellum. The incision is made slightly above the neck. If part of the cranium is removed and not replaced (i.e., to provide decompression from cerebral edema), the procedure is called a **craniectomy.**

STEREOTAXIC SURGERY

Stereotaxic surgery has greatly advanced the practice of neurosurgery by allowing precise location of brain lesions previously considered surgically inaccessible (Figure 6-3). The physical principle in stereotaxic surgery is locating a point in space and defining its position with respect to a frame of reference. Stereotaxic surgery usually is performed on an outpatient basis using local anesthesia, primarily for tumor biopsy, ablative procedures, or implantation of radiotherapeutic devices. A stereotaxic frame with well-defined reference points is attached to the head. A computed tomography (CT) scan is performed, and the lesion is visualized. A computer calculates the lesion's location with respect to the stereotaxic frame, and the incision is marked. A local anesthetic is injected, a burr hole is made, and the dura mater is exposed. Thereafter the prescribed treatment is performed.[80,94,101]

BURR HOLES

A burr hole is a hole made in the skull with a twist drill (Figure 6-1, *A*). Burr holes often are made as an emergency procedure to evacuate a clot or when placing a probe to monitor intracranial pressure.

CRANIOPLASTY

Cranioplasty is the insertion of a synthetic material into the cranium to replace cranial bone that has been removed. This may be done to protect the integrity of the brain or for cosmetic purposes.

INDICATIONS (FOR CRANIOTOMY)

Tumor removal
Vascular surgery
Hydrocephalus
Tumor or lesion biopsy
Repair of cerebral injury

CONTRAINDICATIONS (FOR CRANIOTOMY)

Poor surgical or anesthesia risk

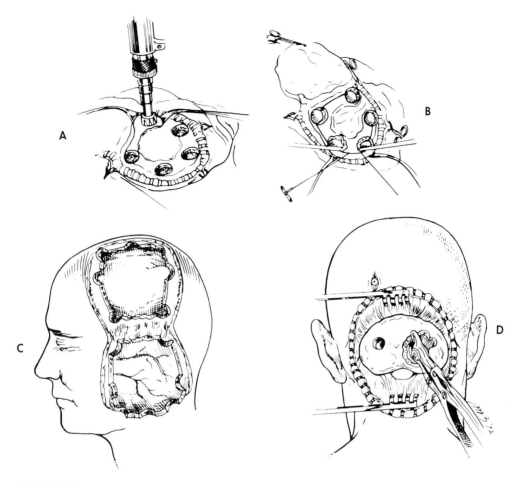

FIGURE 6-1
Techniques of cranial surgery. **A,** Drilling burr holes. **B,** Using Gigli's saw. **C,** Bone flap turned down.
D, Modification for infratentorial craniotomy. (From Barber et al.[16])

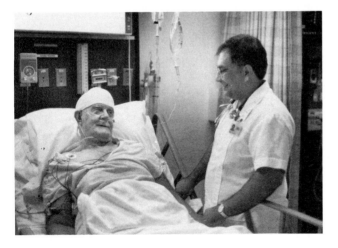

FIGURE 6-2
Postcraniotomy patient with turban placed on head.

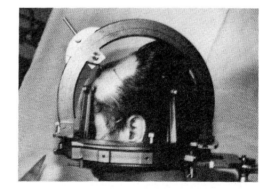

FIGURE 6-3
Stereotaxic frame used for precise location of intracranial lesions and for diagnostic and therapeutic procedures. (Courtesy Radionics, Inc., Burlington, Mass.)

COMPLICATIONS (AFTER CRANIOTOMY)

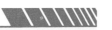

Increased intracranial pressure
Vasospasm
Cerebral infarction
Hydrocephalus
Pneumonia
Pulmonary embolism
Wound infection
Meningitis
Diabetes insipidus
Syndrome of inappropriate secretion of antidiuretic hormone (SIADH)
Seizures
Cranial nerve damage

PREPROCEDURAL NURSING CARE

1. Initiate preoperative instruction for the patient and family:
   a. Explain the purpose and procedure for shaving the patient's head (this is usually done in the operating room).
   b. Explain or review the neurosurgical procedure and postoperative course.
   c. Discuss suggestions for covering the head after surgery.
   d. Teach the patient deep breathing exercises.
   e. Discuss the critical care environment.
   f. Encourage the patient and family to express their fears and concerns.
2. Check operative permission form.
3. Document the patient's baseline neurologic status and all other medical or physical problems.
4. Withhold food and water the night before surgery.
5. Remove all jewelry, glasses, contact lenses, and false teeth.
6. Insert IV line.
7. Administer preoperative medications.

MEDICAL MANAGEMENT

GENERAL MANAGEMENT

Immediate postoperative period: 24-h intensive care monitoring

Hemodynamic and cardiac monitoring: evaluate cardiac rhythm and fluid status. Respiratory: mechanical ventilation may be used if surgical procedure was extensive, level of consciousness is altered, and hyperventilation is necessary. Fluid management: slight state of dehydration is maintained to reduce cerebral edema. Wound care: monitor for excessive drainage; head dressing is wrapped tightly and remains in place for 2-3 days. Laboratory studies: serum electrolytes and CBC are monitored frequently. Physical activity: bed rest. Supratentorial craniotomy: head of bed is kept at 30- to 45-degree angle. Infratentorial craniectomy: head of bed is kept flat or up to a 20-degree angle.

Ongoing postoperative care
Diet: advanced as tolerated. Physical activity: advanced as tolerated. Physical and speech therapy: as needed.

DRUG THERAPY

Preoperative

Anticonvulsants: Phenytoin (Dilantin), may be given preoperatively to patients undergoing supratentorial surgery. Corticosteroids: Dexamethasone (Decadron), methylprednisolone (Medrol).

Postoperative

Corticosteroids: Dexamethasone (Decadron), methylprednisolone (Medrol). Anticonvulsants: Phenytoin (Dilantin), given to patients who have had supratentorial surgery. Stool softeners: Docusate sodium (Colace). H_2 histamine-blocking agent: Cimetidine (Tagamet). Antacids: Magnesium hydroxide (Maalox). Antiinfective agents: Organism specific. Osmotic diuretic (to reduce cerebral edema): Mannitol, IV. Agents used to treat diabetes insipidus: Vasopressin (Pitressin), desmopressin acetate (DDAVP).

1 ASSESS

ASSESSMENT	OBSERVATIONS
Increased intracranial pressure	Restlessness, lethargy; changes in level of consciousness; changes in vital signs (i.e., Cushing's response with increased systolic blood pressure, widening pulse pressure, and decreased pulse rate); pupillary changes; impaired pupillary reflex; papilledema; vomiting; fluctuations in temperature; seizures; worsening of focal neurologic signs; changes in respiratory patterns
Mentation	Personality changes; insidious decrease in mentation; depression; memory deficits; judgment deficits
Focal neurologic disturbances	Gradually increasing weakness; subtle sensory loss; aphasia
Cranial nerve damage	Difficulty swallowing and impaired gag reflex resulting from damage to cranial nerves IX and X (after infratentorial craniotomy); visual disturbances; impaired corneal reflex
Pain	Headaches with steady, persistent, or intractable dull pain; changes in character of headaches
Seizure activity	Tonic-clonic seizures
Fluid balance	Marked polyuria; decreased urine output; marked polydipsia; anorexia; weight gain/loss; signs of dehydration; signs of fluid retention Laboratory studies: decreased/increased urinary specific gravity; increased/decreased serum osmolarity; decreased/increased urine osmolarity; increased/decreased serum sodium
Dressing and wound flap	Excessive bleeding; cerebrospinal fluid (CSF) drainage; elevation of bone flap
Cardiovascular effects	Cardiac dysrhythmias; hypotension; hypertension
Respiratory effects	Crackles, rhonchi; increased secretions; change in respiratory pattern
Meningeal irritation	Nuchal rigidity; irritability; increased sensitivity to light; positive Kernig's sign and Brudzinski's sign
Psychosocial effects	Negative self-esteem; feeling of hopelessness or powerlessness; anxiety; fear

2 DIAGNOSE

NURSING DIAGNOSIS	SUBJECTIVE FINDINGS	OBJECTIVE FINDINGS
Altered cerebral tissue perfusion related to cerebral edema	Complains of increasingly severe headache and increasing anxiety	Restlessness, lethargy; change in level of consciousness; focal neurologic deficits; pupillary changes; change in respiratory pattern; widening pulse pressure; bradycardia; seizures; vomiting

NURSING DIAGNOSIS	SUBJECTIVE FINDINGS	OBJECTIVE FINDINGS
Pain related to headache and incisional pain	Complains of headache, eye pain, incisional pain	Facial grimacing, crying, elevated BP and heart rate, restlessness, irritability
Potential for infection related to surgical procedure, invasive therapy, and immunosuppression	Complains of weakness, chills, and generalized irritability	Elevated temperature; elevated WBC; leakage of CSF; tachycardia
Potential fluid volume deficit related to osmotic diuretic therapy, fluid restriction, or onset of diabetes insipidus (DI)	Complains of thirst and dry mucous membranes; apprehensiveness	Apathy; weight loss; poor skin turgor; dry mucous membranes; increased or decreased urine output; increased or decreased specific gravity; decreased cardiac output, pulmonary capillary wedge pressure (PCWP), and central venous pressure (CVP); tachycardia; hypotension
Potential impaired gas exchange related to altered level of consciousness, effects of anesthesia, altered respiratory patterns, and increased secretions	Complains of shortness of breath; anxiety	Increased restlessness and confusion; change in respiratory pattern; cyanosis; breath sounds: crackles, rhonchi, diminished breath sounds; arterial blood gases: pH < 7.35 or > 7.45; partial pressure of oxygen (Pa_{O_2}) < 80 mm Hg; partial pressure of carbon dioxide (Pa_{CO_2}) > 35 mm Hg
Body image disturbance related to hair loss and possible focal neurologic deficits	Expresses anger, denial, and frustration about altered self-image	Change in approach to social interaction; lack of eye contact; actual or perceived physical disability

Other related nursing diagnoses: Potential fluid volume excess related to onset of syndrome of inappropriate secretion of antidiuretic hormone (SIADH) (see Craniocerebral Trauma); **Potential for injury** related to altered sensory perception, impaired motor function, seizures, and altered thought processes; **Ineffective individual coping** related to physiologic changes and hospitalization.

---

3   PLAN

Patient goals

1. The patient's cerebral perfusion will be improved.
2. The patient will be free of pain.
3. The patient will have no signs or symptoms of infection.
4. The patient will have optimum fluid balance.
5. The patient will have improved ventilation and oxygenation.
6. The patient will accept change in body image.

4 IMPLEMENT

NURSING DIAGNOSIS	NURSING INTERVENTIONS	RATIONALE
Altered cerebral tissue perfusion related to cerebral edema	Assess neurologic status q 1-2 h or prn.	To establish patient's baseline neurologic function, which serves as a guide for quantifying clinical changes.
	Monitor for signs of increasing cerebral edema, change in level of consciousness, focal neurologic signs, change in pupillary size, widening pulse pressure, bradycardia, and change in respiratory rate.	Cerebral edema occurs after cranial surgery; cerebral edema peaks 24-72 h after surgery; brain herniation can occur rapidly if cerebral edema is not treated.
	Monitor blood pressure (BP) and heart rate.	Changes can indicate increased intracranial pressure (ICP) or potential herniation.
	Maintain head position at appropriate angle; maintain head and neck in a neutral position.	Head of bed should be kept at 30- to 45-degree angle after supratentorial craniotomy to facilitate venous drainage; angle should be 0 to 20 degrees after infratentorial craniotomy to prevent pressure on neck muscles and brainstem.
	Instruct the patient to avoid flexion of the hip, isometric exercises, coughing, and straining at stool when possible.	These activities increase intrathoracic and intraabdominal pressure, which can increase ICP.
	Maintain normothermia.	Hyperthermia can change the rate of cerebral metabolism, which can affect ICP.
	Maintain oxygenation, and promote adequate ventilation.	A decrease in arterial oxygen pressure (Pa_{O_2}) and an increase in arterial carbon dioxide pressure (Pa_{CO_2}) increases cerebral blood flow and thus ICP.
	Monitor for seizure activity.	Neurosurgery can precipitate an irritable focus, resulting in seizures, which will increase ICP.
	Plan nursing care to minimize extraneous stimulation.	Even slight stimulation can increase ICP.
	Administer corticosteroids and osmotic diuretics as prescribed.	Osmotic diuretic therapy draws water from the brain cells to reduce cerebral edema; corticosteroids, although controversial, are thought to reduce cerebral edema.
Pain related to headache and incisional discomfort	Assess location, extent, duration of headache and incisional pain q 2 h prn.	Some headache and incisional pain is expected postoperatively. A sudden change or severe pain may indicate elevating intracranial pressure and should be reported to the physician immediately.

5 EVALUATE

PATIENT OUTCOME	DATA INDICATING THAT OUTCOME IS REACHED
Cerebral perfusion is improved.	The patient's level of consciousness is unchanged; there is no evidence of neurologic deficit or seizure activity.
The patient is free of pain.	The patient reports absence of discomfort. Absence of facial grimacing, crying, moaning. Vital signs are within normal limits. Patient participates in appropriate activities.
The patient has no signs or symptoms of infection.	The patient is afebrile; WBC is within normal limits; cultures are negative; and there is no CSF leakage.
The patient's fluid balance is adequate.	Intake and output are balanced; specific gravity is between 1.010 and 1.025; skin turgor and mucous membranes are normal; serum osmolarity, urine osmolarity, serum electrolytes, hemoglobin, and hematocrit are within normal limits; BP and heart rate are normal.
The patient has adequate ventilation and oxygenation.	Breath sounds are normal, arterial blood gases are within normal limits, and the airway is patent.
The patient's self-concept is intact.	The patient openly expresses his feelings of grief and loss, as well as positive feelings about himself; he acknowledges the change in self-concept.

PATIENT TEACHING

1. Involve the family in care, as possible; teach essential aspects of care.
2. Reinforce the physician's explanation of medical management.
3. Explain suture care to the family:
   a. A cap is recommended after head dressing is removed.
   b. After sutures have been removed, hair can be shampooed, but scrubbing around suture line should be avoided.
   c. Hair dryers should not be used until hair has regrown.
4. Explain to the patient and family the importance of reporting the following signs and symptoms:
   a. Increasing headache
   b. Stiff neck
   c. Elevated temperature
   d. New onset of motor weakness or sensory loss
   e. Changes in vision and/or photophobia
   f. Seizures
5. Emphasize the importance of ongoing outpatient care and follow-up visits.
6. Encourage the patient to pursue independent activities, as possible:
   a. Alert the patient to limitations.
   b. Advise him to avoid overprotection.
   c. Stress the need for adaptive devices as indicated.
7. Explain the need for a regular exercise program; teach ROM exercises to the family.
8. Teach the patient the importance of diet as ordered:
   a. Offer supplemental feedings.
   b. Offer small portions; instruct the patient to chew slowly.
9. Teach the patient the importance of safety measures: side rails, ramps, shower chairs, removal of scatter rugs, walker, and canes.
10. Teach the patient the names of medications, dosage, time of administration, and toxic or side effects.
11. Explain the need to avoid over-the-counter medications without first consulting the physician.
12. Encourage the patient to socialize with friends and family.
13. Teach the patient the importance of talking about his anxiety, fear, and feelings about changes in body image.
14. Teach the patient and family about seizures (i.e., safety measures and whom to contact).

Spinal Surgery

A **laminectomy** is a surgical procedure performed to relieve compression of the spinal cord or spinal nerve roots or both. Laminectomies are most commonly performed in the lumbar and cervical regions. During surgery, the patient is placed in the prone position. A midline incision is made, and the paravertebral muscles are retracted. Portions of one or two laminae and the attached ligamentum flavum are removed, exposing the herniated disk. A **discectomy** is the removal of all or part of the herniated intervertebral disk.

Microsurgical techniques have greatly advanced the treatment of intervertebral disk disease. Microsurgery is useful in the treatment of both cervical and lumbar disk disease. It enhances visualization of the operative field and reduces the size of the incision, compared with the traditional laminectomy. Also, less retraction is required, thereby reducing some complications such as dural laceration, cerebrospinal fluid leakage, nerve root damage, and bleeding.

A **spinal fusion** may be performed after a laminectomy to stabilize the vertebral column. Spinal fusion may be indicated when several laminectomies have been performed on vertebrae that have been damaged. A bone graft is taken from the iliac crest of the patient or from a cadaveric donor and inserted in the space between two vertebrae where the disk material was removed. New bone growth occurs, enhancing stabilization.

Surgical treatment of cervical disk disease may involve a posterior cervical laminectomy or an anterior cervical discectomy. The posterior cervical laminectomy is similar in technique to the lumbar laminectomy. The anterior cervical discectomy requires that the patient be placed in the supine position with the neck slightly extended. A small neck incision is made, and the anterior portion of the spine is carefully exposed. The diseased nucleus pulposus is removed.[86]

INDICATIONS

Spinal cord tumor or abscess
Herniated intervertebral disks
Failure to respond to conservative treatment for herniated intervertebral disk
Intolerable pain
Progressive motor and sensory loss
Bowel and bladder dysfunction
Spinal trauma that destabilizes the spinal column and/or causes spinal cord compression

CONTRAINDICATIONS

Based on individual patient

COMPLICATIONS

Paralysis of upper or lower extremities secondary to nerve root injury
Sensory loss
Urinary retention (following lumbar laminectomy)
Paralytic ileus (following lumbar laminectomy)
Cerebrospinal fistula
Arachnoiditis
Hematoma at operative site
Infection
Respiratory distress (following anterior cervical discectomy)
Vocal cord paralysis (following anterior cervical discectomy)

PREPROCEDURAL NURSING CARE

1. Review surgical procedure with patient and patient's family.
2. Explain to the patient that she will be turned in the immediate postoperative period using the log-rolling technique. Have the patient practice log rolling.
3. Discuss the importance of proper body mechanics.
4. Teach the patient deep breathing exercises.
5. Discuss with the patient her current level of pain and treatments or interventions that have been tried.
6. Document the patient's baseline neurologic status and other medical or physical problems.
7. Encourage the patient and family to express their fears and concerns.
8. Check the operative permission form.
9. Withhold food and water the night before surgery.
10. Remove all jewelry, glasses, contact lenses, and false teeth.
11. Insert IV line.
12. Administer preoperative medications.

MEDICAL MANAGEMENT

GENERAL MANAGEMENT

Lumbar spinal surgery[45]

Physical activity: Bed rest for the first 24 h; proper alignment must be maintained, and log-rolling is used to reposition the patient; the head of the bed is flat or slightly elevated; a small pillow may be placed under the head and one under the knees; while side-lying, place a pillow between knees; sitting should be avoided, except for defecation in the first few postoperative days; ambulation should begin on the second postoperative day with short walks and then increase as tolerated (this may vary among physicians). Antiembolic stocking: Should be worn to prevent thrombus and embolus. Diet: Progressed as tolerated. Dressing and wound care: Observe for excessive drainage and hematoma; dressing is removed on approximately the third postoperative day; hemovac drain may be used during the first 24-48 h after surgery.

Cervical spinal surgery (anterior and posterior)[86]

Physical activity: Bed rest is maintained for the first 24 h; the head of the bed should be flat or slightly elevated, and a small pillow may be placed under the head or neck; a cervical collar is worn, and proper alignment must be maintained; ambulation should begin on the second postoperative day and advance as tolerated. Antiembolic stocking: Should be worn to prevent thrombus and embolus. Diet: Advanced as tolerated. Cervical collar: Maintains proper alignment; worn at all times.

DRUG THERAPY

Analgesics: Morphine sulfate; Tylenol no 3; patient-controlled analgesic pump

Stool softeners: Docusate sodium (Colace)

1   ASSESS

ASSESSMENT	OBSERVATIONS
Neurologic effects	
Lumbar laminectomy/ discectomy	Increased postoperative weakness of lower extremities; increased postoperative sensory loss; diminished postoperative reflexes; decreased proprioception
Cervical laminectomy/ discectomy	Increased postoperative weakness of upper extremities and shoulders; decreased proprioception; increased postoperative sensory loss; diminished postoperative reflexes; Horner's syndrome (following anterior cervical discectomy); dysphagia and vocal cord paralysis (following anterior cervical discectomy)
Pain	Sharp, radiating pain through shoulders, legs, thigh, and buttocks; increased BP, heart rate; facial grimacing

ASSESSMENT	OBSERVATIONS
Respiratory effects	Labored respirations, shallow respirations; stridor; change in mental status; pale skin color; edema of trachea (following anterior cervical discectomy); ineffective coughing; hoarseness (following anterior cervical discectomy)
Circulatory effects	Change in BP and heart rate; change in quality of peripheral pulses; increased capillary refill time; numbness, tingling in extremities
Elimination	Absence of bowel sounds; difficulty with urinary elimination; constipation; incontinence
Wound	Excessive bloody wound drainage; hematoma; evidence of CSF drainage

2   DIAGNOSE

NURSING DIAGNOSIS	SUBJECTIVE FINDINGS	OBJECTIVE FINDINGS
Pain related to edema and inflammation of spinal nerve roots	Complains of pain and generalized discomfort	Increased BP and heart rate; facial grimacing; guarding behavior
Potential altered spinal tissue perfusion related to edema and surgical manipulation of spinal nerve roots	Complains of motor weakness, sensory loss, paresthesia	Increased motor weakness, sensory loss, paresthesia; Horner's syndrome (following anterior cervical discectomy); decreased ROM; decreased quality of peripheral pulses; increased capillary refill time
Impaired physical mobility related to imposed physical limitations, pain, and neurologic impairments	Complains of limited ROM and discomfort on movement	Decreased physical activity; limited ROM; loss of neurologic function.
Potential ineffective breathing pattern related to incisional pain, effects of anesthesia, and tracheal edema (following anterior cervical discectomy)	Complains of shortness of breath	Labored respirations; shallow respirations; stridor; increased use of accessory muscles; tracheal deviation; pale skin; change in arterial blood gases; diminished breath sounds
Potential altered urinary elimination related to swelling in operative area, effects of anesthesia, and physical immobility	Complains of abdominal distention and inability to void	Suprapubic distention; inability to void; inadequate urinary output relative to intake; incontinence

→ › ›

NURSING DIAGNOSIS	SUBJECTIVE FINDINGS	OBJECTIVE FINDINGS
Potential altered bowel elimination related to swelling at operative site, immobility, and depressant effect of narcotics	Complains of abdominal discomfort and constipation	Absence of bowel sounds; increased abdominal girth; distention; incontinence
Potential for infection related to surgical incision and complications of cerebrospinal fistula and arachnoiditis	Complains of irritability and headache	Elevated temperature; elevated WBC; increased BP and heart rate; presence on dressing of halolike ring around serosanguineous drainage; presence of glucose in wound drainage (positive Dextro-stix test); headache; nuchal rigidity; positive Brudzinski's and Kernig's signs; photophobia

Other related nursing diagnoses: Potential impaired verbal communication related to laryngeal nerve damage and vocal cord paralysis (following anterior cervical discectomy); **Potential impaired skin integrity** related to use of stabilizing devices and impaired physical mobility.

3 PLAN

Patient goals

1. The patient will have minimum pain or discomfort.
2. The patient will demonstrate adequate spinal tissue perfusion.
3. The patient will have optimum physical mobility.
4. The patient will have effective breathing patterns.
5. The patient will demonstrate adequate urinary elimination.
6. The patient will demonstrate adequate bowel elimination.
7. The patient will be free of infection.

4 IMPLEMENT

NURSING DIAGNOSIS	NURSING INTERVENTIONS	RATIONALE
Pain related to edema and inflammation of spinal nerve roots	Assess pain level, location, and duration; have patient rate pain on scale of 1 to 10.	To determine level of pain; pain may occur secondary to swelling and inflammation of nerve roots.
	Assess patient for sore throat and hoarseness (following anterior cervical discectomy).	Sore throat and hoarseness are common after anterior cervical discectomy secondary to edema and intubation.
	Reinforce the importance of proper body alignment and the need to log-roll patient while in bed; avoid use of large head pillows.	To reduce pain and increase comfort; log rolling decreases muscle tension and maintains spinal alignment.
	Apply stabilizing devices (brace, cervical collar) as prescribed.	To facilitate proper body alignment and reduce pain and muscle spasms.

NURSING DIAGNOSIS	NURSING INTERVENTIONS	RATIONALE
	Reinforce the importance of avoiding prolonged sitting (following lumbar laminectomy).	Sitting can place additional stress on the lumbar region of the spinal column.
	Instruct the patient to avoid straining at stool and to report constipation.	Straining at stool can place additional stress on spinal column.
	Administer narcotics, corticosteroids, throat lozenges, and viscous lidocaine as prescribed.	Pain may be relieved with narcotics; corticosteroids may be prescribed to decrease inflammation at the surgical site; throat lozenges and viscous lidocaine may ease the sore throat following an anterior cervical discectomy.
	Encourage and demonstrate use of relaxation techniques.	To promote relaxation and reduce muscle tension.
Potential altered spinal tissue perfusion related to edema and surgical manipulation of spinal nerve roots	Assess neurologic status q 2-4 h prn; observe for change in motor and sensory status; mark areas of sensory loss with marker; monitor for Horner's syndrome (lid ptosis, constricted pupil, regression of eye in orbit, absence of sweating on that side of face) following anterior cervical discectomy; notify physician of any neurologic changes.	A change in motor and sensory function may indicate damage to nerve roots that may require immediate medical attention; Horner's syndrome may occur after an anterior cervical discectomy as a result of cervical sympathetic nerve damage.
	Assess neurovascular status of upper (cervical spinal surgery) and lower (lumbar spinal surgery) extremities q 2-4 h prn; peripheral pulses, capillary refill time, and extremity color and temperature.	These indicate the extent of tissue perfusion; change in tissue perfusion may indicate nerve root compression and may require immediate medical attention.
	Assess wound for swelling or development of hematoma or both.	Hematoma may develop as a result of abnormal bleeding and may cause further compression; this requires surgical evaluation.
	Use antiembolic stockings.	To facilitate circulation in lower extremities and reduce incidence of thrombi and emboli.
Impaired physical mobility related to imposed physical limitations, pain, and neurological impairments	Assess neurologic deficits.	To determine physical limitations.
	Maintain bed rest at prescribed head angle on firm mattress for the first 24 h.	To reduce pressure to the operative site.
	Reposition patient q 2 h, using log-rolling technique: patient should fold arms across chest, tighten back muscles, and keep shoulder and pelvis straight; a pillow can	Log rolling ensures proper alignment and reduces pain and muscle spasms.

➔ ❯ ❯ ❯

NURSING DIAGNOSIS	NURSING INTERVENTIONS	RATIONALE
	can be positioned between knees; a turning sheet is used, and the patient is gently rolled on her side; sufficient support should be provided to maintain alignment.	
	Maintain proper positioning while in bed; avoid twisting and bending; a cervical collar should be in place at all times after surgery in the cervical region.	Cervical collar maintains proper alignment.
	Sitting should be avoided during the first week after surgery. The patient should be moved from bed to standing position in one smooth movement (following lumbar spinal surgery); use of arms and neck muscles should be avoided following surgery in the cervical region.	To avoid pressure on surgical site and to avoid twisting, bending, and jarring of extremities.
	Advance ambulation as prescribed; follow ambulation/rehabilitation protocol as prescribed.	Controversy exists among surgeons over the level of mobility in the immediate postoperative period.
Potential ineffective breathing pattern related to incisional pain, effects of anesthesia, and tracheal edema (following anterior cervical discectomy)	Assess respiratory rate, use of accessory muscles, breath sounds, and tracheal deviation, inability to handle secretions, and hoarseness (following anterior cervical discectomy).	Pneumonia and atelectasis are potential complications of spinal surgery; following cervical spinal surgery, respirations may be shallow secondary to pain; tracheal edema, dysphagia, and hoarseness may occur following anterior cervical discectomy as a result of hematoma formation and damage to the laryngeal nerve.
	Encourage coughing and deep breathing; be sure the patient is comfortable before coughing.	To facilitate movement of secretions and lung expansion.
	Maintain oxygen at prescribed level.	Supplemental oxygen may be given in the immediate postoperative period.
	Prepare for intubation if signs and symptoms of respiratory distress occur.	Rapid swelling of the upper airway after an anterior cervical discectomy can precipitate respiratory distress.
Potential altered urinary elimination related to swelling in operative area, effects of anesthesia, and physical immobility	Assess voiding pattern; note voiding of small, frequent amounts.	Urinary retention may occur following administration of anesthesia and prolonged immobility; this may be more problematic following surgery in the lumbar region because of the operative site.
	Palpate suprapubic area for distention.	May indicate urinary retention.
	Monitor intake and output.	These indicate fluid volume status.
	Facilitate voiding by positioning patient comfortably and running warm water over hands.	To help patient relax and to stimulate autonomic nervous system.

NURSING DIAGNOSIS	NURSING INTERVENTIONS	RATIONALE
	If patient cannot void adequately, consult with physician regarding intermittent catheterization.	Catheterization may be necessary in the immediate postoperative period.
Potential altered bowel elimination related to swelling at operative site, immobility, and depressant effect of narcotics	Assess for the presence of bowel sounds, abdominal distention, nausea, and vomiting.	Paralytic ileus is a possible complication because of stimulation of the sympathetic nervous system.
	Monitor frequency and consistency of bowel movements.	To determine bowel elimination pattern.
	Use small fracture pan while patient is on bed rest.	To reduce physical discomfort and minimize muscle tension.
	Encourage adequate fluid intake.	To stimulate peristalsis.
	Include high-fiber foods in diet.	To increase bulk, stimulate peristalsis, and decrease straining.
	Encourage physical mobility as prescribed.	To stimulate peristalsis.
	Administer stool softeners and laxatives as prescribed.	To decrease straining.
Potential for infection related to surgical incision and complications of cerebrospinal fistula and arachnoiditis	Assess vital signs and WBC.	Increased heart rate, BP, temperature, and WBC may indicate onset of infection.
	Assess dressing and wound for halolike ring surrounding serosanguineous drainage; assess drainage for glucose with Dextro-stix.	Cerebrospinal fistula can be a complication of spinal surgery, causing CSF drainage. Arachnoiditis (inflammation of the arachnoid layer of the spinal meninges) also is a possible complication of spinal surgery.
	Assess patient for signs and symptoms of meningeal irritation: headache, photophobia, nuchal rigidity, and Brudzinski's and Kernig's signs.	Meningitis can result from a cerebrospinal fistula.
	Notify physician of any of the above symptoms.	Immediate medical treatment is necessary.
	Administer antibiotics as prescribed.	Antibiotics may be prescribed to reduce likelihood of infection.
Knowledge deficit	See Patient Teaching.	

5 EVALUATE

PATIENT OUTCOME	DATA INDICATING THAT OUTCOME IS REACHED
The patient has no pain or discomfort.	Vital signs are within normal limits; the patient has increased participation in physical activities and decreased use of narcotics; muscle tension and facial grimacing are reduced.

→ 〉 〉 〉

PATIENT OUTCOME	DATA INDICATING THAT OUTCOME IS REACHED
The patient demonstrates adequate spinal tissue perfusion.	Neurologic function is maintained or has been improved; ROM is maintained or has been improved; peripheral pulses are palpable, and capillary refill time is less than 3 sec; extremities are warm and pink.
The patient has optimum physical mobility.	The patient has increased participation in activities; maintains proper spinal alignment and uses proper body mechanics; uses stabilizing devices properly.
The patient demonstrates effective breathing patterns.	Respirations are 16-20; lung sounds are present, and breath sounds are clear; there is no tracheal deviation or use of accessory muscles.
The patient's urinary elimination is adequate.	Intake and output are balanced; there is no suprapubic distention, and the patient is voiding adequate amounts of urine. Absence of incontinence.
The patient's bowel elimination is adequate.	Bowel sounds are present, and there is no abdominal distention or pain; the patient is passing flatus, and stools are well formed. Absence of incontinence.
The patient has no infections.	The patient's temperature is normal, and there is no wound drainage; there are no signs of meningeal irritation; WBC is within normal limits.

PATIENT TEACHING

1. Review the surgical procedure and overall rehabilitation program.
2. Instruct the patient on ways to reduce back and neck strain:
   a. Sleep on firm mattress
   b. Use proper body mechanics and maintain good posture
   c. Avoid activities that put added stress on the spine, such as driving, climbing stairs, and bending without flexing the knees
3. Review the use of a stabilizing device if indicated.
4. Encourage periods of rest following activities.
5. Discuss pain management, i.e., use of medications and relaxation techniques.
6. Review the importance of weight control.
7. Review incisional care and signs and symptoms of infection.
8. Review all medications and their potential side effects.
9. Discuss follow-up care.

Transsphenoidal Surgery

Transsphenoidal surgery is the recommended procedure for removing a pituitary tumor or the entire pituitary gland (Figure 6-4). This approach facilitates visual access to the surgical area, which previously was accessible only through an intracranial approach.[30]

Transsphenoidal surgery was performed as early as the 1920s. However, because of inadequate lighting and insufficient equipment, the procedure was abandoned and transfrontal craniotomies were performed. Microsurgical equipment and fluoroscopy have made transsphenoidal surgery the favored approach for tumors within the sella or with moderate suprasellar extension.[35]

The transsphenoidal approach allows the tumor to be removed while leaving the gland intact, thus preserving pituitary function. Other advantages over the transfrontal craniotomy include a lower morbidity and mortality rate, a hidden incision line, and no need to cut the patient's hair.[35]

After general anesthesia has been induced, a horizontal incision is made under the lip at the junction of the gingiva extending from one canine tooth to the other. The maxillary sinus and nasal septum are removed, and nasal mucosa is reflected. The sphenoid sinus is entered by using a drill and nasal speculum. Using fluoroscopy and microscopes, the sella turcica is opened and the dura mater is exposed, providing visualization of the tumor.[35]

After the tumor has been removed, Gelfoam soaked in alcohol may be placed in the cavity to destroy any remaining tumor cells. Defects in the sella diaphragm are packed with muscle or fatty tissue previously obtained from a thigh graft site. The nasal septum is reapproximated, and the nasal cavities are packed with petroleum jelly gauze impregnated with antibiotic ointment. A soft nasal airway may be inserted, and a moustache dressing is applied underneath the nose.[35]

INDICATIONS

Removal of pituitary tumor

CONTRAINDICATIONS

Based on individual patient

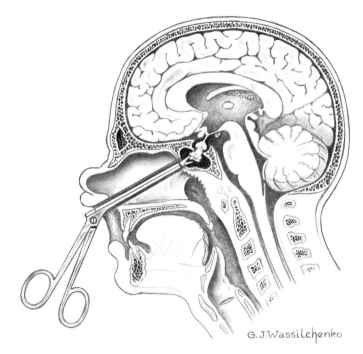

G.J.Wassilchenko

FIGURE 6-4
Transsphenoidal approach for removing a pituitary tumor. (From Rudy.[127])

COMPLICATIONS

Diabetes insipidus
Leakage of cerebrospinal fluid
Diplopia, ptosis, and strabismus
Optic nerve damage
Sinusitis
Laceration of carotid artery

PREPROCEDURAL NURSING CARE

1. Initiate preoperative instruction for the patient and family:
   a. Explain the functions of the pituitary gland.
   b. Briefly explain the surgical procedure.
   c. Instruct the patient on mouth breathing.
   d. Instruct the patient on the importance of avoiding coughing and sneezing.
   e. Instruct the patient on postoperative care of the incision line and mouth care.
   f. Discuss the importance of measuring intake and output.

g. Discuss the importance of reporting persistent postnasal drip.
2. Check the operative permission form.
3. Document the patient's baseline neurologic status, visual acuity, and the presence of diplopia, ptosis, and strabismus.
4. Withhold food and water the night before surgery.
5. Remove all jewelry, glasses, contact lenses, and false teeth.
6. Insert IV line.
7. Administer preoperative medications.

MEDICAL MANAGEMENT

GENERAL MANAGEMENT

Preoperative

Endocrine evaluation: Pituitary tumors often manifest as endocrine problems; careful evaluation of hormonal function before surgery is necessary to prevent postoperative complications. Ophthalmic evaluation: The proximity of the optic chiasm and optic nerve to the hypothalamic-pituitary axis may cause visual disturbances.

Postoperative

Physical activity: Bed rest for the first 24 h; then physical activity is advanced as tolerated. Diet: advanced as tolerated. Fluids: carefully monitored, rate of infusion is dictated by fluid volume status. Laboratory studies: serum electrolytes, serum and urine osmolarities, and CBC q 4-6 h for the first 24 h. Nasal packing or moustache dressing: removed 24-48 h after surgery.

DRUG THERAPY

Diabetes insipidus: Aqueous vasopressin (Pitressin), desmopressin (DDAVP) intranasally.

Hormonal replacement: May be necessary.

Antibiotics: Organism specific.

Corticosteroids: Dexamethasone (Decadron).

1   ASSESS

ASSESSMENT	OBSERVATIONS
Neurologic effects	Change in level of consciousness, motor function, speech, sensory function
Cranial nerve function	Visual acuity; ptosis; strabismus
Pain	Periorbital edema; headache; tenderness over sinuses
Fluid balance	Hypotension; tachycardia; marked polyuria; marked polydipsia; anorexia; weight loss; dehydration; dry skin; poor turgor; apathy; weakness
Laboratory studies	Urine specific gravity of 1.001-1.005; increased serum osmolarity; decreased urine osmolarity; increased serum sodium, increased BUN; increased hematocrit

ASSESSMENT	OBSERVATIONS
Nasal packing	Excessive drainage; persistent postnasal drip; positive glucose in drainage
Respiratory effects	Nasal swelling; airway obstruction; change in respiratory pattern

2 DIAGNOSE

NURSING DIAGNOSIS	SUBJECTIVE FINDINGS	OBJECTIVE FINDINGS
Potential fluid volume deficit related to onset of diabetes insipidus	Complains of thirst and dry mucous membranes; apprehensive	Apathy; weight loss; poor skin turgor; dry mucous membranes; increased urine output and serum osmolarity; decreased urine osmolarity; specific gravity < 1.005; increased serum sodium and hematocrit; very pale urine
Potential for infection related to break in integrity of nasal mucosa and complication of cerebrospinal fluid leak	Increasing headache; neck pain; generalized irritability; complains of postnasal drip and excessive swallowing	Elevated temperature and WBC; nuchal rigidity; photophobia; positive Brudzinski's and Kernig's signs; positive glucose in nasal drainage; positive bacteria on CSF cultures
Altered oral mucosal membrane related to suture line, dehydration, and mouth breathing	Complains of thirst, dry lips, and painful suture line	Breaks or cracks in oral mucosa; extreme redness and swelling at suture line
Sensory-perceptual alteration (visual) related to pressure on optic chiasm and optic nerve	Complains of decreased vision, eye muscle weakness, and double vision	Change in pupillary size and reactivity, visual acuity, and extraocular eye movements

Other related nursing diagnoses: Potential altered cerebral tissue perfusion related to hemorrhage, hematoma, and edema; **Pain** related to headache and blockage of nasal passages; **Potential ineffective breathing pattern** related to nasal swelling and effects of anesthesia.

3 PLAN

Patient goals

1. The patient will have an adequate fluid balance.
2. The patient will have no signs or symptoms of infection.
3. The patient's oral mucosa will have healed.
4. The patient's vision will be unchanged or will have improved.

Carotid Endarterectomy

Carotid endarterectomy is the surgical removal of athero-sclerotic plaques from extracranial vessels. Atherosclerotic plaques can obstruct the lumen of these vessels, decreasing blood flow and thus causing a transient ischemic attack (TIA) or cerebral vascular accident (CVA). The arteries commonly affected are the internal and external carotid arteries and the common carotid artery.[25]

The purpose of the carotid endarterectomy is to restore adequate cerebral circulation in patients who have had a transient ischemic attack so as to reduce the chance of cerebral vascular accident. The procedure involves heparinization and clamping of the artery above and below the area of obstruction. The artery is opened via a small incision along the neck, and the atherosclerotic plaques are removed (Figure 6-5). The artery is then either sutured or patched with an autologous vein or Gortex graft, and the clamps are removed. A small dressing is placed over the neck incision.[25,52]

INDICATIONS

Transient ischemic attacks
Asymptomatic carotid bruit (controversial)

CONTRAINDICATIONS

Based on individual patient

COMPLICATIONS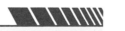

Airway obstruction
Cerebral infarction
Damage to cranial nerves VII, X, XI, and XII
Hypotension/hypertension
Cardiac dysrhythmias
Infection
Vocal cord paralysis

PREPROCEDURAL NURSING CARE

1. Initiate preoperative instruction for patient and family:
   a. Explain the purpose, benefit, and risks of the surgical procedure.
   b. Explain the postoperative course.
   c. Teach deep-breathing exercises.
   d. Discuss the critical care environment.
   e. Encourage the patient and family to express their fears and concerns.

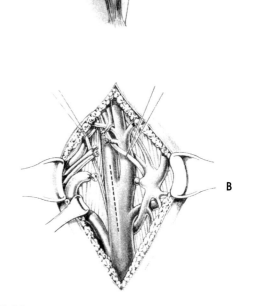

FIGURE 6-5
A, Line of skin incision for carotid endarterectomy. Note relationship to sternocleidomastoid muscle and underlying carotid arteries. **B,** Carotid artery branches are exposed and widely mobilized; facial vein and small veins in region of bifurcation are ligated (dotted line indicates incision). (From the American Association of Neuroscience Nurses: Core curriculum for neurosurgical nursing in the operating room, Chicago, 1980, AANN.[25])

2. Check the operative permission form.
3. Document the patient's baseline neurologic status and all other medical problems.
4. Withhold food and water the night before surgery.
5. Remove all jewelry, glasses, contact lenses, and false teeth.
6. Insert IV line.
7. Administer preoperative medications.

MEDICAL MANAGEMENT

GENERAL MANAGEMENT

Immediate postoperative period: May require 24-h intensive care monitoring.

Arterial line and cardiac monitoring: Monitor for hypotension/hypertension and cardiac dysrhythmias; BP must be closely monitored.

Respiratory: Encourage use of incentive spirometer, coughing, and deep breathing; swelling of surgical site may cause airway obstruction.

Neurologic: Serial neurologic assessments.

Physical activity: Bed rest for 24 h.

Ongoing postoperative care: Diet: advance as tolerated. Physical activity: advance as tolerated.

DRUG THERAPY

Based on patient's individual needs.

1 ASSESS

ASSESSMENT	OBSERVATIONS
Neurologic effects	Change in level of consciousness; hemiplegia; speech deficit; sensory loss; damage to the following cranial nerves: VII (facial droop, inability to close eyelid completely); X (swallowing difficulties, choking, dysarthria, hoarseness); XI (weakness of shoulder muscle, inability to turn head from side to side); XII (weakness of tongue muscle, drooping tongue, dysphagia, upper airway obstruction); obliteration of temporal artery pulses
Cardiac effects	Hypotension; hypertension; cardiac dysrhythmias
Respiratory effects	Change in respiratory rate and pattern; change in baseline arterial blood gases; upper airway obstruction; deviation of trachea; decrease or change in breath sounds
Incision site and wound	Excessive bleeding; hematoma; redness and swelling; drainage
Psychosocial effects	Anxiety; restlessness; fear

2 DIAGNOSE

NURSING DIAGNOSIS	SUBJECTIVE FINDINGS	OBJECTIVE FINDINGS
Potential altered cerebral tissue perfusion related to decreased cerebral blood flow	Complains of dizziness, motor weakness, sensory loss, and difficulty speaking	Change in level of consciousness; hemiplegia; speech deficit; sensory loss; facial paralysis; loss of gag reflex; weakness of shoulder and tongue muscles; loss of temporal artery pulses

➜ ❯ ❯ ❯

PRESSURE WAVES

Intracranial pressure's dynamic state is reflected by the pressure waves produced. These wave forms are most commonly known as A waves, B waves, and C waves (Figure 6-7). **A waves** (or plateau waves), which occur at variable intervals, are spontaneous, rapid increases in pressure between 50 and 200 mm Hg. Plateau waves usually occur in patients with moderate intracranial pressure elevations and last 5 to 20 minutes, falling spontaneously. Factors that can trigger plateau waves include rapid eye movement (REM) sleep, emotional stimuli, isometric muscle contractions, the rebound phase of Valsalva maneuver, hypercapnia, hypoxemia, sustained coughing and sneezing, arousal from sleep, and certain positions such as neck flexion or extreme hip flexion. A waves are known to cause cerebral ischemia and brain damage and can produce paroxysmal or transient symptoms of change in level of consciousness, headache, nausea and vomiting, altered motor function, abnormal pupillary reactions, changes in vital signs (i.e., increased blood pressure, widened pulse pressure, and decreased pulse rate), and respiratory patterns (i.e., ataxic breathing and central neurogenic hyperventilation). Because of the ischemia and these symptoms, A waves are the most clinically significant intracranial pressure wave forms and require immediate intervention to prevent further brain injury.

B waves appear as sharp, rhythmic, sawtoothed waves that occur every 30 seconds to 2 minutes and have pressures up to 50 mm Hg. B waves correlate to changes in respiration, such as Cheyne-Stokes respirations, and they often precede the onset of plateau waves. B waves also can occur in patients with normal intracranial pressure.

C waves are small, rapid, rhythmic waves that occur at a rate of approximately four to eight per minute and increase pressures up to 20 mm Hg. C waves are also called Traube-Herring-Mayer waves. These wave forms correspond to normal changes in the systemic arterial pressure and are not clinically significant.

INDICATIONS

Head trauma
Cerebral hemorrhage

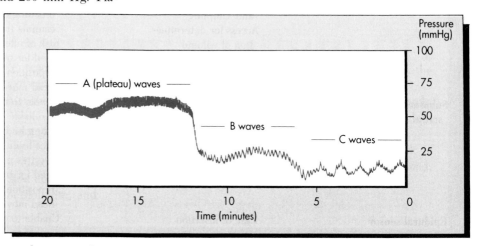

FIGURE 6-7
Intracranial pressure waves. Composite drawing of A (plateau) waves, B waves, and C waves.

Massive brain lesions
Encephalitis
Congenital hydrocephalus
Hydrocephalus resulting in an alteration in cerebrospinal fluid production or absorption
Any other clinical problem resulting in elevation of intracranial pressure

CONTRAINDICATIONS

Based on individual patient

COMPLICATIONS

Infection

PREPROCEDURAL NURSING CARE

1. Explain to the patient and family the purpose of and indications for intracranial pressure monitoring.
2. If the monitoring system is to be implanted at bedside, prepare all required equipment.
3. Assist the neurosurgeon in placing the catheter, bolt and screw, or sensor.

MEDICAL MANAGEMENT

GENERAL MANAGEMENT

Respiratory system: Mechanical ventilation and controlled hyperventilation may be indicated to prevent hypercapnia and hypoxemia.

Cardiac monitoring and arterial blood pressure monitoring: Cardiac dysrhythmias may occur with intracranial pressure; bradycardia may signify impending brain herniation.

Hemodynamic monitoring: Careful monitoring of CO, PCWP, PAS, and PAD is indicated.

Draining of CSF: Done only if intraventricular catheter is used.

Laboratory studies: Arterial blood gases, serum electrolytes, CBC, platelets, serum and urine osmolarities, and anticonvulsant levels.

SURGERY

An ICP monitoring system can be implanted at the bedside on an emergency basis or in the operating room.

DRUG THERAPY

Corticosteroid agents (to reduce cerebral edema): Dexamethasone (Decadron).

Osmotic diuretics (to create osmotic gradient that draws water from the brain into the plasma): Mannitol.

Diuretics (to reduce cerebral edema): Furosemide (Lasix), acetazolamide (Diamox).

Barbiturate therapy: Used to treat uncontrolled intracranial hypertension via continuous IV infusion of barbiturates (Thiopental, Pentobarbital). A barbiturate coma is induced, which requires extreme caution, sophisticated monitoring, and mechanical ventilation.

Muscle relaxants and sedatives: Used to decrease patient's response to noxious stimuli. Requires that the patient be intubated and appropriately monitored.

H$_2$ histamine blocker: Cimetidine (Tagamet), ranitidine (Zantac).

Antacids: Magnesium hydroxide (Maalox).

Antiinfective agents: Organism specific.

Anticonvulsive agents: Phenytoin (Dilantin).

Laxatives: Docusate sodium (Colace).

1 ASSESS

ASSESSMENT	OBSERVATIONS
Loss of intracranial pressure wave form	Transducer may be incorrectly connected; monitoring device could be occluded; air may be present between pressure source and transducer diaphragm

→ > >

CHAPTER 7

Neurologic Rehabilitation

Although information about rehabilitation has been interwoven throughout this book, four areas need further discussion: an overview of rehabilitation itself; adaptation, adjustment, and coping; sexuality; and stabilization and mobility. The other major concerns of rehabilitation are then identified, but the reader is referred to the integrated content elsewhere in the text. Other rehabilitation issues such as driving, home modification for accessibility, and avocational and vocational concerns have not been addressed in this text, so the reader is referred to an appropriate rehabilitation resource from the list on the inside back cover for further information.

OVERVIEW OF REHABILITATION

Rehabilitation is the process by which a person works toward a former level of functioning after experiencing some type of injury or the effects of a disease. Rehabilitation is achieved by relearning skills formerly mastered and by learning new ways to do activities one no longer can accomplish with previously learned skills.

Rehabilitation has both a general focus and a very specialized focus. The general focus is one of the aims of all nursing care. It involves maintaining current function, preventing complications and further deterioration, and restoring function lost by injury or disease. The specialty practice of rehabilitation usually is associated specifically with patients experiencing neurologic trauma or disease, orthopedic conditions, chronic pain and, more recently, cancer and AIDS. The maintenance and preventive functions of acute rehabilitation begin in the hospital, usually after the trauma or the chronic condition has been assessed. Interventions to restore function begin once the patient's condition is medically stable. The quicker the specialized rehabilitation team is notified of the patient's admission and diagnosis, the earlier they can assess the patient and identify specific rehabilitative interventions. Intensive rehabilitation may be necessary in some instances. In this case, the patient may be transferred to a specialized rehabilitation unit within the hospital or to a freestanding rehabilitation center. This intensive phase of rehabilita-

tion may last several weeks to several months, depending on the extent of impairment and the patient's progress toward goals. After discharge, the patient may continue to need long-term therapy, a transitional living center, and/or vocational rehabilitation for several months to several years. Although the goal is to return most patients to their homes, some patients will need the level of care supplied by a skilled nursing facility; or, if adequate supervision is unavailable in the home, a supportive environment of group living may be considered.

GOALS OF REHABILITATION

The major goals of rehabilitation are to help the individual achieve the full potential of independence and function; to help the individual and family adapt to an impairment and change in lifestyle; to maintain current functioning while preventing loss of function and complications; and to help the individual and family achieve a personally acceptable quality of life. Although rehabilitation focuses on the patient's abilities, strengths, and potential and not on the disability, losses are acknowledged and grieved. It is especially important that the primary nurse, as well as other members of the patient's health care team, develop a therapeutic relationship with the patient and members of the family. This trusting relationship facilitates the expression of true feelings and guides the professional's corresponding interventions. Although friendships often develop, the professional relationship should always be maintained.

Table 7-1

PROFESSIONAL REHABILITATION TEAM AND FUNCTIONS OF MEMBERS

Member	Functions
Physical medicine physician (physiatrist)	Develops medical care plan with patient and other health team members; coordinates care with other team members; provides ongoing evaluation of patient's progress toward goals of care; provides medical/surgical care as needed by patient.
Nurses	Provide bedside patient care; develop nursing care plan with and for the patient and family; coordinate care of and with allied health personnel; provide ongoing evaluation of nursing care plan to identify possible problems and recommend changes in care, if needed.
Physical therapists	Provide therapy through various modalities to help patient regain muscle and joint functions; may assist with exercise regimen, ambulation, heat or cold therapies, massage, and others as deemed part of the patient's care plan; teach self-care related to specific treatments, wrappings, use of exercise equipment, and others; provide input to other rehabilitation team members regarding patient's progress toward goals.
Occupational therapists	Teach patient self-care techniques, special exercises, or activities to relearn previous skills or to adapt remaining muscles to necessary skills; evaluate home situation and make recommendations for needed adjustments, if any; provide input to other rehabilitation team members regarding patient's progress toward goals.
Psychiatrist/psychologist	Assesses patient's reactions to present condition; helps patient adapt or adjust to loss of functions, if needed; does psychometric testing to determine patient's need for counseling or other therapy, if any.
Orthotist/prosthetist	Measures and fits patient for specific orthosis, splint, or prosthesis as needed; adjusts orthotic devices as needed; provides input to rehabilitation team members regarding application of orthosis or prosthesis as patient progresses toward goals.
Dietitian	Makes nutritional assessment to determine nutritional needs to maintain protein/calorie balances; monitors daily intake for adequacy and necessary changes; provides input to rehabilitation team regarding patient's progress.
Social worker	Makes financial assessments related to medical insurance, finances, and concerns for long-term care; seeks health care facilities for extended care; provides input to rehabilitation team regarding financial and long-term care arrangements.
Pharmacist	Provides input to rehabilitation team members related to medication regimen for pain and infection control; evaluates patient's responses to medications and recommends changes to rehabilitation team, if needed.
Speech therapist	Helps patient regain or improve communication skills, if needed; provides input to rehabilitation team members regarding special training or equipment needed by patient.
Vocational counselor	Helps patient adjust to disabilities related to work or employment possibilities if adjustments are needed; helps patient make transition from rehabilitation center to home and/or employment setting with regard to disabilities.

From Mourad.[104]

THE REHABILITATION TEAM

Although rehabilitation usually is associated with physical functioning, it also focuses on the cognitive, emotional, psychologic, social, educational, economic, and vocational realms of functioning. This necessitates teamwork among various health care disciplines. Table 7-1 identifies common members of the rehabilitation team and their areas of primary focus. The patient is considered a member of the decision-making team and needs to be included, if possible, in setting goals and choosing interventions, in evaluating progress, and in discharge planning. The continuous involvement of family members or significant others is crucial—not only to support the patient's efforts, but also because of their possible role as future caregivers.

Because much of rehabilitation necessitates learning new information and skills, each member of the rehabilitation team needs a variety of teaching skills and a working knowledge of teaching-learning theory. Rehabilitation patients come from diverse educational, vocational, and experiential backgrounds. Financial and social resources may be sparse or abundant. Each variable lends itself to modifying the patient's learning needs. The patient may need to learn how to direct others in providing care he cannot do for himself; and, in some instances, the patient or family will need to learn how to hire and train personal care attendants.

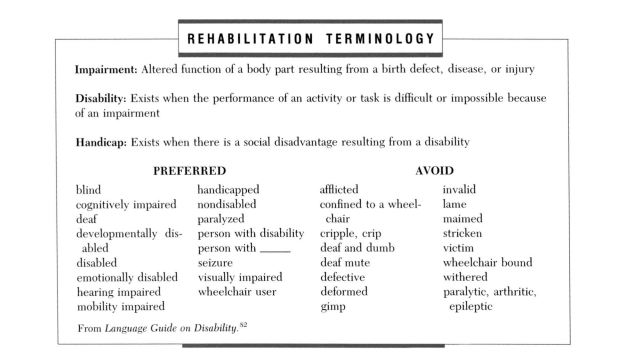

In the box:

REHABILITATION TERMINOLOGY

Impairment: Altered function of a body part resulting from a birth defect, disease, or injury

Disability: Exists when the performance of an activity or task is difficult or impossible because of an impairment

Handicap: Exists when there is a social disadvantage resulting from a disability

PREFERRED		AVOID	
blind	handicapped	afflicted	invalid
cognitively impaired	nondisabled	confined to a wheel-	lame
deaf	paralyzed	chair	maimed
developmentally dis-	person with disability	cripple, crip	stricken
abled	person with _____	deaf and dumb	victim
disabled	seizure	deaf mute	wheelchair bound
emotionally disabled	visually impaired	defective	withered
hearing impaired	wheelchair user	deformed	paralytic, arthritic,
mobility impaired		gimp	epileptic

REHABILITATION NURSING

The specialty of rehabilitation nursing requires an expanded knowledge base concerning the specific types of trauma and disease conditions encountered, rehabilitation techniques, patient and family education, and interprofessional collaboration. Rehabilitation nurses act as consultants, primary caregivers, case managers, administrators, educators, and researchers. The practice setting ranges from critical care settings to rehabilitation centers to home health services. In all settings, the rehabilitation nurse acts as a patient advocate, often coordinating various aspects of care and discharge planning.

THE REHABILITATION MILIEU

Specialized rehabilitation units and rehabilitation centers not only provide intensive therapy but also create a milieu that is accepting, optimistic, encouraging, and supportive. The physical environment must be accessible to wheelchairs; it must have spacious rooms and bathrooms, wide doorways with free-swinging doors, extended sinks, and wheelchair-accessible showers. Special adaptations for the disabled include modified bed, light, and nurse call switches, lowered closet hooks, lowered or tilted mirrors, lowered hand-pressure switches for lights, elevated electrical outlets, lever door handles, lowered windows, and appropriately modified telephones. Safety concerns include lowered temperature of hot water, uncluttered rooms and hallways, shatterproof glass and mirrors, ground fault interrupter outlets, secure bed brakes, and nonslip flooring.

The environment provides adequate privacy but also encourages socialization by having common lounges, dining rooms, recreation areas, and therapy rooms. The physical environment, as well as staff clothing, conveys a more personal, homier atmosphere. Patients dress in their own clothes, and visiting hours stretch from late morning into the evening. The emphasis is away from the appearance and routines of an acute hospital environment, discouraging the sick role of the patient and encouraging independence.

ADAPTATION, ADJUSTMENT, AND COPING

DEFINITIONS

Adaptation and **adjustment** describe the psychosocial process of establishing and maintaining an equilibrium in one's life and environmental situation. **Coping** describes the psychologic and behavioral activities used to master, tolerate, or mini-

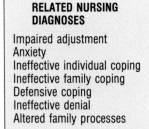

RELATED NURSING DIAGNOSES

Impaired adjustment
Anxiety
Ineffective individual coping
Ineffective family coping
Defensive coping
Ineffective denial
Altered family processes

mize external or internal demands and conflicts. Although the three terms are closely related, adaptation and adjustment usually refer to the internal process, whereas coping usually refers to behaviors to maintain self-concept, emotional stability, and interpersonal relationships and to manage stress. The term "acceptance" usually is avoided, since many believe one never truly accepts the losses caused by disability or chronic disease. To accept would appear passive and imply giving in to fate; yet others consider the choice of terminology only an issue of semantics.[32,46,83]

Shock—lack of or minimal awareness of crisis at hand

Characteristic feelings: numbness, anxiety, fear, overwhelmed
Typical comments: "What happened?", "Oh, my God!", "I've got to get home!"
Interventions: Have someone stay with patient; simply explain what has happened, what is being done, who people are, and where they are; keep patient oriented to time; reassure patient; assign consistent caregiver

Denial—blocking of awareness of painful reality

Characteristic feelings: relief, calmness, indifference, happiness
Typical comments: "I'm fine, why is everyone so glum?", "I'll be up and out of here in a few days!", "I don't need to learn about this—I'll be able to walk when this brace comes off!"
Interventions: Keep goals very short term; inform patient of reasons for care activities and their relationship to the patient's current condition; do not confront patient or argue about reality; involve patient in self-care activities as possible

Developing awareness—beginning awareness of incongruency between what was and current reality

Characteristic feelings: uneasiness, doubt, questioning
Typical comments: "All this therapy, and I still cannot walk!", "Why is everyone here still in wheelchairs?"
Interventions: Encourage interaction with other patients; continue to involve patient in self-care activities; answer questions simply and truthfully; provide patient education as requested and appropriate

Anger—realization of impact of loss; preoccupation with blaming; anger often displaced toward others

Characteristic feelings: anger, guilt, shame
Typical comments: "It's my fault, I shouldn't have been so stupid!", "Why did God do this to me?", "Get out of here. Leave me alone!"
Interventions: Allow expression of feelings; assist staff and family in understanding anger, and instruct them not to "take it personally"; maintain safety of patient and caregivers, set behavior limits if necessary; involve patient in support group and professional counseling as needed

Depression—generalized feeling of despair

Characteristic feelings: hopelessness, sadness, helplessness
Typical comments: "Leave me alone!", "I don't know what I'm going to do," or few comments overall
Interventions: Keep patient involved and attending therapy; allow expression of feelings; provide encouragement, but not false hope; take suicide ideation seriously; refer for counseling if stage is severe or prolonged

Mourning—situation-specific feeling of loss; grieving

Characteristic feelings: overwhelmed, devastated, severe loss, grief
Typical comments: "I can't do my job anymore. What am I going to do?", "I can't stop crying!"
Interventions: Maintain daily routine; continue patient involvement in support group and counseling; allow sufficient time for patient to discuss feelings; acknowledge losses, increase focus on abilities

Adjustment—acknowledgment of reality; desire to manage losses, readjust self-concept, and adapt to environment; may initially "bargain with God"

Characteristic feelings: relief, confidence, satisfaction, happiness
Typical comments: "How can I do my own dressing?", "What equipment do I need?", "How can we adapt our house?"
Interventions: Begin intensive teaching; encourage socialization outside of hospital and rehabilitation environment; teach patient problem-focused and emotion-focused coping behaviors; encourage patient to try newly learned skills in home environment; facilitate patient's identification of community resources

STAGES OF ADJUSTMENT

Seven stages of adjustment have been identified and described in the literature: shock, denial, developing awareness, anger, depression, mourning, and adjustment (see box above). Identification of the stages can help in understanding the patient's behavior and in guiding appropriate interventions. Stages do not necessarily appear in sequence and often overlap. A patient may fluctuate between stages or omit a stage entirely. Caution should be used in labeling a patient's behavior, because the focus should remain on therapeutic interactions and on helping the patient identify, learn, and use successful coping behaviors. The acute process of adjustment can vary in length, depending not only on the patient's nature but also on whether his condition was caused by a traumatic incident or a chronic, progressive disease. Family members often adjust at a rate different from that of the patient, sometimes causing further stress on both parties. Adjustment is a continuous process, extending over a period of years.

Caregivers should reflect on their own feelings during the patient's adjustment process. Nurses should take care not to project their own feelings on the patient, nor should they be judgmental about the patient's or family members' feelings and behavior. Nurses should seek the support of other professionals to discuss how to maintain a therapeutic relationship with the patient and family.

SEXUALITY

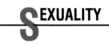

> **RELATED NURSING DIAGNOSES**
> Altered sexuality patterns
> Sexual dysfunction

Sexuality is an important part of everyone's self-image. It includes how a person feels about himself and how he interacts with others. Sexual functioning is the expression of one's sexuality and involves choices in how the sexuality is expressed. Sex usually refers to one's gender and/or the sex act itself. Sexuality and sexual functioning are influenced by age, developmental level, culture, personal values, knowledge, physical and emotional health, sexual patterns and availability of partners, and resources. Factors that may cause sexual dysfunction include a reduced activity tolerance; pain or discomfort; lack of privacy; role changes; knowledge deficit about the effects of an injury, disease, or disability on sexual functioning; value or cultural conflicts; changes in body structures or functioning; mobility or sensory deficits; stress; fatigue; and the effects of medications.

SEXUAL HISTORY AND ASSESSMENT

A sexual history often is taken in several phases, with general information collected at the time of the admission assessment. Information about the person's sexual knowledge, attitudes, function, and current concerns is elicited once a therapeutic relationship has been established. Provide a private, relaxed setting, and ensure professional confidentiality. Clarify any terms if necessary. The person has the right to refuse to answer any questions but may decide to reveal the answers at a later time.

The nurse should be cognizant of and comfortable with her own sexuality, remembering not to make judgments about the patient's sexuality or sexual functioning history, and she should take care not to project her own feelings on the patient and his sexual partner. Patients and sexual partners often have concerns about sexual matters earlier than the concern is actually expressed. This often is due to embarrassment, fear, or the professional's lack of acknowledgment of the patient's subtle hints.

> ### PLISSIT MODEL
>
> **Permission**
>
> Acknowledgment of the person's and/or significant other's question or concern; conveys to them that one is willing to listen and discuss sexual thoughts, feelings, and concerns
>
> **Limited information**
>
> Provision of information about the possible effects of certain conditions, situations, and treatments on sexuality and/or sexual functioning
>
> **Specific suggestions**
>
> Provision of specific suggestions that can address expressed concerns and facilitate sexual functioning or expressions of sexuality
>
> **Intensive therapy**
>
> Intensive sexual counseling by trained professionals; referrals may be necessary for specific interventions or long-term counseling
>
> Adapted from Annon.[7]

PLISSIT MODEL

Once the professional acknowledges to the patient and his partner that sexual concerns are common, the patient often raises many questions. These questions can range from personal desirability and dating skills to explicit sexual functioning and fertility concerns. How to handle menstruation and birth control also are common concerns.

The PLISSIT model (permission, limited information, specific suggestions, intensive therapy) for treating sexual problems can be used (see box above). Each health professional should intervene at the level at which he or she is comfortable and knowledgeable. Most nurses should be prepared to at least provide limited information. Specialty nurses should be able to give specific suggestions. Patient concerns that cannot be addressed should be referred to other professionals who can provide the necessary information or counseling, after getting the patient's permission for the referral.

STABILIZATION AND MOBILITY

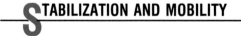

This discussion of stabilization and mobility addresses some of the various techniques and equipment used in the care of patients with neurologic disorders. For example, stabilization of the vertebral column prevents further

> **RELATED NURSING DIAGNOSIS**
> Impaired physical mobility

spinal cord injury after spinal trauma, whereas joint stabilization by an orthosis can facilitate ambulation, help preserve hand function, or prevent joint injury. Mobility can be a major issue for patients who are at high risk for the complications of immobility after a neurologic injury or the increasing impairment of a neurologic disease, as well as for patients whose impaired mobility is a threat to their performance of self-care, work, and leisure activities. Since two of the major goals of rehabilitation are to maintain or improve patient mobility and self-care functioning, special attention is given to how this can be accomplished.

SPINAL STABILIZATION: SURGICAL

Once an unstable vertebral injury has been identified, spinal stabilization is necessary to prevent damage or further trauma to the spinal cord. Internal stabilization of the vertebral bodies is accomplished by spinal fusion and/or the placement of metal instrumentation. A spinal fusion is the surgical placement of cancellous bone plugs or chips, usually from the patient's iliac crest, between affected vertebrae. Wires and glue may be used to secure the bone fragments in place. Spinal fusion usually involves two to six vertebrae, and it limits flexion and rotation of the involved vertebral segment. The actual healing and bone fusion period lasts several months. During this time the area of the fusion must be immobilized by a brace or by a traction and brace combination.

Internal realignment and stabilization of longer segments of the spinal column usually require the use of metal instrumentation, such as Harrington or Leuke rods. These rods can be used alone or in addition to a spinal fusion. A rod is attached to each side of the posterior spinous processes of the vertebrae by screws, wires, and glue. Then the rods are adjusted to provide the proper alignment and stabilization. The type of bracing and the period of immobilization after surgery depend on the type and extent of fusion and stabilization. Spinal stability is confirmed by the radiologist after spinal x-rays are taken. The radiologist and physiatrist or the orthopedic surgeon are in attendance for removal of the brace and positioning the patient during flexion and extension films.

SPINAL STABILIZATION: NONSURGICAL

Nonsurgical spinal stabilization can be done when stability of the spinal column has been confirmed by x-ray. Nonsurgical methods include positioning, traction, and bracing. Positioning and stabilization of the spinal column are critical from the time of injury until some type of stabilization device has been applied. This prevents or minimizes trauma to the spinal cord, thus preventing paralysis. A back board, Meyer cervical orthosis, or a neck brace can be applied at the scene of an accident

when a spinal injury may have occurred. Usually these devices are not removed until a spinal injury has been ruled out or some other type of stabilization device is in place.

Positioning after a spinal fusion involves smoothly log rolling the patient for turning and proper positioning with pillows and foam wedges to maintain spinal alignment. Special beds have been devised to facilitate proper positioning and turning. Three common specialty beds for these purposes are the CircOlectric bed, the Stryker frame, and the RotoRest bed. Special attention is necessary to prevent or quickly detect skin shearing during use of these beds. Use of specialty beds usually requires a physician's prescription.

The CircOlectric bed consists of a bottom mattress and a top-turning stretcher supported between two outside circular frames. During turning, the patient is sandwiched between the mattress and the stretcher while the large circular frame electrically rotates the patient from supine to or from prone, head over feet. After turning, the stretcher can be removed if it is on the top. Cervical or pelvic traction can be maintained at all times. Because the mattress and stretcher are fairly narrow, safety belts should be secure at all times. Safe, proper use of this bed is necessary, since tubing, traction ropes, and electric cords can be obstructed in the turning process. Arm supports and side rails are available.

The Stryker frame has two stretchers, covered with canvas and some padding that are attached to a cart at a pivot device on each end. For turning, the patient is securely sandwiched between the two stretchers, then the apparatus is unlatched and the patient is smoothly, manually rotated from supine to or from prone, side over side. Cervical traction can be maintained during the process. The top stretcher can be removed after turning. Safety straps and/or side rails should always be used. Arm supports are available. Proper use of the bed is critically important to the patient's safety.

The RotoRest bed has numerous foam wedges and bolsters that hold the patient's body snugly in alignment while slowly, constantly rotating side to side electrically. Cervical traction can be maintained during rotation. Safety straps and other devices should be in position at all times. The degree of rotation can be set by the nurse, and the rotation can be stopped at any time and at any angle for providing patient care. Special hatches can be opened and mattress sections removed to permit access to the patient from the underside of the mattress. Special care should be taken to prevent tubing and traction ropes from getting caught during rotation.

TRACTION

Skeletal traction is often used to immobilize and realign cervical and high thoracic fracture sites. A set of skull tongs (i.e., Gardner-Wells, Crutchfield, Vinke, or Barton) is inserted into the skull and connected to traction ropes; prescribed weights are then attached to the ropes. The tongs usually are applied at the bedside using a local anesthetic. Because the procedure can be terrifying to the patient, a mild sedative is sometimes administered. Traction is constantly maintained until prescribed discontinuance, which can be days to weeks later. Pin sites should be inspected and initially cleaned twice daily with a solution that is half hydrogen peroxide and half sterile water, using a sterile cotton swab for each cleansing swipe. The site is rinsed with sterile water on a swab and then dried with another swab. A small amount of antibiotic ointment can be applied around each pin if prescribed. Alcohol can be used to cleanse any drainage on the pins. A small piece of sterile gauze can be wrapped around each pin until drainage subsides in a few days. Pin sites should be inspected daily for signs of infection. Hair should be kept washed, and the back of the scalp should be inspected carefully for skin breakdown.

Once traction has been applied and the vertebrae have been properly realigned, a halo traction brace is commonly applied. A metal halo is attached to the patient by four or more skull pins. Then a lambs' wool-lined vest is put on the patient; the halo is connected to the vest by metal posts so that alignment and traction can be maintained without ropes and weights. The halo brace allows the patient to sit up and stand if there is no paralysis. The pins are cleaned as described above. The pins and halo apparatus should be checked daily for looseness; sandbags should be kept handy to immobilize the neck until the pins can be tightened by a trained professional if looseness is detected. Some halo vests are hinged to allow access for skin care and cardiac compression if necessary, but a full set of appropriate wrenches should be kept with the patient at all times for removal of the front of the vest and/or the halo device in the event of an emergency. (Refer to the "Patient Teaching Guide" on the halo traction device, page 288, for further information to share with the patient.)

SPINAL IMMOBILIZERS

After the skull tongs or halo device has been removed, a cervical collar or brace is applied. As the patient's activities increase, and the neck musculature strengthens, the patient is weaned from the cervical collar at a prescribed rate. If an actual neck brace is used after the tongs are removed, the stability of the spine must be confirmed by x-ray before weaning to a cervical collar.

Although high thoracic injuries may be stabilized with skeletal traction, stable thoracic and lumbar injuries usually require only immobilization while the vertebral fracture heals. Immobilization can be accomplished by flat bed rest, molded plastic or fiberglass jackets or chest shells, or an actual back brace.

POSTURAL HYPOTENSION AFTER IMMOBILIZATION

When a patient has been immobilized for a period of time, especially if the patient is quadriplegic, postural hypotension may be severe. A tilt table can be used to reacclimate the patient to the upright position. Thigh-high support stockings, elastic wraps from toes to groin, and an abdominal binder (to promote better trunk posture and support the abdominal muscles) are also helpful.

ORTHOSES: NONSPINAL

Orthotics available to assist in maintaining proper body alignment and functional positioning include both static and dynamic splints and braces. Hand/forearm splints and hard cones positioned in the paralyzed hand prevent contracture formation. Leg braces provide joint stability for ambulation; Swedish knee cages prevent hyperextension of the knee during ambulation; and an ankle-foot orthosis (AFO) stabilizes the ankle and prevents plantarflexion during ambulation. Although orthoses are prescribed by physicians and usually made by orthotists and some specially trained therapists, physical and occupational therapists assure proper patient and family training in applying and using the orthotic. The nurse should follow through on this training and collaborate with the therapist in determining how the patient can use the device safely.

TRANSFERS

Although various types of transfers can be used in moving the patient from one surface to another, good body mechanics is always necessary. Three- or four-person lifts or a Smooth Mover device results in safe transfer from bed to carts. Hydraulic lifts with various types of slings facilitate bed to chair transfers and weighing patients when they are unable to bear weight on their legs. A sliding board positioned between bed and wheelchair can aid in transferring the patient into and out of bed; or, if the patient has sufficient arm strength and trunk balance, the patient may be able to do this transfer with minimum assistance or even independently. A transfer belt around the patient's waist or chest allows either maximum or minimum help with balance and movement during transfers or ambulation. One of the most important aspects of teaching and learning transfers is consistency of method. Nurses and therapists should collaborate in selecting the safest method for transferring and ambulating each neurologic patient. Special transfers for getting into and out of a car and up or down to the floor should be considered only after team collaboration.

BED MOBILITY

Bed mobility skills include turning, moving up and down in bed, and coming to an upright position. Bed mobility is facilitated by the use of side rails, overhead trapezes, and/or canvas loops. The patient should be taught how to position himself with pillows to prevent skin breakdown, facilitate comfort, and increase self-function. Some patients will need an electric hospital-type bed with adapted hand controls.

WHEELCHAIR MOBILITY

Wheelchair mobility requires not only an accessible environment but also a certain degree of strength, coordination, and judgment. Many types of wheelchairs are available today, from ultralight racing models to electric models equipped with environmental controls and built-in recliners. Although a facility's wheelchair is used until the patient's mobility potential has been determined, each patient is prescribed his own wheelchair on the basis of mobility needs and physical capabilities. A wheelchair that brings the patient to a standing position may be very appropriate. An appropriate wheelchair seat cushion should always be used to prevent skin breakdown.

AMBULATION

Some patients can ambulate with the use of long leg braces and crutches or a walker, but the required energy expenditure may be excessive, leaving little energy to do a task once the patient gets to his destination. These patients therefore may elect to use a wheelchair for most functional activities but may choose to ambulate periodically only for therapeutic reasons.

Ambulation aids include various types of walkers, crutches, and canes—all individually fitted to the patient's height and mobility needs. Gait training by the physical therapist may take several days to several months, interspersed with stretching and strengthening exercises and balance activities. Collaboration among therapists and nurses reinforces teaching and facilitates efficiency.

FUNCTIONAL ELECTRICAL STIMULATION

Functional electrical stimulation (FES), also known as functional neuromuscular stimulation (FNS), involves electrical stimulation of nerves in paralyzed muscles. It is used to control and coordinate movement of these muscles. Electrodes are placed on, in, or near the selected muscles; then a low-level current is administered, causing muscle contraction. The stimulation is controlled and coordinated by a computer-controlled stimulator that is either portable or attached to exercise equipment similar to an exercise bicycle. FES is being tested and used for aerobic exercise, standing, walking, and stair climbing. Refinement of FES over the past decade has enabled persons with complete spinal cord injuries not only to maintain muscle mass and cardiovascular fitness but also to regain the ability to stand and ambulate. Further refinement of the system and its effects and practical use are being tested in research programs across the country.

ELIMINATION

Related Nursing Diagnoses

Colonic constipation
Bowel incontinence
Altered patterns of urinary elimination: functional incontinence, reflex incontinence, stress incontinence, total incontinence, urge incontinence, or urinary retention
Further Information: Refer to pages 131-133

SKIN INTEGRITY

Related Nursing Diagnoses

Impaired tissue integrity
Impaired skin integrity
Further Information: Refer to pages 131-134

SWALLOWING

Related Nursing Diagnoses

Impaired swallowing
Potential for aspiration
Altered nutrition: less than body requirements
Further Information: Refer to pages 65-66

COMMUNICATION

Related Nursing Diagnoses

Impaired communication
Impaired verbal communication
Further Information: Refer to page 179

NEUROBEHAVIORAL MANAGEMENT

Related Nursing Diagnoses

Altered thought processes
Potential for injury
Further Information: Refer to pages 63-65

SELF-CARE AND ACTIVITIES OF DAILY LIVING

Related Nursing Diagnosis

Self-care deficit: feeding, bathing/hygiene, dressing/grooming, toileting, or total self-care deficit
Further Information: Refer to pages 66-67, 78, 130

CHAPTER 8

Patient Teaching Guides

Patient education about neurologic disorders, diagnostic tests, treatment procedures, and ongoing care needs is vital to the patient's health. While the patient may be the focus of the teaching/learning activities, certainly the inclusion of the patient's family members and significant others is important to the supportive or caregiver role each may have. Each member of the professional team caring for the patient has a responsibility to participate in the educational process. Often the same information needs to be shared numerous times and using various teaching methods in order for the patient to adequately learn necessary self-care skills. While some educational encounters may be more formal than others, the opportunity to teach the patient at any appropriate moment should be seized. Written teaching guides, such as those included in this chapter, provide the learner with information and the sequence of procedural steps that can be referred to during both the teaching session and later to refresh one's memory or share with others. Written material should always be reviewed with the patient.

The first step in patient teaching is a thorough assessment of the learner(s) and the situation that requires teaching/learning. Learner attributes include cognitive and physical capabilities; educational level; degree of coping with current health crisis; awareness of own knowledge deficit/readiness to learn; fears and anxieties concerning own abilities; and general feel-

ings about prior learning experiences. A situation/environment assessment includes identification of skills and information to be learned; physical needs of the learner that must first be met; educational resources available; staff teaching skills; and necessary modifications of the environment so it is conducive to learning.

If a nursing diagnosis of a knowledge deficit has been identified, the next step is to identify specific learner goals. Most of these goals are action oriented; for example, the patient will be able to do his own catheterization. Then a teaching plan is developed to meet both short-term and long-term learner goals.

The evaluation of learning is ongoing during the teaching process, since modification of teaching methods and adaptation of techniques are an ongoing process. Adequate time must be set aside for uninterrupted teaching sessions. While the learning of certain information and skills is necessary before a safe home visit or before actual discharge, it is important to remember that new learning needs emerge after discharge. A plan to address these new needs should be a part of subsequent discharge referrals and follow-up visits.

As with all aspects of the nursing process, documentation of the teaching-learning process is necessary. This not only documents the care of a specific patient but also permits the evaluation of an overall educational program.

Acute Head Injury Discharge Sheet

Even though your head injury is not serious enough to require a hospital stay, you must watch for the following signs and symptoms that could signal complications:

- Increased drowsiness
- Difficulty waking (have a family member or friend wake you every 2 hours the first night)
- Slowing heart rate
- Nausea and vomiting
- Continuing or worsening headache
- Stiff neck
- Bleeding or fluid coming from the ears or nose
- Weakness in arms or legs
- Seizures
- Blurring of vision
- Slurred speech
- Problems with memory
- Clumsiness
- Restlessness
- Irritable behavior
- Confusion
- Unusual sensations
- Difficulty walking

If you experience any of these signs or symptoms, call your doctor immediately or go to the emergency room.

Arrange for someone to stay with you for the next 2 to 3 days. Share this Patient Teaching Guide with family and friends. Give them your doctor's name and phone number.

For the next several days:

- Do not drink alcoholic beverages.
- Do not take any medications for a headache, nausea, or muscle soreness without first calling the doctor.
- Avoid driving, contact sports, swimming, taking a tub bath, using power tools, and hunting.

First Aid for a Seizure

It is important that you know how to care for the person when he has a seizure. Seizures can happen anytime, anywhere.

1. If the person loses consciousness, try to prevent or break his fall.
2. Turn the person onto his side.
3. Loosen any tight clothing around the neck. Any object in the immediate area that could cause injury, such as hard or sharp objects, should be removed.
4. Do not put anything in the person's mouth, including your fingers. (There is no danger that he will swallow his tongue.)
5. Let the person lie on his side until the seizure is over. Talk to him, and tell him what happened and where he is.
6. If the person has injured himself or has another seizure right away, call the doctor.
7. The person may be groggy and confused after the seizure. Stay with the person and call the doctor immediately.

Doctor's Name_____

Phone No._____

Special Instructions

_____
_____
_____
_____
_____
_____
_____
_____
_____
_____
_____
_____
_____

Seizure Management

Seizures occur when the brain experiences abnormal electrical activity. This activity alters the brain's function, and the person suffering the seizure will usually experience motor, sensory, or psychic symptoms and/or a change in the level of consciousness. The site in the brain where the seizure takes place determines what kind of seizure is experienced and the person's signs and symptoms.

Kinds of seizures, signs, and symptoms

There are four types of seizures: simple partial, complex partial, generalized tonic-clonic, and absence.

A **simple partial seizure** occurs in the cerebral cortex of the brain. It causes the stiffening or jerking of an arm or a leg on one side of the body. The area affected sometimes also has a tingling sensation. The person does not lose consciousness unless the seizure progresses to a generalized tonic-clonic seizure.

A **complex-partial seizure** occurs in the temporal lobe of the brain. The signs and symptoms of this type of seizure vary from person to person, but each person tends to consistently have the same type of signs and symptoms. The person usually has an aura, a type of sensation that precedes the seizure and acts as a warning. This seizure may cause the person to stare, not respond to questions or give confused answers, move or walk around aimlessly, smack his lips, make chewing motions, fidget with clothing, or appear drunk or drugged. A person may feel emotional or have unusual sensations. The person may struggle if someone tries to restrain his activity. The seizure may last 1 to 3 minutes. The person usually does not remember the seizure and may feel confused afterward.

A **generalized tonic-clonic seizure** extends across the entire brain. There usually is no aura or warning. The person may give a shrill cry as air rushes out of the lungs. The person falls and loses consciousness. The whole body then stiffens, and the muscles begin to spasm and relax, causing jerking motions of the arms and legs. The person may bite his tongue. Breathing is also very jerky, causing the individual to become pale or to blush. The person may urinate or have loss of stool. The seizure lasts 1 to 3 minutes. The person slowly regains consciousness but usually is confused, sleepy, and has a headache. He may have difficulty speaking and weakness of the arms or legs or both. The person will have no memory of the seizure.

Absence seizure has no identified focus in the brain. It lasts only 1 to 10 seconds. The person has a short loss of consciousness and will stare, blink his eyes, or have slight facial twitching. There is no aura, and the person keeps his posture and does not fall. Some people may have several hundred of these seizures a day.

Your doctor will want to examine you and perform some diagnostic tests to discover the cause of your seizures. This will help her determine what treatment and medication to prescribe to prevent your seizures.

The following are some of the tests that you may undergo:

Cerebral angiography shows the blood circulation in your brain and can detect any displacement of cerebral circulation or any hemorrhaging in the brain.

Cerebrospinal fluid analysis can help detect multiple sclerosis, tumors, infection, or an obstruction around the subarachnoid space of the spinal cord.

A *computed tomography (CT) scan* can detect tumors, hematomas, aneurysms, lesions, and edema of the brain.

Electroencephalography (EEG) evaluates the brain's electrical activity and also can help locate abscesses and tumors.

Treatments

Diet. Maintaining adequate energy and glucose levels is very important to the way your brain's neurons function. If you diet or skip meals, the neurons become unstable and begin to malfunction, causing a seizure. Eat regular meals, and snack in between if you begin to feel shaky, faint, or hungry.

Medication. It is very important that you follow your doctor's instructions exactly when you take your anticonvulsant medication. Too much or too little of the drug can cause seizures. If you miss a dose, your doctor will tell you what to do. Make sure you don't take any over-the-counter medication without your doctor's approval.

Periodically your doctor will alter the dosage of your medicine if he finds your blood levels have changed. Don't ever stop taking the medicine unless your doctor says to. Medication can help prevent seizures but can't cure the underlying cause. So even though you haven't had a seizure in years, it doesn't mean you are cured. You may need to continue the anticonvulsant drug for the rest of your life.

Surgery. Sometimes surgery becomes necessary if drug therapy fails to work or if surgery can correct or lessen the severity of the seizure disorder.

Prevention. Some sights and sounds can trigger seizures, such as flashing video, television, or computer screens, and construction noises. Caffeine and alcohol can cause a seizure, as can fatigue and illness. Most of these things can be avoided if you find they trigger seizures.

It is important that you always wear a Medic-Alert bracelet in case you have a seizure in public. If you feel a seizure coming on, lie down in the nearest safe place.

Support groups

Support groups can help you cope with your feelings. These groups are made up of people like you who have experienced seizures and who want to share their experiences. Ask your nurse for the name and address of the local and national Epilepsy Foundation.

Your Seizure Medications:

_____

_____

_____

Your Doctor's Name:

_____

Your Doctor's Phone Number:

_____

First Aid for a Seizure

If you know a person with a seizure disorder, it is important that you know how to care for the person when he has a seizure. Seizures can happen anytime, anywhere.

1. If the person loses consciousness, try to prevent or break his fall.
2. Turn the person onto his side.
3. Loosen any tight clothing around the neck. Any object in the immediate area that could cause injury, such as hard or sharp objects, should be removed.
4. Do not put anything in the person's mouth, including your fingers. (There is no danger that he will swallow his tongue.)
5. Let the person lie on his side until the seizure is over. Talk to him, and tell him what happened and where he is.
6. If the person has injured himself or has another seizure right away, call the doctor.
7. The person may be groggy and confused after the seizure. Be sure that he can resume activities safely before leaving him alone.

Please share this information with your family and friends.

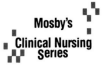
Safety Tips for Persons with Confusion or Impaired Judgment

The person who has confusion or impaired judgment may be unable to remember where dangers lie, or to judge what is dangerous (steps, stoves, medications). Fatigue and inability to make her body do what she wants also can lead to injury. Therefore it is very important that this person live in an environment that has been made as safe as possible. The following are some safety guidelines to use in your home:

- Keep clutter out of the hallway and off stairs or anywhere the person is likely to walk. Remove small rugs that could cause tripping.
- Remove breakables and dangerous objects (matches, knives, guns).
- Keep medications in a locked cabinet or drawer.
- Limit access to potentially dangerous areas (bathrooms, basement) by locking doors if the person tends to wander. Have the person wear an identification bracelet in case she wanders outside.
- Dress the person appropriately for the season.
- Put name labels in clothing. Make sure clothing is not too baggy and that shoes fit well and have nonskid soles.
- Keep the person's bed low. If she falls out, you may want to place the mattress on the floor or install siderails.
- Make sure rooms are well lit, especially in the evening. Night-lights can help prevent falls.
- Have someone stay with the person if she is severely confused or agitated.
- Encourage rest periods if the person tires easily.
- Keep exit doors locked. Consider some type of exit alarm, such as a bell attached to the door.
- Consider a mat alarm under a bedside rug to alert others of the person getting up during the night.

Encourage the person to do the following:
- Rest frequently. Don't let the person get fatigued.
- Avoid crowded places such as shopping malls and stadiums.
- Have someone with the person when she goes outdoors.
- Keep meal times quiet and calm.
- Limit the number of visitors.
- Have the person do one activity at a time.
- Keep activities simple—this will minimize fatigue.
- Plan activities ahead of time.
- Ensure that medications are taken as prescribed.
- Get the doctor's consent before giving the person over-the-counter medications.
- Keep a calendar of activities visible on the wall. Cross off days as they pass.
- Maintain a photo album with labeled pictures of family members, friends, home, and so on.
- Include the person in family activities and conversations.
- Remember to treat the person with respect and maintain his privacy.

Some things to avoid
- Alcohol
- Contact sports
- Horseback riding
- Swimming
- Hunting
- Power tools or sharp implements
- Driving
- Riding recreational vehicles such as bicycles, skateboards, motorcycles, or snowmobiles
- Cooking without supervision

Guidelines for Swallowing Disorders

Neurologic disorders can affect many bodily functions, including the muscles and reflexes used for swallowing. The person with a swallowing disorder has a higher risk of choking and therefore must be very careful when eating or drinking. The following are some guidelines to help the person with a swallowing disorder:

At first a caregiver should supervise mealtimes and make sure the person is drinking and eating correctly. If the person wears dentures, they should be in and should fit well. A calm, unhurried environment for eating will help the person concentrate on the action of swallowing.

Semisolid foods such as applesauce, pudding, and mashed potatoes are easier to swallow than liquids or solids. Thickening powder can be added to liquids for easier swallowing.

The swallowing procedure
1. While eating, make sure you are sitting upright and are leaning slightly forward.
2. Chew your food well.
3. Tilt your head forward and think "swallow."
4. Make sure you swallow the food you have in your mouth before you take another bite. Don't talk with food in your mouth.
5. Brush your teeth after eating.

Choking
Since you are at a greater risk for choking, you, your friends, and family should know the universal sign of choking—hand on throat. Your friends and family should know how to perform the Heimlich maneuver, and you should know how to perform the Heimlich maneuver on yourself. Ask the nurse to instruct you and your family in using the Heimlich maneuver.

Heimlich Maneuver
As long as the person is able to breathe in and out, speak, cough forcefully, and is alert, the Heimlich maneuver is not necessary. Allow the person to continue coughing and trying to clear his or her airway. Proceed with doing the Heimlich maneuver if or when the person has great difficulty with breathing, is unable to speak, loses the ability to cough forcefully, or begins to lose consciousness or the skin becomes dusky or bluish.
1. Stand or sit behind the person choking.
2. Wrap your arms around the person's body.
3. Make a fist with one hand and place the thumb side of the fist against the person's abdomen—midline between the bottom tip of the sternum and the waist.
4. Cover your fist with your other hand.
5. Give several quick inward and upward thrusts.

Family and friends should consider learning CPR (cardiopulmonary resuscitation). Contact your local chapter of the American Red Cross or the American Heart Association for CPR class information.

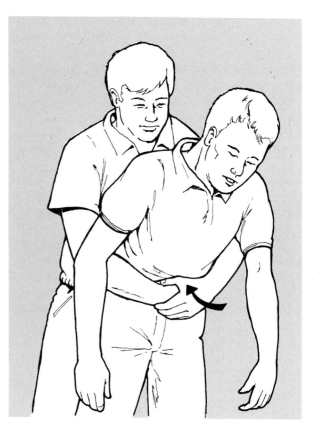

PATIENT TEACHING GUIDE

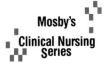

Mosby's
Clinical Nursing
Series

Communicating with Aphasic Patients

Aphasia is the loss of ability to communicate. The person with aphasia may have difficulty understanding spoken or written language or may have trouble expressing herself in spoken or written language. Aphasia usually results from damage in the communication centers of the brain. The location and extent of the damage determine the type of aphasia.

Kinds of aphasia

Nonfluent aphasia. The person with nonfluent aphasia speaks slowly and with difficulty. She may grimace and use hand gestures in attempting to communicate. She also may leave out words and endings of words as she speaks.

Fluent aphasia. The person with fluent aphasia speaks normally or rapidly but may unconsciously substitute words or sounds with incorrect choices. She may say "car" when she means "train" or may say "tan" instead of "can." She doesn't realize she is making these errors and so will not correct herself.

Anomic aphasia. With anomic aphasia, the person may speak quite normally but has great difficulty sometimes in coming up with the name of an object or place.

Conduction aphasia. The person with conduction aphasia has trouble repeating words spoken by someone else. Otherwise speech is nearly normal.

Global aphasia. The person with global aphasia has great difficulty speaking, repeating, or comprehending language.

Receptive aphasia (Wernicke's aphasia). The person with receptive aphasia hears what is said but cannot understand; she can speak but cannot understand or monitor her own speech.

Expressive aphasia (Broca's aphasia). The person with expressive aphasia hears and understands but cannot express her own thoughts.

Communicating with the person with aphasia

When aphasia occurs, it is very important that speech therapy is begun very quickly. Being unable to communicate is very frustrating, and it is important to keep encouraging and helping the person to regain her speech. A professional speech therapist will work with the person, but it is equally important to continue the therapy at home after the patient has been released from the hospital. Here are some speech therapy tips to remember:

1. The calmer and quieter the atmosphere, the more relaxed the person will be. A noisy environment will discourage the person from trying to communicate.
2. Encourage the person to speak, and keep stimulating conversation going throughout the day.
3. Some persons with aphasia say "yes" when they mean "no" and vice versa. You must be able to discern the reliability of her answers.
4. Let the person speak for herself. Don't interrupt—give her plenty of time to complete her thought.
5. Constantly correcting the person's mistakes will cause frustration and probably discourage her from trying to speak. Praise her efforts instead.
6. If the person has trouble understanding what you are saying, use nonverbal gestures such as pointing or facial expressions to communicate. Cards with important words on them, such as "hungry" or "bedpan," may be helpful.
7. Don't pretend to understand the person if you don't. Calmly tell her that you don't understand, and encourage her to use nonverbal communication or to write out what she wants.
8. Don't shout or use baby talk. Neither will help the person understand you.
9. If the person appears tired or upset, don't push communication. Aphasia worsens with fatigue and anxiety.
10. Most importantly, be patient, and treat the person with aphasia as an intelligent adult.

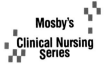

Halo Vest Care at Home

The halo vest is a brace that sometimes is worn after an injury (usually a fracture) to the cervical part of the spine. The vest keeps the head and neck from moving and allows the injured spine to heal.

A person wearing a halo vest needs special care. The halo vest and the pin sites where the screws secure the halo to the head must be inspected and cleaned twice a day. Below is the procedure a caregiver should follow:

Equipment

Cotton swabs
Hydrogen peroxide
Alcohol
Antibiotic ointment if prescribed
Sheepskin or foam padding
Basin of water
Soap
Washcloth
Towel

Procedure

1. Check the pins on the halo traction ring (around the head) to make sure they are secure.
2. Pour hydrogen peroxide on a cotton swab, and wipe carefully around the pin sites. Use a different swab for each pin. Repeat using water on next set of swabs, then dry with additional swabs.
3. Soak a different cotton swab with alcohol, and cleanse each pin of any drainage.
4. If antibiotic ointment has been prescribed, apply it to the pin sites with a cotton swab.
5. Check the pin sites for signs of infection, such as redness, tenderness, swelling, or drainage.
6. Have the person lie down on a bed with his head resting on a pillow (so there is no pressure on the brace). Loosen **one** side of the vest. Gently wash the skin under the vest with soap and water; rinse, and then dry thoroughly. Using a flashlight, check for any redness, chafing, bruising, or any signs that the vest is pressing or rubbing on the skin. If you find indications of pressure, pad the **surrounding** area with sheepskin or foam padding.
7. Fasten the open side of the vest before opening the other side. Wash, rinse, dry, and inspect the other side. Fasten the vest.

8. If the vest lining gets wet, you may cautiously dry it with a hair dryer set on low.

Remember—never open the halo vest while the person is sitting or standing; this will remove the necessary neck support.

Other tips for a person in a halo vest

- Using a cane on steps and uneven ground will aid stability. Flat, sturdy shoes are a must.
- Turn your entire body if you want to look to the side. Mirrors can be attached to the brace to give you a wider range of vision. Avoid activities that may require you to turn your head (such as driving).
- Always keep the set of wrenches to the halo vest with you in case of emergency.
- If you notice a loose pin, infection around a pin site, or have any other problems, contact your doctor immediately.
- Check with your doctor or nurse about how to launder or replace the vest lining when it becomes soiled.
- Mark the proper hole in vest straps, so that when they are rebuckled, the proper fit will be maintained.

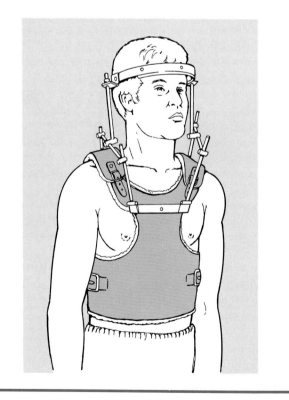

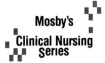
Autonomic Hyperreflexia

Autonomic hyperreflexia is a life-threatening state unique to patients with a spinal cord injury at or above the T6 segment. The condition is caused by a variety of stimuli, most commonly an overly full bladder or rectum. The stimulus triggers an exaggerated reponse of the nervous system, which if left untreated could be fatal.

The symptoms

The symptoms of autonomic hyperreflexia come on suddenly. They include:

- Sudden onset of a severe headache
- Elevated blood pressure
- Pulse rate under 60 beats per minute
- Sweating above the level of injury
- Red splotches on the body above the injury and pale skin below the injury
- Goose bumps, hair raising on arms
- Nasal congestion
- Feelings of anxiety

Treatment
Treatment must begin immediately.

- Raise the person to a sitting position.
- Remove the stimulus causing the hyperreflexia. If the bladder or rectum is full, it must be emptied. A straight catheterization should be performed to drain urine from the bladder. Stool in the rectum should be gently removed manually.

If the above actions do not resolve the symptoms, or if hyperreflexia continues to recur, call the doctor. He may prescribe a medication to lower the blood pressure and prevent future episodes.

Prevention

Prevention is the key to managing autonomic hyperreflexia. Make sure that the person's bladder is not allowed to overfill and that the bowel does not become impacted. Sometimes hyperreflexia occurs because the bowel is being stimulated to evacuate its contents. If this happens frequently, a local anesthetic can be used before the bowel is stimulated.

A person susceptible to autonomic hyperreflexia should always wear a **Medic-Alert** bracelet.

Carry this card in your wallet or purse

Alert

I have a spinal cord injury and may have episodes of autonomic hyperreflexia. I may have the following symptoms: sudden onset of a severe headache; elevated blood pressure; pulse rate under 60 beats per minute; sweating above the level of injury; red splotches on the body above the injury and pale skin below the injury; goose bumps (hair raising on arms); nasal congestion; or feelings of anxiety.

My usual blood pressure is_____

The cause of autonomic hyperreflexia is usually a distended bladder or rectum.

Intervention must be immediate because autonomic hyperreflexia is life threatening

- Catheterize bladder
- Gently remove stool from rectum

Medication may be needed to quickly lower blood pressure while the cause is found and remedied.

Intermittent Self-Catheterization for Men

When the bladder cannot empty itself or cannot do so completely, intermittent catheterization (IC) becomes necessary. This is a procedure that you do yourself. To avoid introducing germs and possibly infection into the bladder, it is important that you are careful to follow a clean procedure. Your doctor will tell you the maximum amount of urine you should have in your bladder and how often you will need to catheterize yourself.

Equipment

Before you begin, make sure you have everything you need:
1. Catheter (and optional extension)
2. Water-soluble lubricant jelly
3. A basin for collecting urine
4. A plastic bag for storing the catheter
5. Premoistened towelettes or a soapy washcloth and rinse cloth

Procedure

Catheterization may be performed while sitting on the toilet, in a wheelchair, in bed, or while standing.
1. Wash your hands thoroughly with soap and water.
2. Wash the penis and surrounding area with soap and water. Rinse with the rinse cloth.
3. Open the lubricant jelly, and squeeze a generous amount onto a paper towel.
4. Open the catheter package, take out the catheter, and roll the first 3 inches or so of the catheter in the lubricant.
5. Put one end of the catheter in the basin or over the seat of the toilet. Hold your penis outward with one hand, and with the other gently insert the catheter through the urinary opening. As you push the catheter in, pull outward on your penis to help the catheter slide in more easily.
6. Continue pushing the catheter in until urine begins to flow; then insert the catheter another 1 to 2 inches. Hold the catheter in place until all the urine has drained into the basin or toilet. To make sure your bladder is completely empty, take some deep breaths or press on your lower abdomen.
7. When the urine flow stops, pinch the catheter

closed and slowly remove it.
8. Empty the basin and rinse it.
9. Wash your hands.
10. Wash the catheter in warm, soapy water and rinse it, both inside and out. Dry it with a clean towel, and place it in a clean plastic bag until the next time you need it. If the catheter appears crusted, rinse or soak it in a solution of half distilled vinegar and half water. Catheters that show wear, become brittle, crack, or do not drain urine well must be replaced.

When to call your doctor

1. If you have any problems inserting the catheter
2. If you have any of the following signs:
   Little or no urine flow
   Pain in the lower back and lower abdomen
   Cloudy or foul-smelling urine
   Bloody urine
   Chills or fever
   Lack of appetite or lack of energy, or both
   Sandlike material (sediment) in the urine
   A red or swollen urinary opening

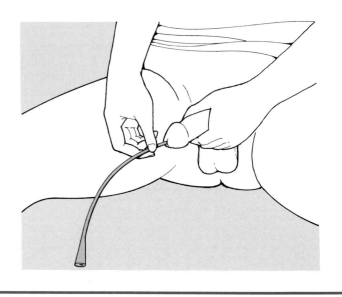

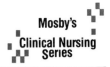
Intermittent Self-Catheterization for Women

When the bladder cannot empty itself or cannot do so completely, intermittent catheterization (IC) becomes necessary. This is a procedure that you do yourself. To avoid introducing germs and possibly infection into the bladder, it is important that you are careful to follow a clean procedure. Your doctor will tell you the maximum amount of fluid you should have in your bladder and how often you will need to catheterize yourself.

Equipment

Before you begin, make sure you have everything you need:

1. Catheter: Use a short female catheter if you are doing catheterization on a toilet. Use a long catheter with an extension tube if you are doing this procedure from a wheelchair.
2. Water-soluble lubricant jelly
3. A basin for collecting urine
4. A plastic bag for storing the catheter
5. Premoistened towelettes or a soapy washcloth and a rinse cloth

Procedure

Catheterization may be performed while sitting on the toilet, in a wheelchair, in bed, or while standing.

1. Wash your hands thoroughly with soap and water.
2. Wash the urinary area (urethral opening) and the surrounding area with soap and water. Use downward strokes, and avoid the anal area. Rinse with the rinse cloth.
3. Open the lubricant jelly, and squeeze a generous amount onto a paper towel.
4. Open the catheter package, take out the catheter, and roll the first 1 inch or so of the catheter in the lubricant.
5. Put one end of the catheter in the basin or over the seat of the toilet. With the index finger and ring finger of one hand, spread the lips of the vulva apart, and with the middle finger locate the urethral opening. With the other hand, gently insert the catheter into the urethra.
6. Continue pushing the catheter in about 2 to 3 inches until urine begins to flow. Hold the catheter in place until all the urine has drained into

the basin or toilet. To make sure your bladder is completely empty, take some deep breaths or press on your lower abdomen.
7. When the urine flow stops, pinch the catheter closed and slowly remove it.
8. Empty the basin and rinse it.
9. Wash your hands.
10. Wash the catheter in warm, soapy water and rinse it, both inside and out. Dry it with a clean towel, and place it in a clean plastic bag until the next time you need it. If the catheter appears crusted, rinse or soak it in a solution of half distilled vinegar and half water. Catheters that show wear, become brittle, crack, or do not drain urine well must be replaced.

Hint: A lighted, free-standing make-up mirror can be useful when first learning this procedure.

When to call your doctor

1. If you have any problems inserting the catheter
2. If you have any of the following signs:
   Little or no urine flow
   Pain in the lower back and lower abdomen
   Cloudy or foul-smelling urine
   Bloody urine
   Chills or fever
   Lack of appetite or lack of energy, or both
   Sandlike material (sediment) in the urine
   A red or swollen urinary opening

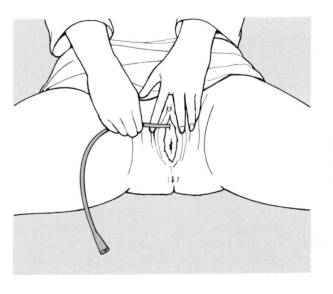

Bowel Management at Home

Because your spinal cord has been injured, your brain cannot send messages to or receive messages from your bowel. You may not be able to tell when your bowel is full, and you may not be able to empty your bowel at will. However, depending on the location of your injury, you may have a bowel that easily responds to rectal stimulation and a well-planned bowel program that includes a proper diet, consistent timing, activity, and medicine.

Diet

To keep your bowel functioning regularly, it is important to eat three well-balanced meals each day. The following is a list of what to include:

- 2 servings from the milk group, which includes milk, cheese, yogurt, cottage cheese, and ice cream
- 2 or more servings from the meat group, which includes beef, pork, fish, poultry, eggs, cheese, and dry peas or beans
- 4 or more servings from the vegetable and fruit group, which includes all fruits and vegetables; it is also recommended that you eat dark green leafy or orange vegetables and fruit three or four times a week
- 4 or more servings from the breads and cereals group, which includes enriched or whole grain products, pasta, and grits

If you are overweight, choose low-calorie foods from the list above. Stay away from foods that you know will upset your stomach, give you gas, or cause diarrhea.

If your stool is too hard or scant, eat more food that is high in fiber, such as raw fruits and vegetables and whole grain breads and cereals with bran. Soft stools may be caused by insufficient fiber in the diet or by a cold or the flu.

Timing

Attempts will be made to return your body to the bowel routine it knew before your injury. If you used to have a stool every day or every other day, then that routine probably will be reestablished. (Bowel movements more than 3 days apart are discouraged because of possible constipation.)

The colon is naturally stimulated to eliminate its contents about 30 minutes after eating. If this fits in with your life-style and the time that your assistant is present (if you employ one), then you may want to choose this routine. Whatever routine you choose, try always to do your program within 15 minutes of your established time.

Activity

You should get as much exercise as possible. Physical activity will improve your muscle tone and stimulate your gastrointestinal tract to move food through the intestines and stool to the rectum. Exercise makes you feel better and improves your appetite, which improves your bowel program.

Your physical activity will depend on how much you can do. Stretch and move every muscle you can. Contract and relax your abdominal muscles by breathing deeply and tightening your abdomen periodically. Do range-of-motion exercises, change your position frequently, and perform as much of your own care as you can. If you can, wash yourself, feed and dress yourself, and do your own transfers and bowel and bladder program.

Medicine and treatment

Sometimes medications such as suppositories and stool softeners are needed to help establish a proper bowel program. Because your bowels can become reliant on laxatives and enemas, it is best to use these medicines only occasionally, when constipation cannot be relieved by other methods.

Rectal stimulation can be used to activate peristalsis and relax the sphincter muscle. The stimulation causes wavelike movement of the intestinal tract, which in turn causes the bowel to eliminate its contents. Your doctor or nurse will give you further instructions on rectal stimulation. Massaging your abdomen from the right side to the left also can help stimulate the intestinal tract.

Things to remember

1. If you can manage it, the best position for your body during a bowel movement is sitting erect with your feet flat on the floor or on a small stepstool. This allows gravity to help the process.
2. Never stay seated on a toilet more than 20 to 30 minutes at a time because of the risk of developing a pressure area.
3. You can substitute a bedside commode for a toilet. Since they are somewhat unstable, you will need to have someone to hold it steady or find a way to stabilize it. If you cannot maintain a sitting position, position yourself on your left side in bed.

Skin Care Tips

Your injury has caused a loss of sensation (feeling) in parts of your body and has made moving these parts difficult or impossible. This can cause problems with your skin. Because you cannot feel discomfort, you don't realize that parts of your skin may not be receiving an adequate blood supply and that skin breakdown may be occurring. Skin breakdown can lead to skin ulcers, a serious problem. Therefore it is important to prevent skin problems. Following are some of the disorders that can result from lack of skin care and tips on how to prevent them.

Pressure areas

Pressure areas are those areas of the body that come in contact with solid things, such as a chair or a bed. The weight of the body pressing against a bed, for example, causes the blood supply to the skin to be cut off. If the pressure is not relieved, an ulcer (sore) may begin to form. Pressure areas can also be caused by clothing that is too tight or wrinkled, belts, elastic bands, tight-fitting shoes, buttons, and ill-fitted equipment, or by lying on articles such as pins, rubber bands, or even crumbs.

To relieve pressure areas when you are in a wheelchair, change your position at least every 15 to 30 minutes. Lean from side to side, forward and backward (make sure the brake is on). When you are in bed, follow a turning schedule that includes your sides, back, and abdomen. Usually you should turn yourself at least every 2 hours. Ask your nurse to help you develop your own turning schedule. You may need to set an alarm clock to wake yourself periodically during the night to turn yourself. No two skin surfaces should rest together. You can use pillows to relieve pressure areas. Your feet and ankles can lie suspended over the end of the bed.

Remember: When you lie on your back, don't let your heels rest on the mattress.

- Always use and maintain special mattresses and wheelchair cushions as directed.
- When you lie on your side, don't let your ankles lie on top of each other or on the mattress.
- When you lie on your stomach, use pillows to protect your hip bones, knees, and toes.

If a pressure area develops, call your doctor, and keep all pressure off the area until it returns to normal.

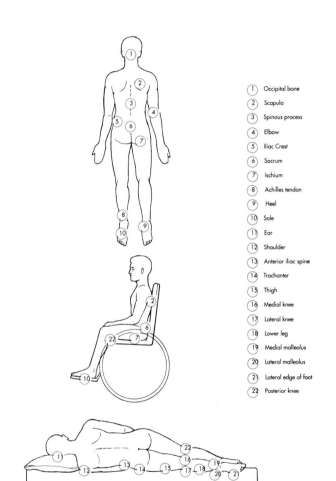

1. Occipital bone
2. Scapula
3. Spinous process
4. Elbow
5. Iliac Crest
6. Sacrum
7. Ischium
8. Achilles tendon
9. Heel
10. Sole
11. Ear
12. Shoulder
13. Anterior iliac spine
14. Trochanter
15. Thigh
16. Medial knee
17. Lateral knee
18. Lower leg
19. Medial malleolus
20. Lateral malleolus
21. Lateral edge of foot
22. Posterior knee

Scratches and abrasions

Scratches and abrasions are caused by uncut or rough fingernails and toenails and by bumping into things that have rough or sharp edges, such as furniture corners or open drawers. Abrasions also can occur from allowing skin to be dragged over a surface, such as sheets or a chair.

To prevent scratches and abrasions, keep your nails trimmed and smooth. Be aware of your environment at all times. Think safety. Check your wheelchair for areas that could cause scratches.

If you do get a scratch or abrasion, wash the area and dry it well. Leave the wound open to air. Do not cover it with a bandage. Do not apply any medication unless your doctor tells you to.

Burns

Burns can come from many sources besides fire. A scalding shower or bathwater, hot car upholstery, sun, cigarettes, electric blankets or pads, hot liquids, pots and pans, and radiators. A hot sidewalk can burn your feet.

Accidents will happen, but you can take steps to prevent burns:
- Always pretest bathwater or showers.
- Place pads, towels, or cushions on car upholstery before sitting.
- Build up a tolerance to the sun—use sunscreen or wear protective clothing.
- Don't use heating pads, electric blankets, or hot water bottles.
- Use pads and wooden trays to carry hot pans.
- Be sure that exposed pipes under sinks are covered with protective insulation.
- Always wear shoes.

If you should get a burn, apply cold water to the area and call your doctor. Use medication on the area only if your doctor prescribes it. Don't break open burn blisters. Keep all pressure off the burned area.

Frostbite

Frostbite occurs when the skin is exposed to extreme cold. Fingers and toes are the areas that are usually affected. You can prevent frostbite by wearing protective clothing in cold weather, including gloves, warm socks, and shoes. Ice packs can cause frostbite and should not be used.

If you do get frostbitten, put the affected part in *lukewarm* water and call your doctor. Never rub the frostbitten area or put it in hot or cold water.

Chafing

When moisture is allowed to remain between two body parts, such as under arms, between thighs, behind knees, between toes, or under breasts, chafing can occur. The moisture may be caused by perspiration, urine, stool, or inadequate towel drying after a bath or shower.

To prevent chafing, wash your skin with mild soap and water, rinse, and dry thoroughly. Whenever possible, expose chafed areas to air. Separate the areas that are touching each other. Do not apply powder, creams, or medication unless your doctor instructs you to.

Bruises

Bruises are caused by bumping into things, falling, or by being hit by moving objects, such as a baseball or Frisbee. Being aware of where things are in your environment will help prevent bruising. If you should be bruised, keep any pressure off the affected area until it is healed. If the area is swollen, call your doctor, for you may have sustained a fracture.

Skin checks

Check your skin at least twice a day. Make sure you check all parts of your body. Use a mirror to check any areas that you can't see easily. Look for red areas, blisters, scratches, rashes, pimples, open areas, or bruises. Keep any pressure off a reddened area until it has healed. Protect blisters from further injury. Never rupture the blister. Contact your doctor or nurse for further advice.

Nail care

It is important to keep your nails and the skin around them in good shape. Check the skin around your nails at least once a week. Look for any changes in color and any cracks, blisters, or swelling. Report any signs of infection to your doctor.

Clean your nails carefully, but don't use metal or sharp objects. Trim nails carefully and smooth them with an emery board. Toenails should be cut straight across. Remove any hangnails by cutting them close to the point of origin. Wear properly fitted shoes. Protect your feet from injury.

CHAPTER 9

Drug Therapy for Neurologic Disorders

INTRACRANIAL PRESSURE/CEREBRAL EDEMA

Diuretics and glucocorticosteroids are the major drug categories used to treat increased intracranial pressure and/or cerebral edema.

DIURETICS

The parenteral osmotic diuretics, including mannitol and urea, induce diuresis by adding to the solutes already present in the tubular fluid; they are particularly effective in increasing osmotic pressure there because very little if any drug is reabsorbed by the tubules. Thus more water is pulled into tubular fluid and less sodium, chloride and water are reabsorbed by the kidneys in an effort to equalize the higher solute content. The excesses are then excreted in the urine.

Indications: Treatment of elevated intracranial and cerebral edema.

Usual dosage: *Mannitol IV:* 0.25-2 g/kg of a 15% to 25% solution over ½-1 h. *Urea IV:* 0.5 to 1.5 g/kg of 30% solution in 5% or 10% dextrose injection over ½-2 h.

Precautions/contraindications: Use with extreme caution in hypervolemia, severe renal function impairment, intracranial bleeding, severe dehydration, severe cardiac decompensation, and frank liver failure.

Side effects/adverse reactions: CNS: Blurred vision, headaches, seizures, confusion, dizziness. **GI:** Nausea, vomiting, diarrhea. **GU:** Difficult urination or an increase in urination. **CV:** Arrhythmias, edema, angina-type chest pains, hypotension or hypertension. **Metabolic:** Fluid and electrolyte imbalance, acidosis. **Pulmonary:** pulmonary congestion. **Other:** Dry mouth, chills, fever, skin rash.

Pharmacokinetics: Onset of action: *IV:* Mannitol and urea within 10-60 min. **Duration of action:** Mannitol 6-8 h, urea 5-6 h. **Route of elimination:** Primarily by the kidneys.

Interactions: May potentiate effects of other diuretics. Diuretic usage may result in hypokalemia, therefore concurrent therapy with digitalis glycosides may increase the risk for arrhythmias and digitalis glycoside toxicity. Urea may increase the excretion of lithium, thus reducing lithium effectiveness.

Nursing considerations: High concentrations of mannitol and/or exposure to low room temperatures may result in crystallization of mannitol. If crystals are observed, the bottle may be warmed in a hot water bath, then cooled to body temperature prior to administration. A final in-line filter should be used with mannitol solutions, especially with mannitol solutions of 15% or greater. Do not add mannitol to other intravenous solutions or medications. Monitor renal function, urine output, blood pressure, respiratory parameters, daily weight and serum electrolytes. Frequently evaluate vital signs to detect any rapidly changing conditions due to alterations in intravascular volume, pulmonary edema or hemoconcentration. If urine output is less than 30-50 ml/h or a weight gain is in excess of 3 pounds/day, contact the physician for instructions.

Assess patient for signs and symptoms of hyponatremia, hypernatremia, hypokalemia, hyperkalemia, and metabolic acidosis. Neurologic status is also closely monitored. Avoid extravasation; inspect intravenous site regularly for tissue inflammation and irritation. Urea infusion rate should not exceed 4 ml/min because a more rapid infusion may result in hemolysis and cerebral vasomotor symptoms. Each urea dose should be freshly prepared and any unused portion discarded.

Furosemide (Lasix)

Furosemide is a potent loop diuretic that inhibits reabsorption of chloride, sodium, and water along the ascending branch of the loop of Henle and perhaps the proximal and distal tubules. It also exhibits a renal vasodilator effect, resulting in less vascular resistance and an increase in renal blood flow. In addition, it increases urinary excretion of calcium.

Indications: Furosemide is used in the treatment of edema and as adjunct therapy in the treatment of hypertension and hypertensive crisis.

Usual dosage: *Oral:* Initial dose range is 20-80 mg. *IM or IV:* The usual dosage range is 20-40 mg. Additional doses are determined according to individual's response to furosemide.

Precautions/contraindications: Use cautiously in neonate and geriatric patients and patients with diabetes mellitus, ascites, hepatic cirrhosis, hearing function impairment, gout, pancreatitis, acute myocardial infarction, history of systemic lupus erythematosus (SLE), and in patients taking digitalis glycosides, other diuretics, or potassium-depleting glucocorticoids. Avoid use in anuria, severe or frank hepatic or renal impairment, hypovolemia, electrolyte depletion, and hypersensitivity to sulfonamides.

Side effects/adverse reactions: CNS: Headache, vertigo, weakness, confusion. **GI:** Anorexia, abdominal cramps or pain, diarrhea, nausea, vomiting. **GU:** Polyuria, renal failure, bladder spasms, glycosuria. **CV:** Orthostatic hypotension, chest pain. **Other:** Ototoxicity, tinnitus, fluid and electrolyte imbalance, and thrombocytopenia.

Pharmacokinetics: Onset of action: Intravenously 5 min., orally ½-1 h. **Duration of action:** *IV:* 2 h; *Oral:* 6-8 h. **Route of elimination:** Primarily via the kidneys.

Interactions: Diuresis, hypotension, and fluid and electrolyte imbalance may be potentiated if administered with other diuretics. Concurrent therapy with potassium-depleting glucocorticoid or amphotericin B increases the risk of hypokalemia. When given in conjunction with coumarin or heparin, a decrease in anticoagulant effect may result, whereas an increased potential for toxicity is present when administered with digitalis glycosides, lithium, and salicylates. Furosemide diuretic effects may be reduced or antagonized by indomethacin and possibly by the other nonsteroidal anti-inflammatory drugs (NSAIDs).

Nursing considerations: *Oral preparations:* Furosemide may be administered with food or milk to reduce potential for gastric distress. Drug doses should be scheduled for morning or early afternoon to avoid nocturia and sleep interference. *IV:* Administer IV dos-

ages slowly, over at least 1-2 min. If high-dose therapy is necessary, administer by intravenous infusion at a rate of 4 mg/min. *IM:* Use Z-track method for injections. Intramuscular injections are painful; therefore IV administration is preferred. Assess and monitor for electrolyte imbalance, rapid weight changes, intake and output, and vital signs. Neonates and the elderly may be especially sensitive to this drug, so monitor closely for both diuretic response and the development of side/adverse effects, especially hypotension and electrolyte alterations.

GLUCOCORTICOSTEROIDS

Dexamethasone (Decadron)

Dexamethasone is a synthetic glucocorticosteroid with antiinflammatory and immunosuppressive effects.

Indications: Dexamethasone is used in the diagnosis of Cushing's syndrome; the treatment of allergies, anaphylaxis, angioedema, serum sickness, urticarial transfusion reactions; and in acute exacerbation of systemic lupus erythematosus (SLE), rheumatic carditis, and nonrheumatic inflammation, and systemic dermatomyositis. It has been used to treat a variety of respiratory, dermatologic, gastrointestinal, neurologic, neurotraumatic (especially cerebral edema associated with metastatic brain tumors, craniotomy or head injuries), and hematologic disorders.

Usual dosage: *Oral:* Intra-articular, intralesional and intravenous, range of 0.5 to 16 mg. *For cerebral edema:* 10 mg IV followed by 4 mg IM every 6 hours. *For shock:* 20 mg followed by 3 mg/kg IV infusion per 24 h or 1-6 mg/kg as a single dose.

Precautions/contraindications: Contraindicated in psychosis, systemic fungal infections, active tuberculosis, and intramuscular use in idiopathic thrombocytopenic purpura. Use cautiously in patients with a history of hypersensitivity, bacteria, fungal or virus infection, cirrhosis, cardiac disease such as congestive heart failure, and in peptic ulcer disease.

Side effects/adverse reactions: CNS: mood changes, headache, disorientation, hallucinations, dizziness, restlessness, seizures, insomnia; **GI:** increased appetite, gastric distress or ulceration, nausea, vomiting, pancreatitis; **CV:** tachycardia, hypotension, thrombophlebitis, arrhythmias; **Other:** fungus infections, osteoporosis, acne, poor wound healing.

Pharmacokinetics: Onset of action: *Oral:* Usually within 6 h; *IV:* Rapid. **Duration of action:** *Oral:* Approximately 2.75 days; *IM:* 6 days. **Route of elimination:** Metabolized in liver, excreted by kidneys.

Interactions: Aminoglutethimide should not be administered with dexamethasone because it decreases the half-life and therapeutic effect of dexamethasone.

Severe hypokalemia may result with concurrent administration of parenteral amphotericin B and potassium-depleting diuretics. The potential for arrhythmias and digitalis glycoside toxicity increases in the presence of hypokalemia. Avoid administration of live virus vaccines or immunizations because they are less effective and may increase the risk of developing a viral disease. Avoid concurrent administration of ritodrine to pregnant women because pulmonary edema in the mother has been reported. Glucocorticoids may increase blood glucose levels; therefore insulin or the oral antidiabetic agent's dosage may need to be increased in diabetic patients.

Nursing considerations: Glucocorticoids may be administered via many routes; therefore carefully read physician's orders and drug labels to select the proper formulation, because all products are not safe for different routes of administration. Monitor input and output record and serum electrolytes, glucose, and protein levels, especially with patients receiving parenteral agents. Monitor patient for rapid weight gain, dyspnea, peripheral edema, increased heart rate, and/or blood pressure. Assess patients for signs and symptoms of hypokalemia and the many side/adverse effects previously reviewed. Intramuscular injections must be administered deeply in the gluteal muscle to prevent tissue atrophy. Avoid deltoid muscle administration and repeated injections into the same site. Advise patients taking oral dexamethasone to take it with food and never on an empty stomach.

ACQUIRED IMMUNODEFICIENCY SYNDROME (AIDS)

Many drug products are under investigation for the prevention and treatment of AIDS-associated infections. This section will review the major (approved) drugs for the treatment of toxoplasmosis, cryptococcus meningitis, cytomegalovirus, and primary HIV infections.

TREATMENT OF TOXOPLASMOSIS

Pyrimethamine (Daraprim) and Sulfadiazine

Pyrimethamine and sulfadiazine are folic acid antagonists that act synergistically to treat this protozoal infection.

Indications: Treatment of central nervous system toxoplasmosis and malaria.

Usual dosage: *Oral:* 50 to 100 mg orally of pyrimethamine daily in combination with 0.5-1.5 g of sulfadiazine q 6 h for 3-6 weeks. *Maintenance:* 25-50 mg of pyrimethamine daily in combination with 250 mg to 1 g of sulfadiazine q 6 h.

Precautions/contraindications: Use cautiously in patients with a history of seizure disorders or impaired hepatic or renal function, and in persons with malabsorption syndrome that affects folate levels, such as in alcoholism and pregnancy. It is contraindicated in patients that are hypersensitive to the drug(s) and in patients with megaloblastic anemia.

Side effects/adverse reactions: CNS: Depression, seizures, malaise. **GI:** Painful and/or inflamed tongue, dry mouth or throat, diarrhea, anorexia, nausea, vomiting. **CV:** Cardiac rhythm disorders. **Other:** Fever, rash, blood dyscrasias.

Pharmacokinetics: Pyrimethamine has a peak effect in 3 h, half-life of 80-123 h but may be as short as 23 h in AIDS patients; sulfadiazine has an onset of action of ½ h, peak effect in 3-6 h, half-life of 8-10 h. **Route of elimination:** Pyrimethamine and sulfadiazine are metabolized in the liver and primarily eliminated by the kidneys.

Interactions: Increased potential for leukopenia and/or thrombocytopenic effects if used concurrently with other anti–folic acid drugs and/or bone marrow depressants.

Nursing considerations: If gastric irritation occurs, take medications with meals or snacks. Encourage maintenance of regular visits to physician for blood counts. In high-dose therapy, patients may be required to have complete blood and platelet counts weekly. To prevent folic acid deficiency induced by these medications, leucovorin (folinic acid) is usually prescribed. To reduce the potential of inducing CNS toxicity in patients with a history of seizure disorders, smaller initial doses of pyrimethamine are recommended.

TREATMENT OF CRYPTOCOCCUS MENINGITIS

Amphotericin B and Flucytosine

The systemic-acting antifungal agents amphotericin B (Fungizone) and flucytosine (Ancobon) are the primary agents used to treat cryptococcus meningitis. Amphotericin B has been theorized to act by binding to sterols in the fungus cell membrane, which eventually leads to loss of cellular potassium and other small cell substances. Thus it is fungistatic or fungicidal, depending on the drug concentration in body fluids and fungus susceptibility. Flucytosine enters fungal cells, where it is converted to fluorouracil, an antimetabolite. This antimetabolite interferes with fungal pyrimidine metabolism and thus exhibits selective toxicity against the fungi.

Indications: Amphotericin B is indicated for the treatment of aspergillosis, blastomycosis, disseminated candidiasis, coccidioidomycosis, cryptococcosis, histoplasmosis, and other susceptible fungal infections. Flucytosine is used in the treatment of serious systemic infections caused by susceptible strains of *Candida* or *Cryptococcus*.

Usual dosage: Amphotericin B intrathecal dose is 25-100 μg initially q 2-3 days, gradually increasing dose by 500 μg as tolerated by the patient. Maximum total dose is 15 mg. Intravenous infusion initial dose is 1 mg in 5% dextrose injection administered over 2-4 h. If tolerated, the dose may be increased in 5-10 mg increments according to patient response and severity of infection. Maximum daily dose is 50 mg.

Flucytosine is administered orally, 12.5 to 37.5 mg/kg body weight q 6 h.

Precautions/contraindications: Amphotericin B has been reported to be nephrotoxic; therefore use with extreme caution in renal function impairment. Reduce flucytosine dose in renal function impairment to avoid drug accumulation and toxicity. Use extreme caution in patients with bone marrow depression or in patients that have previously received cytotoxic drug or radiation therapy as flucytosine may exacerbate bone marrow depression. Hypersensitivity to either drug is a contraindication to their usage.

Side effects/adverse reactions: *Amphotericin B effects*—**CNS:** Fever, shaking chills, headaches; rarely reported: seizures, peripheral neuropathy (reported more often with intrathecal injections). **GI:** Nausea, vomiting, abdominal distress, diarrhea, cramps. **CV:** Arrhythmias, hypotension, hypertension, cardiac arrest. **Hematologic:** Normochromic, normocytic anemia. **Renal:** Increased or decreased urination, renal function impairment. **Other:** Weight loss, pain at injection site with thrombophlebitis, anaphylaxis, flushing, rash, pruritus. *Flucytosine effects*—**CNS:** Less frequently reported: headache, sedation, dizziness, confusion, hallucinations. **GI:** Nausea, vomiting, diarrhea, anorexia, abdominal pain. **Hematologic:** Anemia, leukopenia (sore throat, fever), and thrombocytopenia (increased bleeding episodes, bruising). **Other:** Jaundice, skin rash.

Pharmacokinetics: *Amphotericin B:* Half-life approximately 24 h, peak plasma level between 0.5 and 2 μg/ml after an initial intravenous infusion of 1 to 5 mg/day. **Route of elimination:** Very slowly via the kidneys (amphotericin B is detected in urine for at least 7 weeks after the drug is discontinued). Half-life is 2.5-6 h, time to peak serum level is 1-2 h. **Route of elimination:** Kidneys.

Interactions: Concurrent use of either drug with other bone marrow depressants or radiation therapy may result in an increased bone marrow depressant effect. Also, amphotericin B given in combination with glucocorticosteroids may result in severe hypokalemia. If amphotericin B, which frequently causes hypokalemia, is given concurrently with a digitalis glycoside, digitalis toxicity may result. An increased potential for nephrotoxicity occurs when amphotericin B is given concurrently with other nephrotoxic agents. Use extreme caution and close supervision when any of these combinations are administered concurrently.

Nursing considerations: *Amphotericin B* is diluted with 10 ml of sterile water (without preservatives); then it is added to 5% dextrose injection. To avoid removal of significant amounts of amphotericin B during intravenous infusion, the final in-line filter (if used) should have a mean pore diameter greater than 1 micron. Reconstituted amphotericin B solutions should be protected from light (foil covered) during administration. If administered intravenously, amphotericin B should be given slowly over 6 h. Monitor IV flow rate closely because rapid infusion may cause cardiovascular collapse. If reaction occurs, stop therapy and notify the physician immediately. During the initial IV infusion, monitor vital signs q 15 to 30 min and observe patient closely for adverse effects. Be aware that fever, chills, nausea, and headache occur in 20% to 90% of the patients, usually beginning several hours after starting the infusion and subsiding in 4 h after the drug is discontinued. These drug-induced side effects usually decrease with continued therapy, but when necessary the physician may prescribe use of a prophylactic drug (such as acetaminophen, antiemetic, or corticosteroids) prior to the infusion to reduce the intensity of these effects. Closely monitor intake and output ratio and patterns (such as changes in appearance of urine or quantity of urine); perform blood tests, especially for potassium; renal function tests; and hematologic profiles prior to and during therapy. Frequently check IV site for extravasation, local inflammation, or thrombophlebitis. To reduce the risk of thrombophlebitis, use a scalp vein needle in the most distal vein possible; use alternate veins for administration of infusions, or the physician may prescribe the addition of heparin or hydrocortisone to the infusion. *Flucytosine*—Monitor laboratory tests, especially renal function, hematologic and hepatic function tests, prior to and frequently during therapy. Monitor intake and output ratio and patterns (inpatient setting) and advise patient to report sore mouth or throat, unusual bleeding or bruising, and fever (home setting). To reduce the incidence of nausea and vomiting, instruct the patient to take capsules (if more than one is ordered) over a 15-min period.

ANTIVIRAL AGENTS

The following antiviral drugs are used to treat specific viruses and reduce relapses induced by them. They are not cures and they do not totally eradicate the specific virus.

HERPES SIMPLEX AND HERPES ZOSTER

Acyclovir (Zovirax)

Acyclovir is an antiviral agent that interferes with herpes simplex virus (HSV) and herpes zoster virus

(HZV) by inhibiting DNA viral replication.

Indications: Acyclovir is indicated for the treatment of herpes simplex, herpes zoster, and herpes genitalis.

Usual dosage: *Oral:* For herpes zoster, 800 mg q 4 h while awake, five times daily for 7 to 10 days. At this time, there is no approved oral dosage schedule for herpes simplex. *IV:* Herpes simplex, 5 to 10 mg/kg body weight q 8 h for 7-10 days. Herpes simplex encephalitis, 10 mg/kg body weight q 8 h for 10 days. Herpes zoster in immunocompromised patients, 10 mg/kg of body weight q 8 h for 1 week.

Precautions/contraindications: Use IV acyclovir with extreme caution in dehydrated patients or in patients with impaired renal function. Approximately 1% of the patients receiving IV acyclovir exhibit encephalopathic changes. Therefore use with caution in patients with underlying neurologic abnormalities, severe renal or hepatic impairment, electrolyte imbalance, or significant hypoxia.

Side effects/adverse reactions: *Oral*—CNS: Headache, dizziness; **GI:** Nausea, vomiting, diarrhea, stomach pain. *Parenteral*—CNS: Rarely, confusion, hallucinations, convulsions, tremors, coma. **GI:** Loss of appetite, nausea or vomiting. **Other:** Acute renal failure (if given by bolus injection), pain or inflammation at injection site.

Pharmacokinetics: Half-life: *Oral:* 3.3 h *IV:* 2.5 h. **Peak serum level:** *Oral:* In 1.7 h. *IV:* At the end of administering the infusion, usually 1 h; **Route of elimination:** Via the kidneys.

Interactions: An increased risk for nephrotoxicity occurs when acyclovir is given concurrently with other nephrotoxic medications, especially in the presence of impaired renal function.

Nursing considerations: Prophylactic use of oral acyclovir is reserved for patients that have frequent (more than 6 attacks annually), painful herpes attacks. Drug resistance may develop in immunocompromised patients who receive continuous or repeated acyclovir therapy. Parenteral acyclovir is prepared by adding 10 ml sterile water for injection (without preservatives) to the acyclovir. Shake well to dissolve drug in solution. This solution should be used within 12 h. This is added to a compatible IV infusion solution with a final concentration of 7 mg/ml or less. The diluted solution should be used within 24 h. Acyclovir is for IV infusion only and should be administered over at least 1 h to prevent nephrotoxicity. Closely monitor the IV flow rate and infusion site during administration. Monitor intake and output and maintain proper hydration according to physician's orders to prevent crystallization of acyclovir in the renal tubules. Closely monitor laboratory results, especially blood, liver, and renal function tests, because drug dosage adjustments may become necessary.

TREATMENT OF CYTOMEGALOVIRUS

Ganciclovir (Cytovene, DHPG)

Ganciclovir is an antiviral agent used to treat cytomegalovirus retinitis. It is a prodrug that is structurally similar to acyclovir. Ganciclovir's antiviral action is activated by chemical conversion in the infected cells, which results in an inhibition of viral DNA synthesis.

Indications: Treatment of cytomegalovirus (CMV) retinitis in immunocompromised patients.

Usual dosage: *IV:* Initial dose is 5 mg/kg body weight administered over a minimum of 1 h, q 12 h for 2-3 weeks. Maintenance dose is 5 mg/kg body weight administered over a minimum of 1 h, daily, or 6 mg/kg body weight administered over a minimum of 1 h for 5 days each week.

Precautions/contraindications: Use with extreme caution in renal function impairment (reduce dose), and with absolute neutrophil counts less than 500 cells/mm^3 or platelet counts less than 25,000 cells/mm^3. Contraindicated in cases of known hypersensitivity to acyclovir or ganciclovir.

Side effects/adverse reactions: CNS: Increased nervousness, tremors, mood alterations. **GI:** Anorexia, nausea, vomiting, stomach pain. **Other:** Anemia, granulocytopenia (sore throat and fever), thrombocytopenia (bleeding, bruising), pain at injection site.

Pharmacokinetics: Half-life: Approximately 3 h. **Peak serum levels:** At the end of the intravenous infusion or approximately 1 h. **Route of elimination:** Kidneys.

Interactions: Increased bone marrow depressant effects may occur if ganciclovir is given with other bone marrow depressants or radiation therapy. Concurrent use with zidovudine may result in increased myelosuppression.

Nursing considerations: To avoid drug toxicity, administer ganciclovir over a minimum of 1 h in adequately hydrated patients. In severe neutropenia (absolute neutrophil count [ANC] less than 500 cells/mm^3) or severe thrombocytopenia (platelet count less than 25,000 cells/mm^3), it is recommended that drug therapy be temporarily stopped until bone marrow recovery is noted (ANC is 750 cc/mm^3). Closely monitor complete blood counts, platelet count, and liver and renal function tests, as drug dosage may need to be decreased or stopped, based on test results. Ophthalmologic examinations should be performed weekly during the induction drug therapy and every 2 weeks during the maintenance drug therapy.

TREATMENT OF PRIMARY HIV

Zidovudine (Retrovir, AZT)

Zidovudine is an antiviral agent used in the treatment of AIDS or AIDS-related complex (ARC) or asymptomatic human immunodeficiency virus (HIV). Zidovudine is a virustatic; that is, it inhibits viral DNA replication.

Indications: See previous paragraph.

Usual dosage: *Symptomatic HIV infection:* 100 mg orally q 4 h (600 mg/day). *Asymptomatic HIV infection:* 100 mg orally q 4 h while awake (500 mg/day). Parenterally, 1-2 mg/kg body weight by intravenous infusion over 1 h, q 4 h around the clock until oral therapy is instituted.

Precautions/contraindications: Zidovudine is contraindicated in patients that have had severe, life-threatening allergic reactions to it. Use with extreme caution in patients with impaired renal and hepatic function and in patients with bone marrow depression, that is, granulocyte counts below 1000 cells/mm³ or hemoglobin below 9.5 g/dl.

Side effects/adverse reactions: CNS: Severe headaches, insomnia, paresthesia, sedation, dizziness. **GI:** Loss of appetite, diarrhea, nausea, vomiting, abdominal pain and distress. **Other:** Malaise, weakness, rash, myalgia, fever, chills, sore throat.

Pharmacokinetics: Half-life: 1 h. **Peak serum level:** ½-1½ h. **Route of elimination:** Liver metabolized, excreted by kidneys.

Interactions: Bone marrow depressant effects may be increased if given concurrently with other bone marrow depressants or radiation therapy. If given concurrently with ganciclovir, severe hematologic toxicity has occurred. Zidovudine has an increased serum concentration, extended half-life, and increased potential for toxicity if given concurrently with probenecid.

Nursing considerations: Advise patient to closely adhere to the prescribed medication schedule and course of therapy, to not take other medications concurrently without approval of his physician, to maintain schedule for regular visits to his physician for blood tests, and to avoid sexual contact or practice safe sex to help prevent transmission of the AIDS virus to others. Parenteral zidovudine (intravenous infusion) should be administered over 1 h at a constant rate. Closely monitor all laboratory tests, especially complete blood counts and liver and renal function tests. The care of the patient with AIDS is complex; therefore the nurse should use the nursing process to organize and coordinate patient care and closely follow the guidelines recommended by the Centers for Disease Control (CDC) and its agencies.

SKELETAL MUSCLE RELAXANTS

Baclofen (Lioresal) and Dantrolene (Dantrium)

Baclofen and dantrolene are agents commonly prescribed for the treatment of spasticity resulting from multiple sclerosis, spinal cord diseases and/or injuries.

In addition, dantrolene is also indicated for the treatment of spasticity caused by cerebrovascular accident, cerebral palsy, and as a therapy adjunct in malignant hyperthermia.

Indications: See previous paragraph.

Usual dosage: Baclofen tablet 5 mg three times daily initially. A 5 mg dosage increment increase may be instituted q 3 days as necessary, until the desired effect is achieved. Dantrolene is available in oral and parenteral dosage forms. The oral antispastic dose is 25 mg daily initially. The daily dose may be increased by 25 mg q 4-7 days until the desired effect is achieved or until 100 mg four times daily is reached. Whenever possible, administer the oral dosage form in four divided daily doses. Currently the parenteral dosage form is only indicated for the treatment of malignant hyperthermia. The prophylactic dose by intravenous infusion is 2.5 mg/kg body weight given over 60 min, prior to anesthesia. The minimum therapeutic or treatment dose is 1 mg/kg body weight initially, by rapid IV push. This dose should be repeated until the desired effect is achieved or a maximum cumulative dose of 10 mg/kg body weight is reached. The oral prophylaxis dose is 4-8 mg/kg body weight daily in 3 or 4 divided doses for 48 h prior to surgery. The last dose is given with a minimum of water approximately 3-4 h prior to the scheduled surgery. The postmalignant hyperthermia treatment dose is 4-8 mg/kg body weight per day in four divided doses for 24-72 h. This oral regimen is usually prescribed as a follow-up to parenteral therapy.

Precautions/contraindications: *Baclofen*— Use with caution in geriatric patients because they are usually more susceptible to the CNS toxic effects of this drug. Also use with caution in patients with an existing cerebral lesion(s) or cerebrovascular accident because of the possibility of increasing CNS, respiratory and/or cardiovascular depression, ataxia, and reports of psychiatric disturbances such as hallucinations, confusion, depression, or euphoria. Baclofen may increase blood glucose levels in diabetics and may reduce seizure control in epileptic patients. *Dantrolene* should not be administered to patients with active hepatic disease states, such as in hepatitis or cirrhosis. It should also be used with caution in patients that have impaired cardiac function (dantrolene may cause pleural effusion and pericarditis), impaired liver function (increased risk of hepatotoxicity), preexisting myopathy or neuromuscular diseases (may predispose the patient to respiratory insufficiency), and in patients older than 35 years old (especially females and patients with an increased risk of developing hepatotoxicity).

Side effects/adverse reactions: *Baclofen*—**CNS:** Dizziness, sedation, weakness, confusion, headache, slurred speech, trembling, ataxia, unusual excitement, or unusual tiredness. **GI:** Nausea, constipation. **CV:** Hypotension. The CNS toxic effects following an overdose include visual alterations (blurred or double), seizures, severe muscle weakness, strabismus, vomiting, and respiratory depression.

Dantrolene—**CNS:** Dizziness, sedation, general discomfort, increased weakness. **GI:** Diarrhea, nausea, vomiting. **Other:** Muscle weakness other than muscles affecting respiration; respiratory depression. Chronic oral dosing may result in visual disturbances, chills, elevated temperature, dysphagia, headache, anorexia, slurred speech, uncontrolled urination or frequent urge to urinate, insomnia, and increased nervousness. Physician intervention is usually necessary when the patient has dark or bloody urine, seizures, allergic dermatitis, hepatotoxicity, depression, phlebitis, pleural effusion with pericarditis, difficulty urinating, or severe constipation.

Pharmacokinetics: Onset of action: *Baclofen*—Unpredictable, may range from hours to weeks. *Dantrolene*—Orally for spasticity caused by upper motor neuron disturbances, within 1 week or more; malignant hyperthermia, adjunct to other therapies. **Peak serum level:** Baclofen in 2-3 h; dantrolene, oral, 5 h. **Route of elimination:** Baclofen via the kidneys; dantrolene metabolized in liver, metabolites excreted by the kidneys.

Interactions: Baclofen or dantrolene, if administered concurrently with other CNS depressing drugs, may result in enhanced CNS depressant effects. The concurrent use of other hepatotoxic medications with dantrolene may increase the risk of hepatotoxicity. This risk is higher in females over 35 years old that are also taking estrogens. It is recommended that calcium channel–blocking agents not be administered concurrently with intravenous dantrolene due to the risk of inducing serious cardiac arrhythmias.

Nursing considerations: *Baclofen*—Because this drug decreases seizure threshold, closely monitor for increased convulsions in patients with epilepsy. Observe patient's response to this medication, which may be noted by a decrease in the frequency of spasms and an increase in range of motion and daily physical activities. Assess and monitor intake and output, hepatic function, and vital signs. Inform diabetics of the possible increase in blood glucose levels that may be induced by baclofen. Advise them to report any changes to their physician. Caution patient to avoid driving or potentially hazardous activities until his reaction to baclofen is determined. Also warn patient not to take this medication with alcohol, CNS depressant drugs, or over-the-counter drugs without physician's approval. *Dantrolene*—With the exception of a potential increase in blood glucose serum levels, all other nursing considerations listed for baclofen apply to dantrolene. Moni-

tor closely for hepatotoxicity, especially in female patients over 35 years of age and in patients taking high doses of dantrolene, combinations of antispastic medications, or other hepatotoxic medications. In chronic dantrolene therapy, advise patient to immediately report any signs of jaundice, yellow skin, dark urine, pruritus, abdominal distress, and clay-colored stools. *Parenteral dantrolene:* Monitor vital signs, ECG, serum potassium, and blood and liver tests. Avoid extravasation because this drug is very irritating to tissue. Patients that have had malignant hyperthermia should be advised to carry complete medical information with them that, at a minimum, includes the name of the drug causing the reaction and their physician's name and phone number.

AGENTS USED IN THE TREATMENT OF MIGRAINE HEADACHES

In clinical practice today many agents are used in the treatment of migraine headaches. This section will focus on the use of ergotamine (Ergomar, Gynergen) for the symptomatic treatment, and methysergide maleate (Sansert) and propranolol (Inderal) for the prophylactic treatment, of migraine.

Ergotamine is an alpha-adrenergic blocking agent with a direct effect on vascular smooth muscle. It also has a vasoconstriction effect on dilated cerebral blood vessels and antagonizes serotonin effects in the CNS. Methysergide maleate has an antiserotonin effect that may be related to its effectiveness in preventing migraines. Propranolol's mechanism of action in preventing migraine headaches is unknown, but it may be related to inhibition of both cerebral vasodilation and arteriolar spasms.

Ergotamine (Ergomar, Gynergen)
Indications: Indicated for the treatment of vascular headaches, such as migraine and cluster headaches.

Usual dosage: *Oral:* 2 mg tablets at the onset of an attack, repeated every 30 minutes if necessary, up to a maximum of 6 mg per day or, 10 mg per week. *Sublingual tablets:* at onset of an attack, 1 mg that may be repeated in ½-1 h if needed. If a second dose was necessary, at the onset of the next attack the initial dose should be 2 mg, which may be repeated in ½-1 h if needed. Maximum initial dose is limited to 5 mg with the maximum established per week at 10 mg. *Inhalation:* oral inhalation of one metered spray (360 μg) at onset of attack, which may be repeated q 5 min as necessary until relief is noted. Maximum is 6 sprays in 24 h or 15 metered sprays per week.

Precautions/contraindications: Avoid the use of ergotamine in patients that are considering or have had recent angioplasty or vascular surgery, and in severe hypertension. Use with extreme caution in patients that have a history of an allergic reaction to ergotamine; unstable or vasospastic angina pectoris, coronary artery disease, peripheral vascular disease; impaired renal or hepatic function; and in sepsis or in the presence of a very severe infection. The elderly are very susceptible to ischemic complications and ergotamine-induced hypothermia.

Side effects/adverse reactions: CNS: Dizziness. **GI:** Diarrhea, nausea or vomiting. **CV:** Edema of the lower legs or feet, angina pectoris, cerebral ischemia which presents as anxiety, confusion, and ocular vasospasm.

Pharmacokinetics: Onset of action: Orally variable or usually 1-2 h. **Peak serum level:** ½-3 h. **Route of elimination:** Metabolized in liver, metabolites excreted in bile.

Interactions: Ergotamine should not be given concurrently with other ergot preparations or systemic vasoconstrictor agents, due to the increased risk of inducing peripheral vascular ischemia and gangrene. Also, the vasoconstrictor effects may be increased, which may result in severe hypertension and cerebral hemorrhage. Patients receiving oral contraceptive agents (estrogen and progestin) may be more susceptible to complications due to ergotamine induced vasospasm.

Nursing considerations: Advise patient to (1) take the prescribed dosage form of ergotamine at the first sign of a migraine attack because early treatment may prevent or reduce the full syndrome; (2) contact the physician if migraine attacks increase or are not relieved by the medication; (3) closely follow the dosage schedule and not exceed the maximum amount recommended; (4) report any muscle pain or extremity weakness, cold or numb fingers, nausea, vomiting, or irregular heart rate; (5) be aware that withdrawal from food substances that contain caffeine, tyramine, or other vasopressors like chocolate, fava beans, or food additives or preservatives may trigger a migraine attack. Keeping a food and beverage diary may help in identifying any precipitating substances. Additional factors that may precipitate a migraine include stress, fatigue, insomnia, hormones, and various medications (such as the oral contraceptives and vasodilators).

Methysergide Maleate (Sansert)

Indications: Indicated for prevention of vascular headaches, such as migraine and cluster headaches.

Usual dosage: Oral: 4-6 mg daily, in divided doses.

Precautions/contraindications: Avoid or use with extreme caution in patients with coronary artery disease, unstable or vasospastic angina, severe hypertension, pulmonary disease, rheumatoid arthritis, valvular

heart disease, impaired liver or kidney function, sepsis, or other severe infections and severe pruritus.

Side effects/adverse reactions: CNS: Lightheadedness, depression, sedation, ataxia, insomnia. **GI:** Diarrhea, heartburn, nausea, vomiting, abdominal pain. **CV:** Hypotension, peripheral ischemia, peripheral edema. **Other:** Visual disturbances, CNS excitement, leukopenia, flushing of face, and skin rash.

Pharmacokinetics: Onset of action: 24-48 h. **Duration of effect:** 24-48 h. **Route of elimination:** Primarily via the kidneys.

Interactions: While no significant drug interactions are noted in the USP DI, the nurse should be aware that other vasoconstrictor agents and other ergot alkaloids may enhance vasoconstrictor effects.

Nursing considerations: Methysergide may induce fibrosis; therefore it is recommended that the patient follow a schedule of 6 months on the drug and approximately 1 month drug free. When methysergide is discontinued, the medication should be withdrawn gradually over a 2-3 wk period to prevent rebound headaches. Advise patient to take medication with meals or milk to reduce abdominal distress and to closely adhere to the prescribed dosage. Caution patient about the postural hypotension effects—that is, to make position changes slowly, to lie down if dizziness or faintness occurs, and to avoid driving or performing hazardous tasks until the person's individual reaction to the drug can be determined. The patient should also be instructed to report stomach, back or chest pain, difficulty in breathing, leg pains when walking, cold or numb extremities, elevated temperature, dysuria, and edema.

Propranolol (Inderal)

Indications: Propranolol is indicated for the chronic treatment of angina pectoris, prophylaxis and treatment of cardiac arrhythmias, hypertension, hypertrophic cardiomyopathy, prophylaxis of myocardial reinfarction, prophylaxis of vascular headaches, thyrotoxicosis, anxiety, and tremors.

Usual dosage: For vascular headaches, 20 mg taken orally four times daily initially, increasing dose gradually as necessary until desired effect is achieved or a maximum of 240 mg is reached.

Precautions/contraindications: Avoid the use of propranolol in overt cardiac failure, cardiogenic shock, second or third degree heart block, and in hypotension when the systolic blood pressure is less than 100 mm Hg. Use cautiously in patients with diabetes mellitus, history of allergies, asthma, or emphysema, hyperthyroidism, or mental depression.

Side effects/adverse reactions: CNS: Slight drowsiness, dizziness, depression, insomnia. **GI:** Diarrhea.

CV: Bradycardia. **Other:** Numbness of fingers and/or toes, increased weakness, and decrease in sexual functioning.

Pharmacokinetics: Time to peak effect: 1-1½ h. **Half-life:** 3-5 h. **Route of elimination:** Kidneys.

Interactions: Concurrent administration with insulin or the oral antidiabetic agents may result in hypoglycemia or hyperglycemia. Propranolol may also mask symptoms of developing hypoglycemia, such as elevation in pulse rate and blood pressure. Administration of propranolol with calcium channel blocking agents, clonidine, or guanabenz may potentiate the antihypertensive effect, resulting in excessive hypotension.

Nursing considerations: Carefully screen patients for allergies, asthma, or other obstructive pulmonary type disease states because propranolol may induce bronchospasm and increase the severity and duration of anaphylactic reactions to allergens. Whenever possible, avoid concurrent drug administration. Advise patient to take propranolol consistently, before meals and at bedtime. The presence of food may alter the absorption of propranolol. Patients with diabetes should be closely monitored. Instruct patient to report excessive sweating, hunger, or fatigue or the inability to concentrate, because insulin or the oral antidiabetic drug dosage may need to be adjusted. When propranolol is to be discontinued, gradually reduce the dose over a 1-2 wk period because abrupt discontinuation of this drug can result in a withdrawal-type syndrome—that is, trembling, severe headache, malaise, tachycardia, rebound hypertension, myocardial infarction, and life-threatening arrhythmias. Caution patient about performing tasks that require alertness because propranolol may induce drowsiness and dizziness.

ANTICHOLINESTERASE DRUGS

Ambenonium chloride (Mytelase), Edrophonium (Tensilon), neostigmine (Prostigmin), and Pyridostigmine (Mestinon)

These are cholinergic agents that prevent the destruction of acetylcholine by inhibiting acetylcholinesterase. Acetylcholine facilitates transmission of nerve impulses across the myoneural junction, thus improving cholinergic responses in myasthenia gravis.

Indications: These agents are used as antimyasthenic agents, as an antidote for tubocurarine and other nondepolarizing neuromuscular blocking agents, and for the prevention and treatment of postoperative gastrointestinal ileus and/or urinary retention. Edrophonium, due to its short duration of action, is primarily indicated for the differential diagnosis of myasthenia gravis.

Usual dosage: *Edrophonium chloride as a diagnostic aid:* Initially administer 2 mg IV over ½ min, followed by 8 mg if no response is noted after 45 seconds. To differentiate a cholinergic crisis from myasthenia crisis, 1 mg IV initially followed by another 1 mg if the first dose does not further aggravate the condition. *Antimyasthenic dosages:* ambenonium chloride 5 mg orally initially 3-4 times daily, adjusting dosage as needed at 1-2 day intervals. Neostigmine 15 mg orally q 3-4 h. Dose and frequency may be adjusted according to the patient's response. Maintenance dose is 150 mg orally administered in divided doses over a 24-h period. *Parenteral neostigmine for antimyasthenic use:* 500 µg (0.5 mg) IM or SC. Additional doses are determined by the patient's response. Pyridostigmine 60-120 mg orally q 3-4 h, adjusting dose as necessary. Maintenance dose is 600 mg orally per day.

Precautions/contraindications: Ambenonium is longer acting than the other drugs; therefore concurrent administration with other anticholinesterase or cholinergic drugs is contraindicated. Ambenonium, edrophonium, neostigmine, and pyridostigmine are contraindicated for use in patients with known sensitivity to the drug and in patients with peritonitis or mechanical obstruction of the gastrointestinal or urinary tract. Edrophonium and pyridostigmine are contraindicated for use in patients with bronchial asthma. These agents should be used with caution in patients with epilepsy, asthma, bradycardia, cardiac arrhythmias, peptic ulcers, and hyperthyroidism.

Side effects/adverse reactions: GI: Diarrhea, nausea, vomiting, abdominal cramps or pain, and increased mouth secretions. **Other:** Increased sweating. Pyridostigmine produces significantly less side/adverse effects, especially the bradycardia, increased salivation and gastrointestinal disturbances reported with neostigmine.

Pharmacokinetics: Neostigmine requires larger oral doses than parenteral because it is poorly absorbed from the GI tract. **Onset of action:** *Oral:* 20-30 min for ambenonium and pyridostigmine; within 1 min for edrophonium IV or 2-10 min IM; 45-75 min for neostigmine. **Duration of action:** 3-8 h for ambenonium; about 10 min for edrophonium IV or 5-39 min IM; 2-4 h for neostigmine; and 3-6 h for pyridostigmine. **Route of elimination:** Via the kidneys.

Interactions: Avoid concurrent administration with other cholinesterase inhibitors (such as demecarium, echothiophate, and soflurophate) because additive toxicities may result. In addition, when the anticholinesterase agents are given with guanadrel, guanethidine, mecamylamine, or trimethaphan, the antihypertensive and antimyasthenic effects may be antagonized or decreased. Drug antagonist effects may also occur if these drugs are given concurrently with procainamide or quinidine.

Nursing considerations: Monitor pulse, respiration, and blood pressure during drug dosage adjustment. If parenteral dosage forms are utilized, monitor intake and output and check for urinary retention. Parenteral atropine sulfate should be available for use if a cholinergic crisis occurs. Teach patient to keep a diary of drug administration (each dose) and the onset of myasthenic symptoms or drug side effects to assist his physician in establishing an appropriate drug dose and schedule. Time of muscular weakness is an important indication to distinguish between cholinergic or myasthenic crisis. Usually muscle weakness that occurs within an hour of drug administration is a cholinergic crisis, whereas muscle weakness occurring 3 hours later is more apt to be due to myasthenic crisis.

AGENTS TO TREAT DIABETES INSIPIDUS

Desmopressin (DDAVP) and Vasopressin (Pitressin)

These are vasopressor and antidiuretic hormones that conserve water in the kidneys. Vasopressin is a natural hormone released by the posterior pituitary, whereas desmopressin is a synthetic version of vasopressin. A deficiency of vasopressin results in diabetes insipidus.

Indications: Desmopressin and vasopressin are indicated for the central treatment and/or prevention of diabetes insipidus caused by insufficient antidiuretic hormone.

Usual dosage: *Parenteral desmopressin:* Antidiuretic dose is 2-4 µg IV or SC daily, administered in two divided doses (morning and evening). *Nasal form of desmopressin:* Initially 10 µg intranasal at bedtime. If necessary, the dose may be increased nightly in increments of 2.5 µg until the desired response is achieved. Maintenance intranasal dose is 10-40 µg daily, given as a single dose or in 2-3 divided doses daily. *Vasopressin:* Injection (aqueous) is administered in 5-10 units IM or SC, 2 or 3 times daily.

Precautions/contraindications: The use of desmopressin or vasopressin is contraindicated in patients with known hypersensitivity or anaphylaxis to the drugs. Desmopressin should be used with caution in patients with coronary artery insufficiency and hypertension. Vasopressin should not be used, or, if used, used with extreme caution in patients with coronary artery disease. It is recommended to avoid use of vasopressin in chronic nephritis with nitrogen retention. It should also be used with caution in the presence of concurrent disease states, epilepsy, asthma, migraine, and heart failure.

Side effects/adverse reactions: Side effects or adverse effects with desmopressin and vasopressin are usually infrequent or rare and are dose related. *Desmopressin:* **CNS:** Headache. **GI:** Stomach cramps, nausea. **CV:** Slight hypertension with IV administration; if given rapidly, hypotension may result. **Other:** Flushing and pain in the vulva area. The intranasal dosage form may cause a runny or stuffy nose. If hyponatremia or water intoxication occurs, the patient may experience coma, confusion, sedation, persistent headache, convulsions, difficulty in urination, and a rapid weight gain. *Vasopressin* (dose-related effects): **CNS:** Dizziness, feeling of pounding in head, tremors. **GI:** Abdominal distress, gas production, diarrhea, sweating, nausea, vomiting. **Other:** Pale appearance. Rare adverse effects include allergic reaction, angina pectoris or myocardial infarction, and the water intoxication syndrome as described previously with desmopressin.

Pharmacokinetics: Onset of action: *Desmopressin:* Intranasal, within 1 hour. **Half-life:** *Desmopressin:* Two phases—8 and 75 min. *Vasopressin*—10-20 min. **Duration of action:** *Desmopressin*—Intranasal, 6-24 h. *Vasopressin*—2-8 h. **Route of elimination:** *Desmopressin:* Via the kidneys; *Vasopressin*—Metabolized in liver and kidneys, excreted by kidneys.

Interactions: No significant drug interactions are reported with desmopressin or vasopressin, although carbamazepine, chlorpropamide, or clofibrate may potentiate the antidiuretic effect and demeclocycline, lithium, or norepinephrine may decrease the antidiuretic effect of desmopressin.

Nursing considerations: *Desmopressin:* Monitor pulse rate and blood pressure when drug is given IV or IM, monitor intake and output ratios, check for edema and weight gain. Follow physician's orders closely concerning allowable fluid intake because adjustments may be necessary to reduce the risk of inducing water intoxication and hyponatremia. Initial therapy is usually administered in the evening with dosage increases as necessary until the patient is free from nocturia. When nocturia is controlled, if the patient has a daily urine volume greater than 2 liters, a morning dose of desmopressin is usually ordered. This dose is monitored and adjusted until the urine volume does not exceed 1.5-2 liters in 24 hours. Teach patient the proper method of using the intranasal dosage form with the flexible catheter so that the spray is delivered deep in the nasal cavity and not in the patient's throat. Desmopressin dosage forms should be refrigerated unless instructed otherwise by the manufacturer. *Aqueous vasopressin:* Prior to therapy record blood pressure, patient's weight, intake and output patterns and ratios. Be aware that even small doses of this drug may cause coronary insufficiency or angina or precipitate a myocardial infarction in the elderly; therefore appropriate equipment and medications should be available and the patient should be closely monitored. Monitor the patient's alertness and responses frequently during therapy. The onset of confusion, headaches, and lethargy may signal the onset of water intoxication.

ANTICONVULSANTS

While the exact mode and site of action of the anticonvulsants are unknown at the molecular level, a proposed mechanism of action is the stabilization of cell membranes by altering cation transport (sodium, potassium, calcium) either by increasing sodium efflux or by decreasing sodium influx into the cells. Pharmacologically, the main effect is (1) to increase the motor cortex threshold to reduce its response to incoming electric or chemical stimulation or (2) to depress or reduce the spread of a seizure discharge from its focus (origin) by depressing synaptic transport or decreasing nerve conduction. Carbamazepine (Tegretol), phenobarbital, phenytoin (Dilantin), and valproic acid (Depakene) are reviewed in this section.

Carbamazepine (Tegretol)

Indications: For the treatment of epilepsy in patients that are refractory or have not responded to phenytoin, phenobarbital, or primidone; for partial seizures with complex symptomatology; for generalized tonic-clonic seizures; for psychomotor seizures; and for mixed seizure patterns. This drug is also used in the treatment of pain associated with true trigeminal neuralgia.

Usual dosage: *Oral:* Initially 200 mg twice a day, increased by 200 mg/day weekly in divided doses until the desired response is noted. Maximum daily dose is 1200 mg/day.

Precautions/contraindications: Carbamazepine is contraindicated for use in patients with a history of bone marrow depression, drug hypersensitivity, or a history of hypersensitivity to any tricyclic antidepressant (such as amitriptyline, desipramine, or imipramine). It should also not be administered concurrently with any MAO-inhibiting drugs. Use with caution in patients with a history of psychosis or adverse hematologic reactions to drugs, and in the elderly.

Side effects/adverse reactions: CNS: Vertigo, drowsiness, dizziness, headache, confusion, visual hallucinations, lethargy, hostility, stupor. **GI:** Nausea, vomiting, dry mouth, diarrhea, anorexia. **Other:** Myalgia, arthralgia, leg cramps, photosensitivity, altered skin pigmentation, alopecia, and increased sweating, hyponatremia, activation of latent psychosis, blurred vision, diplopia, hives, pruritus, rash, oculomotor disturbances, and edema.

Pharmacokinetics: Onset of action: Variable, from hours to days. **Half-life:** In chronic dosing, 8-29 h. Therapeutic serum concentration: 4-12 μg/ml. **Route of elimination:** Primarily via the kidneys.

Interactions: When carbamazepine is given concurrently with adrenocorticoids or glucocorticoids, a decrease in response to corticosteroid therapy may result. If given with oral anticoagulants, a decrease in anticoagulant effect may result. When administered with other anticonvulsant drugs, monitor closely because a decrease in serum level and anticonvulsive effect may occur. Cimetidine, diltiazem, or verapamil may produce an increase in carbamazepine serum levels, which may result in toxicity.

Nursing considerations: Blood, liver, and renal studies should be performed before initiation of carbamazepine therapy and at periodic intervals during therapy. During therapy the patient should be closely monitored and taught to report fever, sore throat, mouth ulcers, bleeding gums, nose bleeds, and easy bruising because they may be the early signs and symptoms of potential hematologic problems. Ophthalmologic examinations and complete urinalysis are also recommended before therapy and at periodic intervals afterward. Photosensitivity reactions have been reported; therefore advise the patient to stay out of direct sunlight, especially during the midday hours. He should also be instructed to wear protective clothing, sunglasses, and a sun-blocking agent when outdoors. Teach patient to take medication with meals and to store carbamazepine in a dry area and not in the bathroom or near the kitchen sink. Heat or moisture may reduce the carbamazepine's potency and effectiveness.

Phenobarbital

Indications: For the treatment of tonic-clonic seizures, simple partial seizure pattern, and convulsions or seizures associated with status epilepticus, tetanus, eclampsia, meningitis, and exposure to toxic chemicals.

Usual dosage: *Oral:* 60 to 250 mg per day as a single dose or in divided doses. *Parenteral:* 100-320 mg IV, may be repeated if necessary up to a total daily dose of 600 mg. In status epilepticus, IV (slow) 10-20 mg/kg body weight; repeat if necessary.

Precautions/contraindications: Phenobarbital is contraindicated in patients with a history of hypersensitivity to barbiturates or porphyria, or in patients with severe impairment of liver function or respiratory disease. Avoid use of phenobarbital or use with extreme caution in patients with mental depression or a history of drug abuse and dependence.

Side effects/adverse reactions: CNS: Drowsiness, dizziness, tiredness, hangover-type effects, headaches, confusion, depression, or paradoxic excitement in children or in elderly patients; increased irritability and nervousness. **GI:** Nausea, vomiting, constipation. **Other:** Rashes, hives, fever, sore throat, lip or mouth sores; pain in chest, muscles, bones, or joints.

Pharmacokinetics: Onset of action: *Oral:* From 20-60 min; *IV:* Up to 5 min. **Peak effect:** Maximum CNS depression following IV administration occurs in approximately 15 min. **Therapeutic serum level:** 10-40 μg/ml. **Route of elimination:** Metabolized in the liver, excreted by the kidneys.

Interactions: The effects of anticoagulants, adrenocorticoids, and corticosteroids may be decreased because of enhanced metabolism produced by phenobarbital. Enhanced CNS depressant effects and respiratory depression reported when phenobarbital is administered with alcohol, anesthetics, and other CNS depressant–type drugs (sedatives, hypnotics, or narcotics). Unpredictable effects are reported when phenobarbital is given concurrently with other anticonvulsants, especially phenytoin and valproic acid.

Nursing considerations: If used for long-term treatment, blood tests and liver function tests should be monitored periodically. It takes several weeks of phenobarbital administration before the maximum antiepilepsy effects are achieved. When using IV phenobarbital, it requires 15-30 min before peak levels are reached in the brain. Therefore, to avoid severe barbiturate induced depression and toxicity, a minimal dose should be administered and the effect evaluated before a second dose is given. The rate of IV administration should not exceed 60 mg/min. To discontinue long-term therapy with phenobarbital, withdraw the drug slowly to prevent precipitation of a seizure or status epilepticus.

Phenytoin (Dilantin)

Indications: Treatment of epilepsy, that is, tonic-clonic and simple or complex partial seizures. Also used to control status epilepticus and for the prevention and treatment of seizures in neurosurgery.

Usual dosage: *Oral:* 100 mg three times daily, increasing dose as necessary at 7-10 day intervals. *Parenteral:* By direct IV 10 to 15 mg/kg body weight, administered at a rate of up to 50 mg/min. Maintenance dose by direct IV is 100 mg q 6-8 h.

Precautions/contraindications: Phenytoin is contraindicated in patients with sinus bradycardia, sinoatrial block, second and third degree block, or Adams-Stokes syndrome, and in patients with hypersensitivity to hydantoin products. Use phenytoin with extreme caution in patients with hypotension and severe myocardial insufficiency.

Side effects/adverse reactions: CNS: Drowsiness, dizziness, increased irritability, slurred speech, behav-

ioral changes. **GI:** Constipation, nausea, vomiting, **Other:** Hirsutism, gingival hyperplasia, nystagmus, hand trembling, skin rash, ataxia, blood dyscrasias.

Pharmacokinetics: Half-life: *Oral:* Approximately 22 h. *IV:* 10 to 15 h. **Therapeutic serum level:** Between 10 and 20 μg/ml. **Route of elimination:** Metabolized in the liver, excreted via the kidneys.

Interactions: When phenytoin is given concurrently with adrenocorticoids, corticosteroids, estrogens, and oral contraceptives, a decrease in therapeutic effects of these medications may occur. An increased serum level and/or toxicity may occur with the following drugs when given concurrently with phenytoin: chloramphenicol, cimetidine, disulfiram, isoniazid, oxyphenbutazone, or sulfonamides. Because many drug interactions have been reported with phenytoin, the addition or deletion of any drugs used concurrently with phenytoin should be closely monitored.

Nursing considerations: Complete blood and platelet counts and liver function tests should be performed initially and periodically during therapy, depending on the needs of the patient. In long-term therapy, dental examinations for teeth cleaning and reinforcement of good dental hygiene are recommended every 3 months. If suspension dosage form is ordered, the nurse must shake the container vigorously before measuring out the dose in a graduated or exact measuring device, such as an oral syringe. Patients have been undermedicated and later overmedicated because of improper shaking of this suspension. Intravenous phenytoin is an irritant to veins and is incompatible with many solutions and medications; therefore it is recommended that the intravenous line be flushed with normal saline before and after drug administration. Consult with the prescribing physician before changing from one phenytoin dosage form to another or changing from one brand of phenytoin to a different brand. Problems with bioavailability have been reported that may result in a loss of seizure control or toxic phenytoin blood levels.

Valproic Acid (Depakene)

Indications: Valproic acid is used for the treatment of simple and complex absence seizures, including petit mal, and as adjunctive therapy in clients with multiple seizure types, including absence seizures.

Usual dosage: *Oral monotherapy:* 5 to 15 mg/kg body weight, increasing dose as necessary by 5-10 mg/kg at weekly intervals. *Polytherapy:* The oral initial dose is 10-30 mg/kg, increasing dose as necessary by 5-10 mg/kg at weekly intervals. Maximum daily dose is usually 60 mg/kg/day.

Precautions/contraindications: Valproic acid is contraindicated for use in any patient with liver disease or significant liver dysfunction, or in patients with known hypersensitivity to this drug. Monitor patients closely, especially during the first 6 months of therapy because serious and fatal hepatotoxicities have been reported during this time period. Avoid use of drug in women who are or may become pregnant as it has been reported to cause teratogenic effects. Use drug with caution in patients with a history of bleeding disorders and renal disease.

Side effects/adverse reactions: CNS: Dizziness, sedation, headaches, increased irritability, mood alterations, tremors, ataxia. **GI:** Stomach cramps, anorexia, nausea, gas, vomiting, diarrhea. **Other:** Changes in menstrual cycles, alopecia, rash, hepatotoxicity, hyperammonemia, diplopia, nystagmus and other visual changes, pancreatitis, and thrombocytopenia.

Pharmacokinetics: Peak serum level: *Oral capsules/syrup:* 1-4 h; *Delayed release dosage forms:* 3-4 h. **Half-life:** Variable, 6-16 h. **Therapeutic serum level:** 50-150 μg/ml. **Route of elimination:** Metabolized in the liver, excreted by the kidneys.

Interactions: When valproic acid is given concurrently with alcohol, anesthetics (general), or CNS depressant drugs, a potentiation in CNS depressant–type effects may result. When valproic acid is administered with oral anticoagulants, aspirin, dipyridamole, or sulfinpyrazone, an increased risk of bleeding and hemorrhage may result. Concurrent administration with other anticonvulsants should be closely monitored because variable responses have been reported.

Nursing considerations: Administer drug after meals to avoid gastric irritation. Advise patient to avoid chewing or crushing the tablets or capsules because it can cause local irritation to the mouth and throat. (Syrup form is available for patients unable to swallow.) Divalproex sodium is often prescribed for patients unable to tolerate the GI irritation produced by valproic acid. The patient should be instructed to report any visual disturbances, rash, diarrhea, light-colored stools, spontaneous bleeding and/or bruising, jaundice, and protracted vomiting. Warn patient to avoid alcohol and other CNS-depressant drugs. Also avoid driving or handling dangerous machinery until the individual's response to the drug can be determined. Warn patient not to stop or alter dosage of medication without physician consultation.

CHOLINERGIC DRUGS

Cholinergic drugs act as mediators of the parasympathetic nervous system; that is, they produce effects in the body similar to those produced by acetylcholine.

Bethanechol Chloride (Urecholine)

Indications: Bethanechol is indicated for the treatment of postoperative nonobstructive and postpartum nonobstructive urinary retention. It is also used to treat neurogenic atony of the urinary bladder.

Usual dosage: *Oral:* 5-10 mg initially, repeating dose at 1-2 h intervals until desired response is achieved. Usual dose is 10-50 mg three or four times daily. *SC:* 5 mg three or four times a day.

Precautions/contraindications: The use of bethanechol is contraindicated (or, if used, use with extreme caution) in patients with active or latent bronchial asthma, severe bradycardia, or GI obstruction or when muscle activity or condition of the GI or urinary tract may be questionable, such as after recent bladder surgery, anastomosis or gastrointestinal resection, or in coronary artery occlusion or disease, hyperthyroidism, severe hypotension, peptic ulcer disease or acute inflammatory lesions in the GI tract, peritonitis, or severe vagotonia.

Side effects/adverse reactions: CNS: Headache. **GI:** Belching, diarrhea, nausea, vomiting, abdominal discomfort or pain. **CV:** Postural hypotension. **Other:** Blurred vision, increase in frequency of urination, increased production of saliva, increased sweating and flushing of skin. Adverse reactions, such as severe cholinergic overstimulation that leads to bloody diarrhea, bronchoconstriction, shock, circulatory collapse, or sudden cardiac arrest, require immediate medical attention.

Pharmacokinetics: Onset of action: *Oral:* Within ½-1½ h; *SC:* Within 5-15 min. **Time to peak effect:** *Oral:* Within 1 h; *SC:* Within 15-30 min. **Duration of action:** *Oral:* Up to 6 h; *SC:* About 2 h.

Interactions: Avoid concurrent administration with other cholinergic and anticholinesterase inhibitors because additive toxicities may result. The effects of bethanechol may be antagonized if given concurrently with procainamide or quinidine. Also avoid concurrent administration with ganglionic blocking agents such as mecamylamine, pentolinium, and trimethaphan because a dangerous fall in blood pressure might occur.

Nursing considerations: Monitor pulse rate, blood pressure, and intake and output closely after drug administration. **Do not give this drug by any route except the SC route—cardiac arrest has been reported when drug was accidentally given IM or IV.** Use only when other cholinergic drugs have been discontinued. Administer oral doses on an empty stomach or with food if GI symptoms are troublesome. (Food and milk will decrease drug absorption.) Monitor for toxic signs and symptoms and discontinued drug if they occur. Evaluate therapeutic response by an absence of urinary retention and abdominal distention.

CORTICOSTEROIDS

Corticosteroid is the generic name for all the synthetic and natural adrenal cortex hormones. This section will focus on selected related substances; that is, corticotropin or ACTH (a hormone released from the pituitary gland to stimulate the synthesis of adrenal steroids), plus prednisone and methylprednisolone.

Indications: They are used in replacement therapy for adrenocortical insufficiency and also to treat severe allergic reactions; neurologic disease; anaphylactic reactions not responsive to other therapies; collagen disorders such as systemic lupus erythematosus, carditis, and system dermatomyositis; adjunct treatment to neoplastic diseases; nephrotic syndrome; and in many other illness or disease states.

Usual dosage: *Corticotropin for injection:* diagnostic aid for adrenal-pituitary function, 10-25 USP units in 500 ml dextrose 5%; injection administered over 8 h. Therapeutic dose is 40-80 USP units (IM) daily. For acute exacerbations of multiple sclerosis, the dose is 80-120 USP units daily for 2-3 weeks. *Prednisone oral:* 5-60 mg as a single dose or in divided doses. For acute exacerbations of multiple sclerosis, 200 mg orally daily for 7 days, then 80 mg every other day for 30 days. *Methylprednisolone oral:* 4-48 mg daily in divided or single dose. In multiple sclerosis, 160 mg orally daily for 7 days, then 64 mg every other day for 30 days. *Parenteral (Solu-Medrol):* 10-40 mg IM or IV, repeat as necessary. High-dose "pulse" therapy dose is 30 mg/kg IV given over 30 min. Dose may be repeated q 4-6 h as necessary. For acute exacerbations of multiple sclerosis, 160 mg IM or IV daily for 7 days, then 64 mg every other day for 30 days. While not an approved indication in the United States, this product has been used to treat acute spinal cord injury at a dose of 30 mg/kg given over 15 minutes, followed in 45 minutes by an infusion of 5.4 mg/kg/h for 23 additional hours.

Precautions/contraindications: The corticosteroids should not be used when the following conditions are present: adrenocortical hyperfunction, ocular herpes simplex, osteoporosis, and recent surgery. Use with extreme caution in patients with AIDS, recent intestinal anastomoses, cardiac disease or congestive heart failure, hypertension, psychosis, vaccinia or varicella, impaired renal function, systemic fungus infections, peptic ulcer, gastritis or esophagitis, diabetes mellitus, tuberculosis, or myasthenia gravis.

Side effects/adverse reactions: CNS: Increased irritability, restlessness, insomnia. **GI:** Increase in appetite, gastric distress. **Other:** Allergic reactions, cataracts, and diabetes mellitus. Chronic dosing may result in acne or skin problems, avascular necrosis, Cushing's syndrome, edema of lower extremities, menstrual irregularities, nausea, vomiting, hypokalemia, osteoporosis, pancreatitis, peptic ulcers, intestinal perforation, muscle weakness, striae, tendon rupture, tissue atrophy (frequent SC dosing), and wounds that do not heal.

Pharmacokinetics: Absorption: Fairly rapid with oral and parenteral dosage forms. **Duration of action:** Drug, dose, route and site dependent. **Metabolism:** In the liver. **Route of elimination:** Via the kidneys. Cortisone and prednisone are inactive corticosteroids that require liver metabolism to the active metabolites of hydrocortisone and prednisolone, respectively.

Interactions: Numerous interactions are reported with corticosteroids. Several significant interactions include concurrent administration with parenteral amphotericin B, which may result in severe hypokalemia and may also decrease the adrenal gland response to corticotropin. The corticosteroid-induced hypokalemia may increase the potential for toxicity (dysrhythmias) with digitalis products and reduce the effectiveness of concurrently administered diuretics. The nurse is referred to a current reference source or the package insert for additional drug interactions.

Nursing considerations: Obtain baseline weight before therapy and weigh daily. Monitor intake and output daily. Also monitor laboratory tests for hematologic values, serum electrolytes, and serum and urine glucose levels. Carefully assess for severe fluid and electrolyte imbalances. Note that a myasthenic crisis may be induced if these drugs are administered to patients with myasthenia gravis. Patients who take corticosteroid preparations and who require surgery should receive a preoperative dose of a rapid-acting corticosteroid. The drug is continued postoperatively in decreasing doses for several days. When prescribed as a single dose, the dose should be administered in the morning, before 9 AM if possible. Adrenal activity is at its peak at this time; thus less adrenal suppression will result. To discontinue corticosteroid therapy in patients that have been receiving chronic therapy, the preferred method is to taper and withdraw the drug gradually. Withdrawal should be carried out under close supervision to avoid adrenal insufficiency.

ANTIDYSKINETIC DRUGS

Antidyskinetic drugs are used to treat defects in voluntary body movement, such as idiopathic Parkinson's disease, postencephalitic parkinsonism, and symptomatic parkinsonism that follows injury to the nervous system. Amantadine is also used to treat drug-induced extrapyramidal reactions. While the mechanism of action of the antidyskinetic drugs is not completely understood, these drugs appear to be dopamine agonists; that is, they increase the release of dopamine in the brain. The drugs reviewed in this section include amantadine (Symmetrel), carbidopa-levodopa (Sinemet), pergolide mesylate (Permax), and selegiline (Eldepryl).

Indications: See previous section.

Usual dosage: *Amantadine: Oral:* 100 mg one or two times daily. Maximum daily dose is 400 mg. *Carbidopa-levodopa: Oral:* 10 mg carbidopa with 100 mg levodopa three or four times daily, or 25 mg carbidopa with 100 mg levodopa three times daily. Adjust dosages as necessary at 1 to 2 intervals. *Pergolide tablet:* 0.05 mg daily for 2 days, increased by 0.1 to 0.15 mg daily every third day over the next 12 days. Then dosage increases are 0.25 mg/day every third day until desired response is achieved. This drug is administered in divided doses, three times daily. The mean therapeutic daily dose is 3 mg; maximum daily dose is 5 mg. During titration, concurrent levodopa-carbidopa may be carefully decreased. *Selegiline tablet:* 5 mg at breakfast and at lunch (higher doses are not recommended). This drug is indicated for patents that are not responding to levodopa-carbidopa. After 2 to 3 days of selegiline therapy, a reduction in the levodopa-carbidopa dose should be attempted.

Precautions/contraindications: Each drug is contraindicated for use in patients with a known hypersensitivity to the drug. *Amantadine:* Use with caution in patients with edema, congestive heart failure, history of epilepsy, or other seizure disorders, or with impaired renal function. *Levodopa-carbidopa* is contraindicated for use in patients taking monoamine oxidase (MAO) inhibitors and in patients with narrow angle glaucoma, undiagnosed skin lesions, or a history of melanoma. It should also be used with caution in patients with bronchial asthma, emphysema, severe pulmonary and cardiac disease states, history of myocardial infarction with persistent arrhythmias, peptic ulcer disease, psychosis, or impaired renal function. *Pergolide* is contraindicated for use in patients hypersensitive to ergot derivatives. *Selegiline* is contraindicated for use in patients with a history of peptic ulcer disease. Also, because it is a nonselective MAO inhibitor, the maximum recommended daily dose of selegiline is 10 mg/day.

Side effects/adverse reactions: *Amantadine:* **CNS:** Impaired concentration, dizziness, headaches, increased irritability, nightmares, insomnia, hallucinations, confusion, ataxia, depression. **GI:** Anorexia, nausea, vomiting, constipation, dry mouth. **CV:** Postural hypotension. **Other:** Livedo reticularis. *Levodopa-carbidopa:* **CNS:** Depression, mood changes, nervousness, confusion, headaches, trouble in sleeping, nightmares. **GI:** Nausea, vomiting, anorexia, dry mouth, diarrhea, constipation. **CV:** Postural hypotension, hyper-

tension (rare). **Other:** Tremors, uncontrollable body movements, blurred vision, muscle twitching, flushing of skin. *Pergolide:* **CNS:** Confusion, dyskinesias, hallucinations. **GI:** Stomach distress, nausea, diarrhea, dry mouth, anorexia, vomiting. **CV:** Hypotension, hypertension. **Other:** Urinary tract infections, flu-type symptoms, low back pain, rhinitis, chills, facial edema. *Selegiline:* **CNS:** Mood changes, insomnia, hallucinations, headaches. **GI:** Abdominal distress/pain, nausea, vomiting, dry mouth, gas. **CV:** Angina, dysrhythmias, slow heartbeat, severe hypertension, postural hypotension. **Other:** Asthma, peripheral edema, extrapyramidal side effects, difficult urination.

Pharmacokinetics: Onset of action: amantadine, within 48 h; levodopa-carbidopa, pergolide and selegiline, not listed. **Half-life:** amantadine, 11-15 h; levodopa-carbidopa, 1-2 h; pergolide, not listed; selegiline: 2-20 h. **Route of elimination:** amantadine, levodopa-carbidopa, pergolide and selegiline via the kidneys.

Interactions: *Amantadine:* Avoid concurrent administration with alcohol (increases CNS side effects), anticholinergics (additive anticholinergic effects, especially confusion, hallucinations, and nightmares), and CNS stimulation medications (additive CNS stimulation effects that present as increased nervousness, insomnia, or cardiac arrhythmias). *Levodopa-carbidopa:* Avoid concurrent administration with inhalation anesthetics (arrhythmias), phenytoin, haloperidol or phenothiazines (decreases effects of levodopa), MAO inhibitors (hypertensive crisis), selegiline (may increase dyskinesias). *Pergolide:* None significant. *Selegiline:* avoid concurrent administration with levodopa (may enhance dyskinesias, hypotension, hallucinations, confusion), meperidine (MAO inhibitor interaction, which may result in excitability, rigidity, hypertension, respiratory depression, seizures, coma), foods with high tyramine content (such as aged cheeses, fava beans, smoked or pickled meat, poultry or fish) as severe hypertension may result.

Nursing considerations: *Amantadine:* If insomnia is a problem, advise the patient to take the last daily dose of amantadine several hours earlier. Be aware that CNS side effects most commonly occur within the first few days of initial therapy or after a daily dosage is increased. Symptoms sometimes subside when the drug is given in two divided doses. In parkinsonism, amantadine usually reduces saliva production and the signs and symptoms of akinesia and rigidity, but it usually has little effect if any on tremors. Generally, the maximum therapeutic effect occurs within 2-3 weeks of therapy.

If drug effectiveness declines after 6-8 weeks of treatment, inform physician because dosage adjustment or switch to another medication may be necessary. Caution patient about postural hypotension and the specific precautions to take when changing positions (change positions slowly, especially from a recumbent to a standing position; lie down immediately if dizzy; and so on.) *Levodopa-carbidopa:* Administer drug with food or meals to reduce gastrointestinal disturbances. Monitor vital signs during dosage adjustments and report any changes in blood pressure, pulse rate, and respiratory rate. Monitor for the early signs of overdose—that is, muscle twitching and spasmodic winking. If they occur, contact physician promptly. Monitor patient for behavior and mood changes. Be aware that maintenance therapy should include at least 70-100 mg of carbidopa daily. If less carbidopa is administered, the patient is more likely to have nausea and vomiting. The combination of levodopa and carbidopa needs careful dose selection and titration to achieve maximum benefits; for dosing recommendations see a current package insert or reference guide. In diabetic patients, levodopa can produce false positive reactions (Clinitest tablets) or false negative test results (Clinistix, Tes-Tape) for uri-nary glucose. Frequent monitoring of blood glucose levels is recommended. *Pergolide:* Administer drug with meals to reduce gastrointestinal side effects. Warn patient that dizziness occurs more commonly after initial doses; therefore advise them to take first dose at bedtime or while lying down. Advise patient on postural hypotension and the appropriate interventions to take when changing body positions (see amantadine). Dizziness and nausea that occur with initial therapy usually resolve with continued therapy. If they continue, a dosage reduction may be necessary. *Selegiline:* Caution patient not to take more medication than prescribed because an increase may increase drug side effects. Advise patient on postural hypotension and the suggested interventions to take when changing body positions (see amantadine). Caution patient to avoid consumption of alcoholic beverages, foods with a high tyramine content (see interactions), and large quantities of caffeine-containing food or drinks (chocolate, coffee, tea, cola). Advise patient not to take any new medicines (prescription or OTC) without consultation with his physician.

CEREBROSPINAL FLUID

Parameters	Normal	Abnormal	Possible cause
Pressure (initial readings)	100-180 mm Hg	<60 mm Hg	Faulty needle placement Dehydration Spinal block along subarachnoid space Block at foramen magnum
		>200 mm Hg	Muscle tension Abdominal compression Brain tumor Subdural hematoma Brain abscess Brain cyst Cerebral edema (any cause) Hydrocephalus Benign intracranial hypertension
Color	Clear, colorless	Cloudy	Increased cell count Increased microorganisms
		Yellow xanthochromic	Caused by red blood cell pigments High protein content
		Smoky	Presence of red blood cells
Red blood cells	None	Blood tinged	Traumatic tap
		Grossly bloody	Traumatic tap Subarachnoid hemorrhage

White blood cells	0-6 mm^3	>10 mm^3
		(Cell counts range from below 100 to many thousands, depending on causative factor; all are abnormal findings.)
			Occurs in many conditions:
			  Bacterial infections of meninges
			  Viral infections of meninges
			  Neurosyphilis
			  Tuberculous meningitis
			  Metastatic neoplastic lesions
			  Parasitic infections
			  Acute demyelinating diseases
			  Following introduction of air or blood into subarachnoid space

Protein*	15-45 mg/dl
	(1% of serum protein)
		<10 mg/dl
		>60 mg/dl
			Little clinical significance
			Occurs in many conditions:
			  Complete spinal block
			  Guillain-Barré syndrome
			  Carcinomatosis of meninges
			  Tumors close to pial or ependymal surfaces, or in cerebellopontine angle
			  Acute and chronic meningitis
			  Meningeal hemorrhage
			  Demyelinating disorders
			  Degenerative diseases

Glucose	50-75 mg/dl (approximately 60% of blood glucose level)	<40 mg/dl	Acute bacterial meningitis Tuberculous meningitis Meningeal carcinomatosis
		>100 mg/dl	Diabetes
Chloride	700-750 mg/dl	<625 mg/dl	Hypochloremia Tuberculous meningitis
		>800 mg/dl	Not of neurological significance; correlate with blood levels of chloride

From Rudy.[127]
*Blood in the cerebrospinal fluid will raise the protein level.

References

1. Adams B, Clancey J, and Eddy M: Malignant glioma: current treatment perspectives, *J Neurosci Nurs* 23:1, 1991.

2. Adler R: Trigeminal glycerol chemoneurolysis: nursing implications, *J Neurosci Nurs* 21:6, 1989.

3. American Heart Association: *1990 Stroke facts*, Dallas, 1991, American Heart Association.

4. American Nurses' Association Division on Medical-Surgical Nursing Practice and Association of Rehabilitation Nurses: *Standards of rehabilitation nursing practice*, Kansas City, Mo, 1986, American Nurses' Association.

5. American Nurses' Association Executive Committee Council on Medical-Surgical Nursing Practice and Association of Rehabilitation Nurses: *Rehabilitation Nursing: Scope of Practice—Process and Outcome Criteria for Selected Diagnoses*, Kansas City, 1988, American Nurses' Association.

6. Andrus C: Intracranial pressure: dynamics and nursing management, *J Neurosci Nurs* 23:2, 1991.

7. Annon JS: The PLISSIT model: a proposed conceptual scheme for the behavioral treatment of sexual problems, *J Sex Educ Ther* 2(1):211-215, 1976.

8. Anthony CP and Kolthoff NJ: *Textbook of anatomy and physiology*, St. Louis, 1975, Mosby–Year Book.

9. Anthony CP and Thibodeau GA: *Structure and function of the body*, ed 7, St. Louis, 1984, Mosby–Year Book.

10. Anchie J: Plasmapheresis as a treatment for myasthenia gravis, *J Neurosurg Nurs* 13:1, 1981.

11. Arsenault L: Delayed onset symptomatic hydrocephalus related to aqueductal stenosis, *J Neurosurg Nurs* 15:5, 1983.

12. Arsenault L: Selected postoperative complications of cranial surgery, *J Neurosurg Nurs* 17:3, 1985.

13. Baker AB, editor: *Clinical neurology*, ed 2, New York, 1983, Harper & Row, Publishers.

14. Ballinger PW: *Merrill's atlas of radiographic positions and radiologic procedures*, ed 7, St. Louis, 1990, Mosby–Year Book.

15. Baloh RW and Honrubia V, editors: *Clinical neurophysiology of the vestibular system*, Philadelphia, 1979, FA Davis.

16. Barber J, Stokes L, and Billings D: *Adult and child care*, ed 2, St. Louis, 1977, Mosby–Year Book.

17. Barker E: Brain tumor, frightening diagnosis, nursing challenge, *RN*, September, 1990.

18. Bates B: *A guide to physical examination*, ed 4, Philadelphia, 1990, JB Lippincott.

19. Bell J: Understanding and managing myasthenia gravis, *Focus Crit Care* 16:57-65, 1989.

20. Bires B: Head trauma: nursing implications from prehospital through emergency department, *Crit Care Nurs Quar*, June 1987.

21. Blass J: Alzheimer's disease, *DM* 31:4, 1985.

22. Bobath B: *Adult hemiplegia: evaluation and treatment*, ed 2, London, 1981, William Heinemann Medical Books.

23. Bradbury K and Bauer M: Brain graft surgery: a new treatment for Parkinson's disease, *Crit Care Nurs* 10:8, 1990.

24. Bressman S and Fahn S: Parkinson's disease, *Hosp Med*, December 1987.

25. Bronstein KS, Popovich JM, and Stewart-Amidei C: *Promoting stroke recovery: a research-based approach for nurses*, St. Louis, 1991, Mosby–Year Book.

26. Burgess K: Neurological disturbance in the patient with intracranial neoplasm: sources and implications for nursing care, *J Neurosurg Nurs* 15:4, 1983.

27. Burns EM and Buckwalter KC: Pathophysiology and etiology of Alzheimer's disease, *Nurs Clinics North Am* 23:11-27, 1988.

28. Burns KR and Johnson PJ: *Health assessment in clinical practice*, Englewood Cliffs, NJ, 1980, Prentice-Hall.

29. Campbell V: Neurologic system. In Thompson, JM, et al: *Mosby's manual of clinical nursing*, ed 2, St. Louis, 1989, Mosby–Year Book.

30. Camunas C: Transsphenoidal hypophysectomy, *AJN* 10:1820-1823, 1980.

31. Canobbio MM: *Cardiovascular disorders*, St. Louis, 1990, Mosby–Year Book.

32. Carpenito LJ et al.: *Nursing diagnosis: application to clinical practice*, ed 3, Philadelphia, 1989, J.B. Lippincott.

33. Chase M and Whelan-Decker E: Nursing management of a patient with a subarachnoid hemorrhage, *J Neurosurg Nurs* 16:1, 1984.

34. Chipps E: Myasthenia gravis: the patient in crisis, *Crit Care Nurs* 11:7, 1991.

35. Chipps E: Transsphenoidal surgery for removal of pituitary tumors, *Crit Care Nurs.* In press.

36. Clancey J and Abruzzi L: Nursing interventions for patients with pituitary tumors, *J Neurosurg Nurs* 10:24-28, 1978.

37. Clanin NJ: *Basic principles of skin and wound management*, Evanston, Ill, 1989, Rehabilitation Nursing Foundation.

38. Conn HF and Conn RB Jr.: *Current diagnosis*, Philadelphia, 1980, WB Saunders.

39. Conway-Rutkowski BL: *Carini and Owens' neurological and neurosurgical nursing*, ed 8, St. Louis, 1982, Mosby–Year Book.

40. Cutler WP: *Degenerative and hereditary diseases*, ed 7, Washington, DC, 1983, Scientific American Medicine.

41. Davenport-Fortune P and Dunnum L: Professional nursing care of the patient with increased intracranial pressure: planned or "hit or miss," *J Neurosurg Nurs* 17:6, 1985.

42. DeLisa JA et al: *Rehabilitation medicine: principles and practice*, Philadelphia, 1988, JB Lippincott.

43. DeMeyer W: *Techniques of the neurologic examination*, ed 3, New York, 1980, McGraw-Hill.

44. Delgado J and Billo J: Care of the patient with Parkinson's disease: surgical and nursing interventions, *J Neurosurg Nurs* 20:3, 1988.

45. Devoti A: Lumbar laminectomy, *J Neurosurg Nurs* 15:3, 1983.

46. Dittmar SS et al: *Rehabilitation nursing: process and application*, St Louis, 1989, Mosby–Year Book.

47. Doenges M et al: *Nursing care plans: guidelines for planning patient care*, ed 2, Philadelphia, 1990, FA Davis.

48. Eliasson SG et al, editors: *Neurological pathophysiology*, ed 2, New York, 1978, Oxford University Press.

49. Escourolle R and Poirier J: *Manual of basic neuropathology*, ed 2, Philadelphia, 1978, WB Saunders.

50. Flaskerud J: AIDS: neuropsychiatric complications, *J Psychosoc Nurs* 25:12, 1987.

51. Flynn E: Cerebral vasospasm following intracranial aneurysm rupture: a protocol for detection, *J Neurosci Nurs* 21:6, 1989.

52. Fode N: Carotid endarterectomy: nursing care and controversies, *J Neurosci Nurs* 22:1, 1990.

53. Folstein MF, et al: "Mini-mental state": a practical method for grading the cognitive state of patients for the clinician, *Journal of Psychiatric Research* vol 12, 1975, Pergamon Press, Ltd.

54. Frankel HL, Hancock DO, Hyslop G, et al: Value of postural reduction in the initial management of closed injuries of the spine with paraplegia and tetraplegia, *Paraplegia* 7:179-192, 1969.

55. Gee G and Moran T: *AIDS: concepts in nursing practice*, Baltimore, 1988, Williams & Wilkins.

56. George M: Neuromuscular respiratory failure: what the nurse knows makes the difference, *J Neurosci Nurs* 20:110-117, 1988.

57. Gerk MK and Kassel N: Cerebral vasospasm: update and implications, *J Neurosurg Nurs* 12:3, 1980.

58. Goetz C, Jankovic J, and Paulson G: Update on Parkinson's disease, *Patient Care*, April, 1989.

58a. Govoni E and Hayes JE: *Drugs and nursing implications*, ed 6, Norwalk, Conn, 1988, Appleton & Lange.

59. Grant L: Hydrocephalus: an overview and update, *J Neurosurg Nurs* 16:6, 1984.

60. Grimes DE: *Infectious diseases*, St. Louis, 1991, Mosby–Year Book.

61. Grundy JH: *Assessment of the child in primary health care*, New York, 1981, McGraw-Hill.

62. Guyton AC: *Textbook of medical physiology*, ed 7, Philadelphia, 1986, WB Saunders.

63. Hagen C, Malkmus D, Durham P: Levels of cognitive functioning. In *Rehabilitation of the head injured adult: comprehensive physical management*, Downey, Calif, 1979, Professional Staff Association of Rancho Los Amigos Hospital.

64. Hartshorn J: Immunosuppressive treatment of multiple sclerosis, *J Neurosurg Nurs* 16:5, 1984.

65. Hickey J: *The clinical practice of neurological and neurosurgical nursing*, Philadelphia, 1986, JB Lippincott.

66. Reference deleted in galleys.

67. Hodges K: Meningioma, astrocytoma, and germinoma: case presentation of three intracranial tumors, *J Neurosci Nurs* 21:2, 1989.

68. Holland N, McDonnell M, and Wiesel-Levison: Overview of multiple sclerosis and nursing care of the MS patient, *J Neurosurg Nurs* 13:1, 1981.

69. Horvath M: Myasthenia gravis: a nursing approach, *J Neurosurg Nurs* 14:7-14, 1982.

70. Hummel S: Cerebral vasospasm: current concepts and pathogenesis and treatment, *J Neurosci Nurs* 21:4, 1989.

71. Ignatavicius DD, Bayne MV, et al: *Medical-surgical nursing: a nursing process approach*, Philadelphia, 1991, WB Saunders.

72. Jennett B and Teasdale G: *Management of head injuries*, Philadelphia, 1981, FA Davis.

73. Jennett B, Teasdale G, Braakman R et al: Predicting outcome in individual patients after severe head injury, *Lancet* 1:1031-1034, 1976.

74. Jennett B and Bond M: Assessment of outcome after severe brain damage: a practical scale, *Lancet* 1:480-484, 1975.

75. Johnson B et al: *Standards of critical care*, ed 3, St. Louis, 1988, Mosby–Year Book.

75a. Jones D, Adinolfi A, and Gallis HA: *Care of the patient with HIV infection*, Glaxo Inc, Chapel Hill, NC, 1989, Health Science Consortium.

76. Kaye D and Rose LF: *Fundamentals of internal medicine*, St. Louis, 1982, Mosby–Year Book.

77. Kelly B and Mahon S: Nursing care of the patient with multiple sclerosis, *J Rehab Nurs* 13:5, 1989.

78. Kess R: Suddenly in crisis: unpredictable myasthenia gravis, *AJN* 14:7-12, 1982.

79. Kirkland J and Williams A: Trigeminal neuralgia: approaches to nursing care, *J Neurosurg Nurs* 15:3, 1983.

80. Krause E, Lamb S, Ham B, Larson D, and Gutin P: Radiosurgery: a nursing perspective, *J Neurosci Nurs* 23:1, 1991.

81. Kruger L: Complications of transsphenoidal surgery, *J Neurosci Nurs* 19:179-183, 1985.

82. *Language guide on disability*, Sacramento, 1988, California Governor's Committee on Employment of the Handicapped.

83. Lazarus RS and Monat A: *Stress and coping: an anthology*, New York, 1977, Columbia University Press.

84. Leech RW and Shuman RM: *Neuropathology: a summary for students*, New York, 1982, Harper & Row, Publishers.

85. Levy R, Bredesen D, and Rosenbaum M: Neurological complications of AIDS, *AFP* February, 1990.

86. Liddel D: Anterior cervical discectomy: a basis for planning nursing care, *J Neurosci Nurs* 18:1, 1986.

87. Lisak PR and Batachi RL: *Myasthenia gravis*, Philadelphia, 1982, WB Saunders.

88. Lord J and Coleman E: Chemotherapy for glioblastoma multiforme, *J Neurosci Nurs* 23:1, 1991.

89. Lundgren J: *Acute neuroscience nursing: concepts and care*, Boston, 1986, Jones & Bartlett, Publishers.

90. MacDonald E: Aneurysmal subarachnoid hemorrhage, *J Neurosci Nurs* 21:5, 1989.

91. Maida M: Chymopapain for herniated lumbar disc disease, *J Neurosurg Nurs* 15:3, 1983.

92. Malasanos L, Barkauskas V, and Stoltenberg-Allen, K: *Health assessment*, ed 4, St. Louis, 1990, Mosby–Year Book.

93. Manifold S: Aneurysmal SAH: cerebral vasospasm and early repair, *Crit Care Nurs* 10:8, 1990.

94. Marinari B: Stereotaxis, *J Neurosurg Nurs* 16:3, 1984.

95. Marshall SB, Marshall L, Vos H, and Chesnut R: *Neuroscience critical care: pathophysiology and patient management*, Philadelphia, 1990, WB Saunders.

96. Martin E and Hummelgard A: Traumatic aneurysms, *J Neurosci Nurs* 18:2, 1986.

97. McArthur J and McArthur J: Neurological manifestations of AIDS, *J Neurosurg Nurs* 18:5, 1986.

98. McCance KL, Huether SE, et al. *Pathophysiology: the biologic basis for disease in adults and children*, St. Louis, 1990, Mosby–Year Book.

98a. McEvoy GK, editor: *AHFS Drug Information*, Bethesda, Md, 1991, American Society of Hospital Pharmacists.

98b. McKenry L and Salerno E: *Mosby's pharmacology in nursing*, ed 18, St Louis, 1992, Mosby–Year Book.

99. Meeker M and Rothrock J: *Alexander's care of the patient in surgery*, ed 9, 1991, Mosby–Year Book.

100. Mitchell PH et al: *AANN's neuroscience nursing: phenomena and practice*, Norwalk, Conn, 1988, Appleton & Lange.

101. Mitchem HL: A CT guided stereotactic apparatus: new approach to biopsy and removal of brain tumors, *J Neurosurg Nurs* 16:5, 1984.

102. Morgante L, Madonna M, and Pokoluk R: Research and treatment in multiple sclerosis: implications for nursing practice, *J Neurosci Nurs* 21:5, 1989.

103. Morris J: Thymectomy: a recommended procedure for myasthenia gravis, *J Neurosurg Nurs* 13:226-233, 1981.

103a. *Mosby's Medical, Nursing, and Allied Health Dictionary*, ed 3, St. Louis, 1990, Mosby–Year Book.

104. Mourad LA: *Orthopedic disorders*, St. Louis, 1991, Mosby–Year Book.

105. Muldar D, White K, and Herman C: Thymectomy: surgical procedure for myasthenia gravis, *AORN* 43:3, 1986.

106. Mumma CM et al: *Rehabilitation nursing: concepts and practice—a core curriculum*, ed 2, Evanston, Ill, 1987, Rehabilitation Nursing Foundation.

107. Newmann D and Bailey L: An overview of neurogenic pulmonary edema, *J Neurosurg Nurs* 12:4, 1980.

108. Nikas D: Critical aspects of head trauma, *Crit Care Nurs Q* 10(1): 1987.

109. Noroian EL: Myasthenia gravis: a nursing perspective, *J Neurosci Nurs* 18:74-80, 1986.

110. *Nursing 91 Drug Handbook*, Springhouse, Pa, 1991, Springhouse Corporation.

110a. Olin BR, editor: *Facts and comparisons*, St. Louis, 1991, JB Lippincott.

111. Pagana K and Pagana T: *Diagnostic testing and nursing implications: a case study approach*, ed 3, St. Louis, 1990, Mosby–Year Book.

112. Pallett PJ and O'Brien MT: *Textbook of neurological nursing*, Boston, 1985, Little, Brown, & Co.

113. Passo S: Malformations of the neural tube, *Nurs Clin North Am* 15:5, 1980.

114. Patrick ML et al: *Medical-surgical nursing: pathophysiological concepts*, Philadelphia, 1986, JB Lippincott.

115. Perlstein L and Ake JU: AIDS: an overview for the neuroscience nurse, *J Neurosci Nurs* 19:6, 1987.

116. Petersdorf RG, editor: *Harrison's principles of internal medicine*, ed 10, New York, 1983, Mc-Graw-Hill.

117. Pfister S and Bullas J: Acute Guillain-Barré syndrome, *Crit Care Nurs* 10:10, 1990.

118. Prendergast V: Bacterial meningitis update, *J Neurosci Nurs* 19:2, 1987.

119. Price S and Wilson L: *Pathophysiology: clinical concepts of disease processes*, ed. 4, St. Louis, 1992, Mosby–Year Book.

120. Raimond J and Taylor J: *Neurological emergencies: effective nursing care*, Rockville, Md, 1986, Aspen Systems Publications.

121. Raney D: Malignant spinal cord tumors: a review and case presentation, *J Neurosci Nurs* 23:1, 1991.

122. Riggins RS and Kraus JF: The risk of neurologic damage with fractures of the vertebrae, *J Trauma* 17:126-133, 1977.

123. Robbins SL and Cotran RS: *Pathologic basis of disease*, ed 2, Philadelphia, 1977, WB Saunders Co.

124. Rosenblum M, Levy R and Bredesend D: *AIDS and the nervous system*, New York, 1988, Raven Press.

125. Rothner AD, editor: *Recent developments in the treatment of epilepsy*, Chicago, 1983, Abbott Laboratories.

126. Rowland L, ed: *Merritt's textbook of neurology*, ed 8, Philadelphia, 1989, Lea & Febiger.

127. Rudy E: *Advanced neurological and neurosurgical nursing*, St. Louis, 1984, Mosby–Year Book.

128. Rutledge B: Aneurysm wrapping: principles applicable to the neuroscience nurse, *J Neurosci Nurs* 21:6, 1989.

129. Scherer P: Coma assessment, *Am J Nurs* 86(5):541, 1986.

130. Seeley R, Stephens T, and Tate P: *Anatomy and physiology*, St. Louis, 1989, Mosby–Year Book.

131. Seidel HM et al.: *Mosby's guide to physical examination*, ed 2, St. Louis, 1991, Mosby–Year Book.

132. Shatkin J, Bolt B, and Norton D: Teaching program for patients with low back pain, *J Neurosci Nurs* 19:5, 1987.

132a. Skidmore-Roth L: *Mosby's 1990 Nursing Drug Reference*, St. Louis, 1990, Mosby–Year Book.

133. Speers I: Cerebral edema, *J Neurosurg Nurs* 13:2, 1981.

134. Staller A: Systemic effects of severe head trauma, *Crit Care Nurs Q* 10(1): 1987.

135. Stillman M: Transsphenoidal hypophysectomy for pituitary tumors, *J Neurosci Nurs* 13:117-122, 1981.

136. Stone N: Amyotrophic lateral sclerosis: a challenge for constant adaptation, *J Neurosci Nurs* 19:3, 1987.

137. Taylor JW and Ballinger S: *Neurological dysfunctions and nursing interventions*, New York, 1980, McGraw-Hill.

138. Thelan LA, Davie JK, and Urden LD: *Textbook of critical care nursing: diagnosis and management*, St. Louis, 1990, Mosby–Year Book.

139. Thompson JM et al.: *Mosby's manual of clinical nursing*, ed 2, St. Louis, 1989, Mosby–Year Book.

140. Ulrich S et al.: *Nursing care planning guides*, ed 2, Philadelphia, 1990, WB Saunders.

140a. *United States Pharmacopeia Dispensing Information (USP DI)*, vols 1 and 2, Rockville, Md, 1991, United States Pharmacopeial Convention.

141. Ventura MG and Masser PG: Defining death: developments in recent law. In Rogers MC and Traystman RJ, editors: *Critical care clinics: a symposium on neurologic intensive care*, vol 1, no 2, Philadelphia, 1985, WB Saunders.

142. Vernon M: Parkinson's disease, *J Neurosci Nurs* 21:5, 1989.

143. Walleck C: Intracranial hypertension: interventions and outcomes, *Crit Care Nurs Q* 10(1): 1987.

144. Walleck C: Head trauma in children, *Nurs Clin North Am* 15:125, 1980.

145. Weeks D: Washing the blood, *RN*, May 1991.

146. Whitney C and Daroff R: An approach to migraine, *J Neurosci Nurs* 20:5, 1988.

147. Willis D: Intracranial astrocytoma: pathology, diagnosis, and clinical presentation, *J Neurosci Nurs* 23:1, 1991.

148. Wilson S and Thompson J: *Respiratory disorders*, St. Louis, 1990, Mosby–Year Book.

149. Wyngaarden JB and Smith L, editors: *Cecil's textbook of medicine*, Philadelphia, 1985, WB Saunders.

150. Yarkony GM: *Experience of federal SCI centers*, Chicago, 1991, Rehabilitation Institute of Chicago.

151. Zegeer L: Nursing care of the patient with brain edema, *J Neurosurg Nurs* 14:5, 1982.

Index

DATE DUE

DEC 1 4 2012			

ACG 1082

NEUROLOGIC ORGANIZATIONS

Alzheimer's Disease and Related Disorders Association
4709 Golf Road, Suite 1015
Skokie, IL 60076
(708) 933-1000

American Cancer Society
90 Park Avenue
New York, NY 10016
(212)599-3600

American Heart Association
7272 Greenville Avenue
Dallas, TX 75231
(214) 373-6300

American Paralysis/Spinal Cord Hotline
Patients with spinal cord injury (SCI) and their families can learn what programs and facilities are available to them in their own communities. The hotline has toll-free lines active 24 hours a day to offer information, referral, peer support, and hope for those who have SCI-related problems.
800-526-3456
800-638-1733 (in MD)

American Speech, Language, Hearing Association
10801 Rockville Pike
Rockville, MD 20852
(301) 897-5700

Amyotrophic Lateral Sclerosis Association
21021 Ventura Blvd.
Suite 321
Woodland Hills, CA 91364
(818) 990-2151

Architectural and Transportation Barriers Compliance Board
1111 Eighteenth Street, NW
Suite 501
Washington, DC 20036
(202) 653-7834

Association for Brain Tumor Research
3725 North Talman
Chicago, IL 60618
(312) 286-5571

Epilepsy Foundation of America
4351 Garden City Drive, 5th Floor
Landover, MD 20785
(301) 459-3700

Guillain Barré Syndrome Foundation International
PO Box 262
Wynnewood, PA 19096
(215) 667-0131

Independent Living for the Handicapped
1301 Belmont Street, NW
Washington, DC 20009
(202) 797-9803

Information Center for Individuals with Disabilities
Fort Point Place, 1st Floor
27-43 Wormwood Street
Boston, MA 02210-1606
(617) 727-5540

The Library of Congress Division of the Blind and Physically Handicapped
1291 Taylor Street, NW
Washington, DC 20542
(202) 707-5100

Mainstream, Inc.
1030 15th Street, NW
Suite 1010
Washington, DC 20005
(202) 898-0202

Myasthenia Gravis Foundation, Inc.
53 W. Jackson Blvd., Suite 660
Chicago, IL 60604
(312) 427-6252

National AIDS Inter-Faith Network
300 I Street, NE, Suite 400
Washington, DC 20005
(202) 546-0807

National AIDS Network Hotline c/o American Social Health Association
PO Box 13827, RTP, NC 27709
1-800-342-AIDS
1-800-342-7514

National Association for Home Care
519 C Street NE
Washington, DC 20002
(202) 547-7424

National Easter Seal Society
70 E. Lake Street
Chicago, IL 60601
(312) 726-6200

National Foundation March of Dimes
1275 Mamaroneck Avenue
White Plains, NY 10605
(914) 428-7100

National Head Injury Foundation
333 Turnpike Road
Southborough, MA 01772
(508) 485-9950

National Institute of Neurological and Communicative Disorders and Stroke
Building 31/Rm. 8A52
9000 Rockville Pike
Bethesda, MD 20892
(301) 496-9746

National Institute of Neurological Disorders and Stroke (NINDS)
Office of Scientific and Health Reports (pamphlets on stroke)
Building 31/Rm. 8A16
9000 Rockville Pike
Bethesda, MD 20892
(301) 496-5751

National Institute of Neurological Disorders and Stroke (NINDS)
Division of Stroke and Trauma (grant applications)
Federal Building/Room 1016
7550 Wisconsin Avenue
Bethesda, MD 20892
(301) 496-4188

National Multiple Sclerosis Society
205 E. 42nd Street, Third Floor
New York, NY 10017
(212) 986-3240

National Rehabilitation Information Center
8455 Colesville Road, Suite 935
Silver Spring, MD 20910
(301) 588-9284

National Spinal Cord Injury Association
600 W. Cummings Park, Suite 2000
Woburn, MA 01801
(617) 935-2722

National Stroke Association
300 East Hampden Avenue, Suite 240
Englewood, CO 80110-2654
(303) 762-9922